MEDICAL
MYCOLOGY
A SELF-INSTRUCTIONAL TEXT

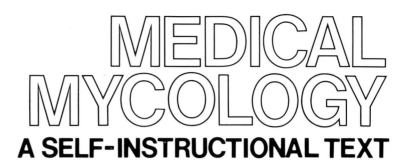

MEDICAL MYCOLOGY
A SELF-INSTRUCTIONAL TEXT

MARTHA E. KERN, D.A., M.S., M.T. (A.S.C.P.), C.L.S. (N.C.A.)
DIRECTOR, INSTITUTE FOR MEDICAL COMMUNICATION
SILVER SPRING, MARYLAND
AND
CHIEF MYCOLOGIST
SOUTHERN MARYLAND HOSPITAL CENTER
CLINTON, MARYLAND

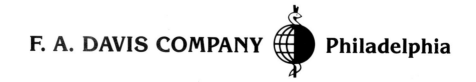

F. A. DAVIS COMPANY • Philadelphia

F. A. Davis Company
1915 Arch Street
Philadelphia, Pennsylvania 19103

LIBRARY OF CONGRESS CATALOGING IN PUBLICATION DATA

Kern, Martha.
  Medical mycology.

  Includes bibliographies and index.
  1. Medical mycology—Programmed instruction.
I. Title.
QR245.S56   1985   616.9'69'0077   84-9580
ISBN 0-8036-5293-3

PREFACE

Fungi have always been a plague to man. Of the 200,000 or more species that exist, approximately 100 of them consistently produce human mycoses. Most pathogenic fungi elicit chronic infections of the superficial, cutaneous, and subcutaneous tissues, causing unsightly but not lethal diseases. In the past, systemic infections were infrequent and usually confined to patients with naturally deficient immune mechanisms or debilitating disease. Recently, however, with increased use of immunosuppressive drugs, antibiotics, and chemotherapy, disseminated life-threatening mycoses are more frequently observed. In addition to classic systemic pathogens, the causative agents are often opportunistic fungal contaminants that previously held no significant disease association.

A competent laboratory mycologist must be aware of the changing etiologic role of fungi. Without proper specimen collection, processing, and culture methods, potential pathogens may be completely missed, with fatal consequences to the patient.

Just as important, the technologist must be able to correctly identify causative organisms within a time frame useful to the clinician and the patient. Since many fungi require a long growth period, a thorough, accurate examination of the specimen direct mount is imperative. It provides a rapid presumptive diagnosis upon which the physician can act. For final mycologic identification, relatively few physiologic tests are available. Differentiation between morphologically similar fungi basically depends on the technologist's experience and judgment. To someone just entering the field, the melange of subtleties in appearance may prove very frustrating.

Many volumes containing fungal descriptions and procedures have been written. Unfortunately, most of them are too detailed and technically oriented to be appropriate for the beginning mycology student. In addition, laboratory technology and microbiology training curricula are so condensed that little time is available for mycologic instruction. The purpose of this book is to provide a basic and practical course in laboratory mycology that can be used for self-teaching or as an adjunct for instructors. The volume also fits the needs of clinical mycology laboratories. Each module contains text with drawings, photographs, and charts. Incorporated into the text are a series of self-study examinations that encourage the reader to actively participate in the learning process. Each unit also contains prerequisites, behavioral objectives, a content outline, follow-up activities, and selected references. All modules except Module 4 contain a Supplemental Rationale section which includes material that is valuable to know but not absolutely necessary for day-to-day laboratory work. The reader must proceed through Modules 1 (Basics of Mycology) and 2 (Laboratory Procedures for Fungal Culture and Isolation) and then study the remaining units, depending on his or her area of particular interest.

MEK

v

ACKNOWLEDGMENTS

There are many wonderful people whose help made this text possible. Michael T. Singer, D.D.S., did most of the photography. He withstood a lot of frustration and retakes and, yet, was always encouraging. If not for him, this book would not have become a reality.

The personnel of the mycology laboratory at Walter Reed Army Medical Center, in particular Joan Brisker, B.S., were extremely generous with their supplies and equipment. Joan additionally provided new stock cultures and good advice. William J. Rauch, M.S., took the remaining photographs and edited the manuscript. I was in a real bind and could not have finished without his help and patience.

Other generous people are Bill H. Cooper, Ph.D., and Chapman H. Binford, M.D., who sent articles and words of encouragement; Kyung J. Kwon-Chung, Ph.D., for donation of a *Paracoccidioides* culture; and Michael R. McGinnis, Ph.D., who gave advice on conidiogenesis. Thanks also to the text readers and review-ers, Eugene R. Kennedy, Ph.D., John C. Rees, Ph.D., Benedict T. DeCicco, Ph.D., Jerome G. Buescher, Ph.D., Kenni B. Beam, M.S., M.T. (A.S.C.P.) S.M., Bonita S. Rosenberg, Russel F. Cheadle, M.S., M.T. (A.S.C.P.), and Herbert Layman, for their constructive comments. I am also grateful to the various publishing companies and authors for giving permission to reproduce their photographs and charts in the book.

Acknowledgment must definitely be given to the staff at F.A. Davis, especially Wendy Bahnsen, Lenoire Brown, and Sally Burke, who did a superior job of coordinating the text with the numerous charts, drawings, and photographs.

Most of all, thanks to my family for giving me the guidance to seek higher levels of learning and the awareness to appreciate what I have attained.

MEK

CONTENTS

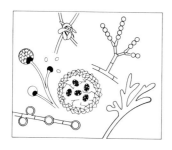

MODULE 1

BASICS OF MYCOLOGY

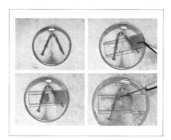

MODULE 2

LABORATORY PROCEDURES FOR FUNGAL CULTURE AND ISOLATION

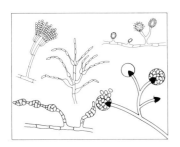

MODULE 3

COMMON FUNGAL CONTAMINANTS

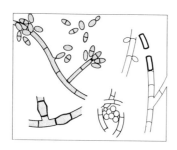

MODULE 4

SUPERFICIAL AND DERMATOPHYTIC FUNGI

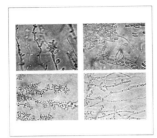

MODULE 5

YEASTS

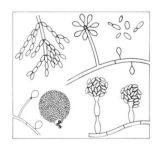

MODULE 6

ORGANISMS CAUSING SUBCUTANEOUS MYCOSES

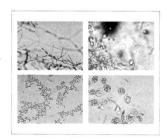

MODULE 7

ORGANISMS CAUSING SYSTEMIC MYCOSES

LIST OF FIGURES

MODULE 1. BASICS OF MYCOLOGY

MODULE 2. LABORATORY PROCEDURES FOR FUNGAL CULTURE AND ISOLATION

MODULE 3. COMMON FUNGAL CONTAMINANTS

MODULE 4. SUPERFICIAL AND DERMATOPHYTIC FUNGI

MODULE 5. YEASTS

MODULE 6. ORGANISMS CAUSING SUBCUTANEOUS MYCOSES

MODULE 7. ORGANISMS CAUSING SYSTEMIC MYCOSES

LIST OF TECHNIQUES
AND PROCEDURES

LIST OF CHARTS

MODULE 1. BASICS OF MYCOLOGY

MODULE 2. LABORATORY PROCEDURES FOR FUNGAL CULTURE AND ISOLATION

MODULE 3. COMMON FUNGAL CONTAMINANTS

MODULE 4. SUPERFICIAL AND DERMATOPHYTIC FUNGI

MODULE 5. YEASTS

MODULE 6. ORGANISMS CAUSING SUBCUTANEOUS MYCOSES

MODULE 7. ORGANISMS CAUSING SYSTEMIC MYCOSES

LIST OF COLOR PLATES

ABBREVIATIONS USED IN THIS TEXT

BHI   brain heart infusion agar

BHIAB   brain heart infusion agar with blood

BHIAB-C&C   brain heart infusion agar with blood, cycloheximide, and chloramphenicol

CM-T80   corn meal-Tween 80 agar

CSF   cerebrospinal fluid

DMSO   dimethyl sulfoxide

KOH   potassium hydroxide

KOH-DMSO   potassium hydroxide-dimethyl sulfoxide

LPCB   lactophenol cotton blue

NALC   N-acetyl-L-cysteine

PDA   potato dextrose agar

SDA   Sabouraud dextrose agar

SDA-C&C   Sabouraud dextrose agar with cycloheximide and chloramphenicol

TOC   Tween 80-oxgall-caffeic acid

MEDICAL MYCOLOGY

A SELF-INSTRUCTIONAL TEXT

INTRODUCTION: HOW TO USE THIS TEXT

Medical Mycology: A Self-Instructional Text was written specifically for the beginning student of mycology. The more common fungi and funguslike bacteria encountered in a medical laboratory are well represented, with emphasis on subtle differences between similar-appearing organisms. This text will be useful for reaching a final identification in most situations. However, comprehensive books on the subject should always be maintained for those instances when more detailed information is required, for example, in speciating unusual strains of *Aspergillus*.

This text is written in a self-teaching context; to receive the most benefit from it, be sure to read the prerequisites, behavioral objectives, and content outline at the front of each module before delving into the main body of the chapter. The prerequisites stress a good microbiology background and completion of Modules 1 and 2. The intent is to provide a thorough understanding of basic terms and techniques, so that vocabulary used in succeeding chapters will be familiar. The objectives are vital; besides supplying important points to consider while reading through the text, they present ways to correlate various pieces of information. Objectives also aid in correctly answering study questions interspersed in the chapter. A content outline is provided, which shows how each topic fits into the overall picture. This is especially useful in Module 1, where the large number of new terms may be confusing if not kept in perspective.

Upon examining the main portion of each chapter, look up the charts, photos, drawings, and so forth referred to in the text. Usually the chart or figure is located very close to the first place of mention, but color photographs are all in the back of the book. Much essential information is contained in these learning aids, and if they are carefully studied, a more complete comprehension of the subject will be attained. Especially useful are Charts 1-3 to 1-13 and page 63, which provide a means of rapidly identifying a fungal isolate. New words are in boldface when initially used, and the definition follows the term. These terms may also be found in the Glossary (Appendix C). Since mycology has undergone many nomenclature changes recently, old fungal genera and diseases are in parentheses behind the new ones. Appendix B provides a list of synonyms and currently accepted names. Recipes and procedures are highlighted in gray boxes following the appropriate test discussions. In this manner, formulas do not clutter up the text, yet all information regarding each test is in one vicinity.

After reading each module section, quiz your retention and understanding by completing the study questions; these will identify weak areas that require further concentration. Look up the answers in Appendix A, and correctly complete any missed questions before proceeding. At the end of each module is a final exam, which should be worked in the same way. Most chapters continue with a Supplemental Rationale segment that contains topics such as taxonomy, general flow charts for identification, mycoses based on body site, animal inoculations, serology, and disease descriptions. These additional readings are intended for learners who wish a more comprehensive review of mycology; they are followed by study questions that incorporate information from the entire module.

Although mycology can be complex, it is fascinating if understood. It is hoped that this book will contribute toward that end.

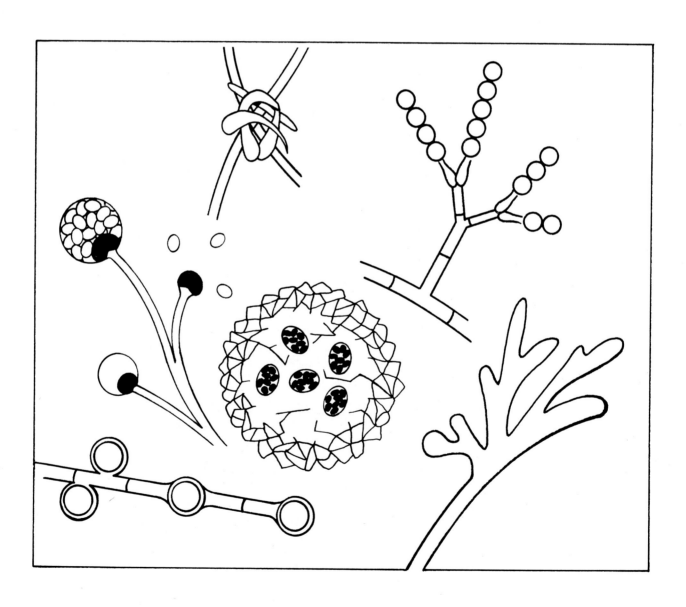

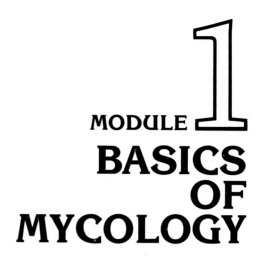

MODULE 1
BASICS OF MYCOLOGY

PREREQUISITES. The learner must possess a good background knowledge in clinical microbiology.

BEHAVIORAL OBJECTIVES. Upon completion of this module, the learner should be able to:

1. Correctly recognize, from fungal cultures, photographs, or drawings:

Hyphae	Chlamydoconidia	Ascocarp
Mycelium	Annellide	Cleistothecium
Aseptate hyphae	Annelloconidium	Basidiospore
Septate hyphae	Macro/microconidia	Basidium
Vegetative hyphae	Poroconidium	Zygospore
Aerial hyphae	Conidiophore	Cottony texture
Favic chandeliers	Phialide	Velvety texture
Nodular organs	Phialoconidium	Granular texture
Racquet hyphae	Sporangiospore	Glabrous texture
Spiral hyphae	Sporangiophore	Rugose topography
Yeasts	Sporangium	Umbonate topography
Arthroconidia	Columella	Verrucose topography
Blastoconidia	Ascospore	
Pseudohyphae	Ascus	

2. Define:

Fungus	Sessile	Cutaneous mycosis
Mycology	Intercalary	Subcutaneous mycosis
Dimorphism	Terminal	Systemic mycosis
Conidiogenous	Superficial mycosis	

3. Given a fungal culture, accurately describe its texture, topography, and front and reverse color.

4. Given the sexual reproduction of a fungus, discuss its taxonomic subdivision, including possible types of asexual reproduction, hyphal septation, and two medically important representative genera.

5. State whether infected material from a specific body site represents a superficial, cutaneous, subcutaneous, or systemic mycosis.

6. Given a fungal structure, state if it is reproductive or nonreproductive, and if it is the former, briefly describe how it reproduces.

7. Given an unknown fungus, correctly identify it by using Charts 1-3 to 1-13.

CONTENT OUTLINE

I. Introduction
II. Microscopic morphology
  A. General information
    1. Hyphae
      a. Aseptate hyphae
      b. Septate hyphae
      c. Vegetative versus aerial hyphae
      d. Nonreproductive vegetative hyphae
        (1) Favic chandeliers
        (2) Nodular organs
        (3) Racquet hyphae
        (4) Spiral hyphae
    2. Yeasts
    3. Dimorphism
    4. Study questions
  B. Reproduction
    1. Asexual reproduction
      a. Conidia
        (1) Blastoconidia
        (2) Poroconidia
        (3) Phialoconidia
        (4) Annelloconidia
        (5) Macroconidia
        (6) Chlamydoconidia
        (7) Arthroconidia
      b. Sporangiospores
      c. Study questions
    2. Sexual reproduction
      a. Ascospores
      b. Basidiospores
      c. Zygospores
III. Colonial morphology
  A. Texture
    1. Cottony or woolly texture
    2. Velvety texture
    3. Granular or powdery texture
    4. Glabrous texture
  B. Topography
    1. Rugose topography
    2. Umbonate topography
    3. Verrucose topography

C. Color
IV. Final exam
V. Supplemental Rationale
   A. Taxonomy
   B. Key to identification of clinically important fungi
   C. Types of mycoses based on body site
   D. Study questions

FOLLOW-UP ACTIVITIES

1. **Students may observe fungal colonies and microscopic preparations and identify various structures in each.**

2. **Students may perform a literature search to find the taxonomic classification schemes that have enjoyed prominence in the last ten years.**

REFERENCES

AINSWORTH, GC: *The Fungi*, Vol. IV B. Academic Press, New York, 1979.

ALEXOPOULOS, CJ AND MIMS, CW: *Introductory Mycology*, ed 3. John Wiley & Sons, New York, 1979.

BENEKE, ES AND ROGERS, AL: *Medical Mycology Manual*, ed 4. Burgess Publishing Co., Minneapolis, 1980.

COLE, GT AND SAMSON, RA: *Patterns of Development in Conidial Fungi*. Pitman Publishing, London, 1978.

KONEMAN, EW, ROBERTS, GD AND WRIGHT, SF: *Practical Laboratory Mycology*, ed 2. Williams & Wilkins, Baltimore, 1978.

McGINNIS, MR: *Laboratory Handbook of Medical Mycology*. Academic Press, New York, 1980.

ROSS, IK: *Biology of the Fungi*. McGraw-Hill, New York, 1979.

INTRODUCTION

In order to be a successful cook, you must know the names of ingredients and utensils. In order to learn medical mycology, you must of course be familiar with the vocabulary. This module presents the basic terminology used in medical mycology, as well as various forms of reproduction observed in fungi. As you follow through this module, refer to the content outline to get a clearer idea of how each item fits into the whole.

Mycology is the study of **fungi,** which are organisms that contain true nuclei (are eukaryotic), are devoid of chlorophyll, and absorb all nutrients from the environment, especially from decaying organic matter. Fungi are observed in two ways: under the microscope and as a colony on an agar plate.

MICROSCOPIC MORPHOLOGY

General Information

Microscopically, fungal cells are observed either as hyphae (molds) or as yeasts.

HYPHAE

Hyphae are long strands of cells which may intertwine to form a mat, called a **mycelium.**

Aseptate Hyphae (Fig. 1-1)

Hyphae may be **aseptate,** meaning they have no cross walls, as in the taxonomic subdivision Zygomycotina. In the past, the point was often overlooked that zygomycetous organisms are *usually* aseptate rather than com-

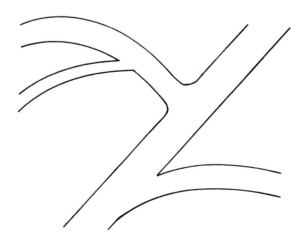

FIGURE 1-1. Aseptate hyphae.

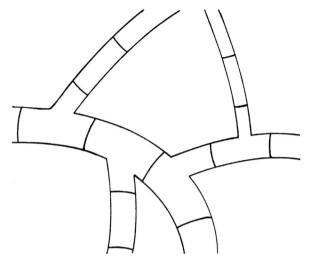

FIGURE 1-2. Septate hyphae.

pletely so: cross walls may be evident at damaged areas and near reproductive structures. These hyphae are wide and ribbonlike, measuring 6 to 10 μm in diameter.

Septate Hyphae (Fig. 1-2)

Most hyphae are **septate,** with cell cross walls very evident, as in the subdivisions Ascomycotina, Basidiomycotina, and Deuteromycotina. These hyphae are 3 to 4 μm in diameter. For the taxonomic classification, see the Supplemental Rationale section of this module.

Vegetative versus Aerial Hyphae (Fig. 1-3)

In a cross-section of a mold culture, the **vegetative,** or food-absorbing, portion of the mycelium is under the surface of the agar. The **aerial** hyphae extend above the agar surface and may support reproductive structures, commonly called conidia, at their tips. Color Plates 1 and 2 show the distinct color differences some-

times observed between the aerial hyphae, on the front side of the colony, and the vegetative hyphae, on the reverse side.

Nonreproductive Vegetative Hyphae

Vegetative hyphae may possess some very distinct nonreproductive characteristics, which may aid in speciation.

FAVIC CHANDELIERS (Figs. 1-4 and 1-5)

Favic chandeliers resemble the antlers of a buck deer, with the ends of the hyphae blunt and branched. Favic chandeliers are diagnostic for identifying cultures of *Trichophyton schoenleinii,* an organism that causes ringworm.

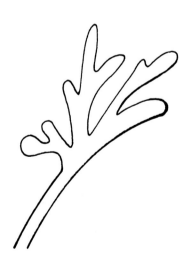

FIGURE 1-4. Favic chandeliers, *Trichophyton schoenleinii,* lactophenol cotton blue (LPCB) stain, ×450

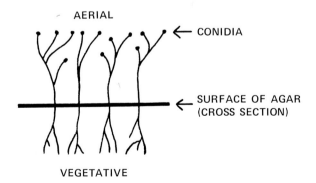

AERIAL

← CONIDIA

← SURFACE OF AGAR (CROSS SECTION)

VEGETATIVE

FIGURE 1-3. Cross view—vegetative and aerial hyphae.

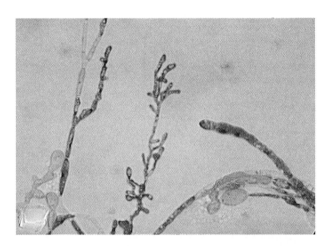

FIGURE 1-5. Favic chandeliers.

NODULAR ORGANS (Figs. 1-6 and 1-7)

Nodular organs are knots of twisted hyphae.

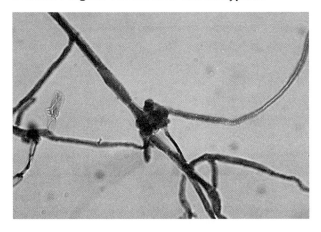

FIGURE 1-6. Nodular organ, *Microsporum ferrugineum,* LPCB stain, ×450.

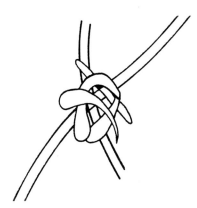

FIGURE 1-7. Nodular organ.

RACQUET HYPHAE (Figs. 1-8 and 1-9)

The name **racquet hyphae** is given because the hyphae resemble tennis racquets placed end to end.

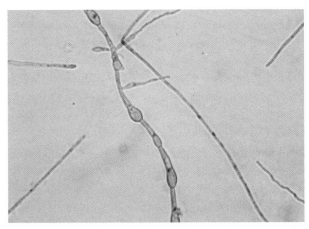

FIGURE 1-8. Racquet hyphae, *Trichophyton ajelloi,* LPCB stain, ×450.

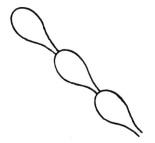

FIGURE 1-9. Racquet hyphae.

SPIRAL HYPHAE (Figs. 1-10 and 1-11)

Spiral hyphae may be flat or may turn like a corkscrew. They are commonly observed in older fluffy cultures of *Trichophyton* species.

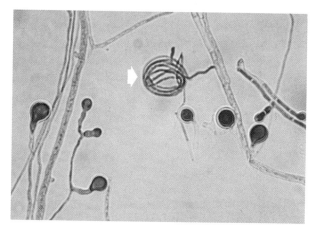

FIGURE 1-10. Spiral hyphae, *Chrysosporium* sp., LPCB stain, ×450.

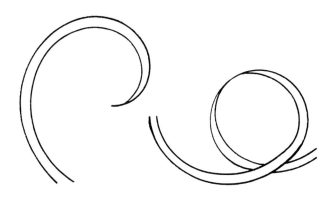

FIGURE 1-11. Spiral hyphae.

YEASTS

Yeasts consist of individual oval to round cells, which frequently bud to form daughter cells (Fig. 1-12).

DIMORPHISM

Most fungi exist only as molds or as yeasts. Some fungi, however, may exhibit **dimorphism,** meaning that they possess two distinct phases. At room temperature (25°C), they grow as molds (mold phase); at body temperature (37°C), they change and grow as yeasts (yeast or tissue phase). Conversion from one form to the other is one of the primary aids in identifying these fungi. Most of the dimorphic organisms produce serious and often fatal systemic disease.

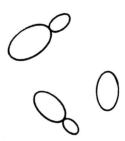

FIGURE 1-12. Budding yeasts.

STUDY QUESTIONS

1. Circle true or false:

   T F Fungi resemble plants in that both contain chlorophyll.

2. A patient's sputum specimen contains a dimorphic fungus. If the sputum is put on a slide and a coverslip added, what would you expect to observe—hyphae or yeasts?

3. Circle the correct answer:
   Knots of twisted hyphae are called mycelium/nodular organs.

4. Circle the letter of the correct answer:
   Figure 1-13 is a drawing of:
   A. Racquet hyphae
   B. Nodular organs
   C. Yeasts
   D. Favic chandeliers
   E. Aerial hyphae

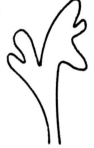

FIGURE 1-13. Study question demonstration.

STOP HERE UNTIL YOU HAVE COMPLETED THE ANSWERS.

Look up the answers in the back of the book. If you missed more than two of them, go back and review the Supplemental Rationale section. Correctly complete any missed questions.

Reproduction

Fungi exhibit just about every type of reproduction. They multiply both asexually and sexually. Depending on the circumstances, fungi may use more than one of these methods to multiply.

ASEXUAL REPRODUCTION

Asexual reproduction is so called because there is merely nuclear and cytoplasmic division, or mitosis, just as with normally growing, nonreproducing cells. **Sex-** ual reproduction involves fusion of two nuclei into a zygote.

Conidia (Singular, Conidium)

The field of **conidiogenesis,** or conidium formation, has undergone drastic changes in the last few years, and the vocabulary becomes very complicated and confusing. At present, fungi are classified by this ontogeny, so some of the more important terms must be reviewed. Chart 1-1 **(on page 19 at end of module)** sums up the essentials. **Conidia** may originate **blasti-**

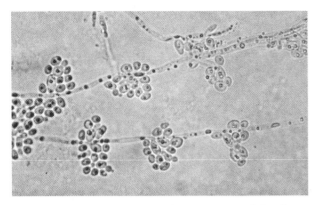

FIGURE1-14. Blastoconidia and pseudohyphae, Candida albicans, ×450.

cally, meaning the **conidiogenous** (parent) cell enlarges, then a septum separates the enlarged portion into a daughter cell. Or they may develop **thallically,** in which a septum forms first, and the growing point ahead of it becomes the daughter. The prefix **holo** in front of these words indicates that all wall layers of the parent cell are involved in daughter conidium development, while the prefix **entero** means that only the inner cell wall layers are included. **Arthric** conidiogenesis is a subheading under thallic; arthric daughter cells fragment within the hyphal strand before dispersing.

BLASTOCONIDIA (BLASTOSPORES)

Blastoconidia, produced by budding, may be seen in molds, such as *Cladosporium*, or in yeasts, such as

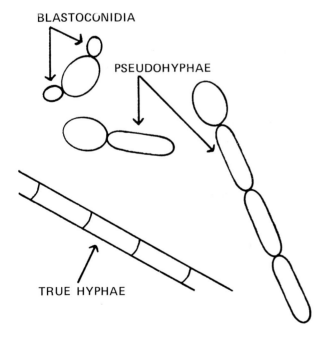

FIGURE 1-15. Blastoconidia, pseudohyphae, and true hyphae.

Candida. In some yeast species, these blastoconidia elongate to form **pseudohyphae,** which often align end to end (Fig. 1-14). Pseudohyphae may be differentiated from true hyphae in that the former are constricted at the point of alignment (Fig. 1-15).

POROCONIDIA

Poroconidia, seen in *Drechslera,* are formed by the daughter pushing through a minute pore in the parent cell. The parent may be in a long stalk **(conidiophore),** or it may be a specialized conidiogenous cell (Fig. 1-16).

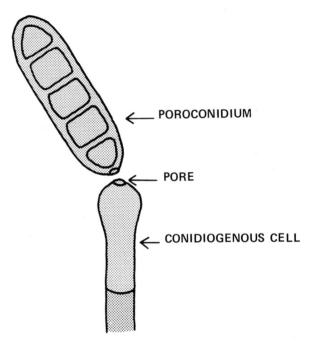

FIGURE 1-16. Poroconidium, pore, and conidiogenous cell.

PHIALOCONIDIA

Phialoconidia, elicited from a tube- or vase-shaped conidiogenous structure termed a **phialide,** may be illustrated in *Penicillium.* The first phialoconidium is holoblastic, but the rest develop enteroblastically. In *Penicillium* (Fig. 1-17) and *Aspergillus,* the phialides were formerly called sterigmata; this old word is now reserved for organisms in the taxonomic subdivision Basidiomycotina. Phialides may exhibit a terminal cup-shaped **collarette.** The supporting conidiophore may be simple or it may be elaborately branched (Fig. 1-18).

ANNELLOCONIDIA

Annelloconidia, observed in *Scopulariopsis,* are grown from inside a vase-shaped conidiogenous **an-**

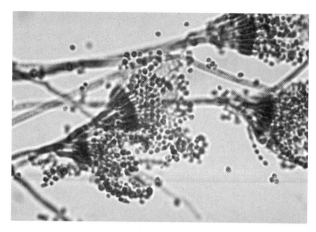

FIGURE 1-17. Phialides and phialoconidia on elaborate branching conidiophores, *Penicillium* sp., LPCB stain, ×450.

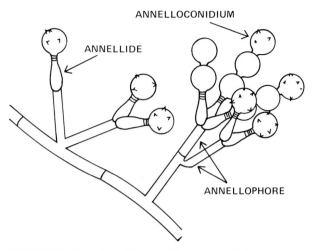

FIGURE 1-19. Annelloconidium, annellide, and annellophores.

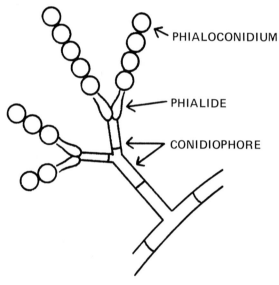

FIGURE 1-18. Phialoconidium, phialide, and conidiophore.

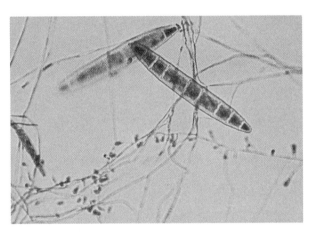

FIGURE 1-20. Macroconidia and microconidia, *Microsporum vanbreuseghemii*, LPCB stain, ×450.

nellide. The first annelloconidium is holoblastic, while the rest are enteroblastic. As each conidium is released, a ring of parent outer cell wall material remains behind, giving a distinct saw-toothed appearance to the sides of the annellide. The supporting structure is termed an **annellophore,** and it may be simple or it may be elaborately branched (Fig. 1-19).

MACROCONIDIA (Figs. 1-20 and 1-21)

A **macroconidium** (macroaleuriospore) arises by conversion of an entire hyphal element into a multicelled conidium. A **microconidium** (microaleuriospore) is produced in the same manner, except the new conidium remains aseptate. The terms macroconidia and microconidia are not used unless both types are apparent

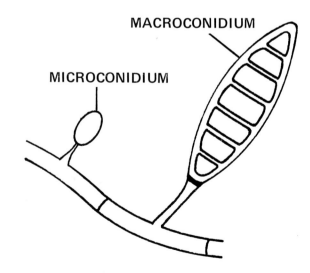

FIGURE 1-21. Macroconidium and microconidium.

in the same culture, when there is a need to differentiate them. Macroconidia may be thick- or thin-walled, spiny or smooth, and club-shaped or oval. They may be **sessile,** arising on the sides of the hyphae, or supported by conidiophores, and they are observed individually or in clusters. Microconidia are usually one celled and round, oval, or club-shaped. They may be sessile or supported alone or in clusters by a conidiophore.

CHLAMYDOCONIDIA (Figs. 1-22, 1-23, and 1-24)

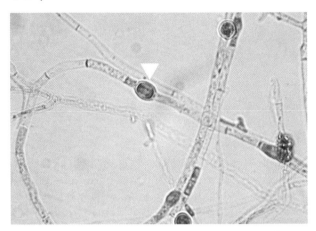

FIGURE 1-22. Intercalary chlamydoconidium, *Gliocladium* **sp., LPCB stain, ×450.**

Chlamydoconidia, thick-walled survival conidia formed during unpleasant environmental conditions, will germinate and produce conidia when a better climate occurs. They may be observed at the hyphal tip **(terminal),** on the sides (sessile), or within the hyphal strand **(intercalary).**

In the past, these structures were termed chlamydospores, and they were grouped together with the

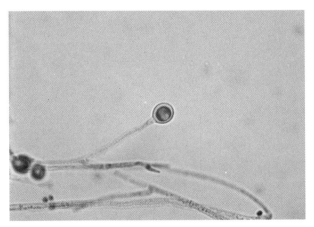

FIGURE 1-23. Terminal chlamydoconidium, *Gliocladium* **sp., LPCB stain, ×450.**

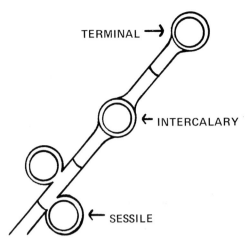

FIGURE 1-24. Terminal, intercalary, and sessile chlamydoconidia.

similar-appearing forms seen in yeasts such as *Candida albicans.* However, the yeast **chlamydospores** are thick-walled vesicles and not conidia, since they neither germinate nor produce conidia when mature. In this text, yeast vesicles will be called chlamydospores, while the word chlamydoconidia applies to germinating structures.

ARTHROCONIDIA (ARTHROSPORES)

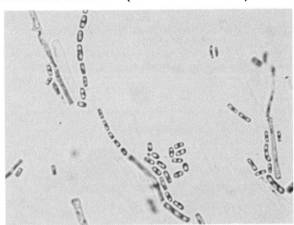

FIGURE 1-25. Arthroconidia, *Geotrichum candidum,* **LPCB stain, ×450.**

Arthroconidia (Fig. 1-25) fragment from the hyphae through the septation points. They separate within the parent hyphal strand before dispersing. Arthroconidia may form adjacent to each other within the hyphae, or they may be separated by alternating empty spaces, **disjunctor cells,** giving a checkered appearance. It is important to determine if the arthroconidia are adjacent or alternate, as *Coccidioides immitis* is partly identified by the presence of disjunctor cells. Arthroconidia mature to be thick-walled and barrel-shaped or rectangular (Fig. 1-26).

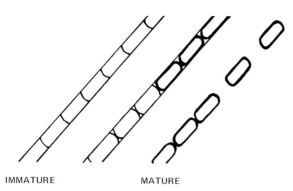

IMMATURE   MATURE

FIGURE 1-26. Arthroconidia.

SPORANGIOSPORES (Figs. 1-27 and 1-28)

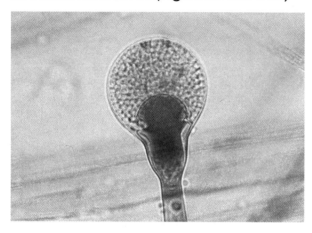

FIGURE 1-27. Sporangium filled with sporangio-spores, *Absidia* sp., LPCB stain, ✕450.

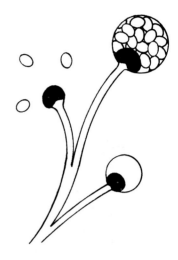

FIGURE 1-28. Sporangia containing a columella and sporangiospores.

Sporangiospores are formed by internal cleavage of the contents of a sac called a **sporangium** (plural, sporangia). The sporangium is supported on a base, or **columella,** and it in turn is supported by a stalklike **sporangiophore.** New sporangia may be empty, while older ones are filled with spores. When the sporangium dissolves and disperses its contents, the columella remains. Sporangiospores are observed in the taxonomic subdivision Zygomycotina.

STUDY QUESTIONS

1. See Figure 1-29. What type of reproductive structure is observed? Circle the letter of the correct answer:

   A. Macroconidium

   B. Phialoconidium

   C. Microconidium

   D. Sporangiospore

   E. Blastoconidium

2. Circle true or false:

   T F Arthroconidia reproduce by fragmentation.

3. Circle true or false:

   T F Chlamydospores of *Candida albicans* will germinate to form new conidia when mature.

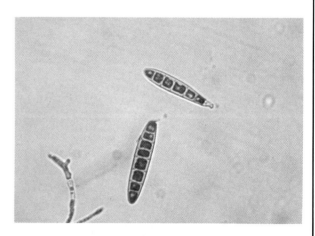

FIGURE 1-29. Study question demonstration, LPCB stain, ✕450.

4. Circle the letter of the correct answer.

   The conidiogenous cell in Figure 1-30 is a(an):

   A. Phialide
   B. Sporangium
   C. Poroconidium
   D. Annellide
   E. Chlamydoconidium

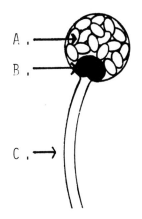

FIGURE 1-31. Study question demonstration.

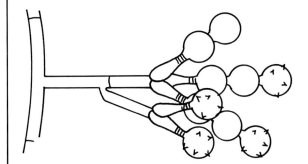

FIGURE 1-30. Study question demonstration.

6. From Figure 1-31, fill in the blanks:

   A. _____

   B. _____

   C. _____

5. Circle the letter of the correct answer.

   Blastoconidia that have elongated are termed:

   A. Mother cells
   B. True hyphae
   C. Chlamydospores
   D. Conidia
   E. Pseudohyphae

STOP HERE UNTIL YOU HAVE COMPLETED THE ANSWERS.

Look up the answers in the back of the book. If you missed more than one, go back and repeat the section on asexual reproduction. Correctly complete any missed questions before proceeding.

SEXUAL REPRODUCTION

Those fungi that have a sexual stage are called the **Perfect Fungi.** Those whose sexual stage does not exist or has not yet been discovered are in the taxonomic subdivision Deuteromycotina, or **Fungi Imperfecti.** The commonly observed sexual mechanisms in medically important fungi follow.

Ascospores (Figs. 1-32, 1-33, and 1-34)

The nucleus from a male cell, called an **antheridium,** passes through a bridge into the female cell, an **ascogonium.** The male and female cells may be from the same, self-compatible colony or from two colonies of opposite mating types. Once the male and female nu-

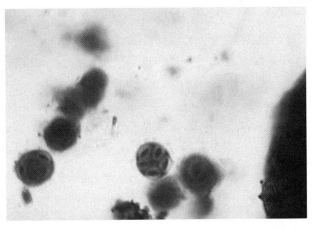

FIGURE 1-32. Ascus with ascospores, *Aspergillus* sp., LPCB stain, ×1000.

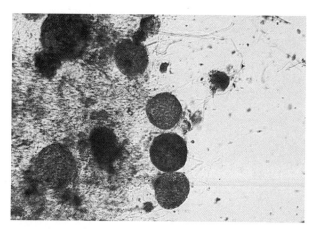

FIGURE 1-33. Cleistothecia, *Aspergillus* sp., LPCB stain, ×100.

clei fuse to form a **zygote,** the female cell becomes an **ascus** (plural, asci). The diploid zygote nucleus divides by meiosis to form four haploid nuclei, which in turn divide by mitosis to form eight nuclei. Each new nucleus walls off inside the ascus to form an **ascospore.**

Some ascomycetous fungi, for example, the yeast *Saccharomyces cerevisiae,* exhibit unprotected asci, while others, for example, the mold *Pseudallescheria boydii,* produce asci within a somatic saclike structure called an **ascocarp.** The ascocarp observed in medically important fungi is completely enclosed and is termed a **cleistothecium.** Ascospores are formed by the subdivision Ascomycotina.

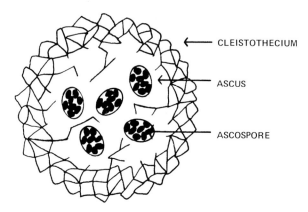

CLEISTOTHECIUM

ASCUS

ASCOSPORE

FIGURE 1-34. Cleistothecium, ascus, and ascospore.

Basidiospores

A binucleate mycelium is formed by fusion of two compatible hyphae or yeast cells, usually with the aid of clamp connections:

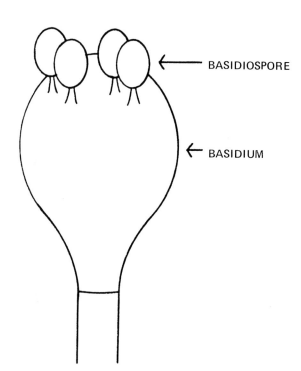

BASIDIOSPORE

BASIDIUM

FIGURE 1-35. Basidiospore and basidium.

The terminal cell of the resulting mycelium enlarges into a club-shaped structure called a **basidium.** The two nuclei within the basidium fuse to form a zygote, then undergo meiosis to produce four haploid nuclei. Four little protrusions **(basidiospores)** (Fig. 1-35) extend out from the end of the basidium, and each haploid nucleus travels into a basidiospore. Some Basidiomycetes, such as mushrooms, produce a protective **basidiocarp** to lodge the basidia and basidiospores. The only really important Basidiomycete in medical mycology is *Filobasidiella neoformans,* the sexual stage of *Cryptococcus neoformans.* Basidiospores are formed by the subdivision Basidiomycotina.

Zygospores

Two compatible hyphae each form an arm **(zygophore)** extending toward the other. The hyphae may be from a self-compatible colony or from two colonies of opposite mating types. When the zygophores meet, they fuse to form a thick-walled, protective **zygosporangium** (Figs. 1-36 and 1-37) within which a **zygospore** develops. Zygospores are formed by the taxonomic subdivision Zygomycotina.

COLONIAL MORPHOLOGY

Although many fungi do not have a colonial morphology characteristic enough to allow identification without

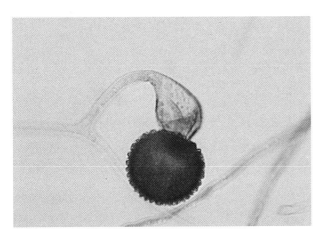

FIGURE 1-36. Zygosporangium, *Zygorhynchus* sp., LPCB stain, ×450.

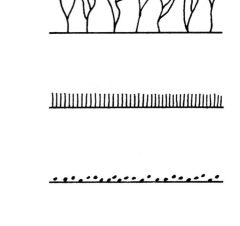

FIGURE 1-38. Colonial textures.

additional criteria, some are very distinct. Certain general terms are used to describe fungal colonies.

Texture

The colonial **texture** describes the height of the aerial hyphae. The textural terms are relative and are best described in a cross-sectional drawing (Fig. 1-38).

COTTONY OR WOOLLY TEXTURE

Cottony or **woolly** colonies produce a very high, dense aerial mycelium (Color Plate 3).

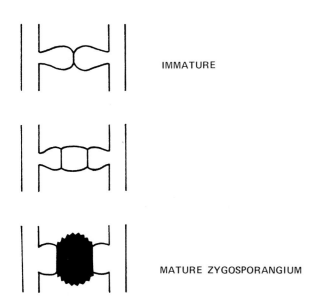

IMMATURE

MATURE ZYGOSPORANGIUM

FIGURE 1-37. Zygosporangium.

VELVETY TEXTURE

Velvety colonies produce a low aerial mycelium which resembles the fabric velvet (Color Plate 4).

GRANULAR OR POWDERY TEXTURE

Granular or **powdery** colonies are flat and crumbly because of the dense production of conidia. The granular texture is rougher, like granulated sugar, and the powdery texture is like flour (Color Plate 5). These two terms are often used interchangeably.

GLABROUS TEXTURE

Glabrous or **waxy** colonies have a smooth surface because they produce no aerial mycelium (Color Plate 6). Usually yeasts form a glabrous macroscopic appearance.

Topography (Fig. 1-39)

Colonial **topography** describes the various designs of hills and valleys seen on fungal cultures. The topography is often masked by the aerial hyphae; therefore, this characteristic is better observed on the reverse side of the colony. A colony may possess no topography, that is, it is flat.

RUGOSE TOPOGRAPHY

Rugose colonies have deep furrows irregularly radiating from the center of the culture (Color Plate 7).

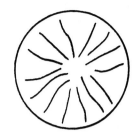

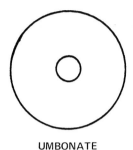

RUGOSE

UMBONATE

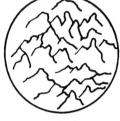

VERRUCOSE

FIGURE 1-39. Colonial topographies.

UMBONATE TOPOGRAPHY

Umbonate colonies possess a buttonlike central elevation. They may be accompanied by rugose furrows around the button (Color Plate 8).

VERRUCOSE TOPOGRAPHY

Verrucose colonies exhibit a wrinkled, convoluted surface (Color Plate 9).

Color

Be as specific about the colony colors as possible. For example, instead of describing a culture as brown, use words such as beige, tan, khaki, or mahogany. If there are concentric rings of different colors, describe each one. Be sure to characterize both the front and reverse sides of the culture.

FINAL EXAM

1. **From drawings A through L on page 17, fill in the blanks:**

   A. _____

   B. _____

   C. _____

   D. _____

   E. _____

   F. _____

   G. _____

   H. _____

   I. _____

   J. _____

   K. _____

   L. _____

2. **See Color Plates 10 and 11. Describe the texture, topography, and front and reverse colors of this colony.**

   STOP HERE UNTIL YOU HAVE COMPLETED THE ANSWERS.

   Look up the answers in the back of the book. If you missed more than two, go back and repeat this module. Correctly complete any missed questions before proceeding.

SUPPLEMENTAL RATIONALE

Taxonomy

The taxonomy of fungi has undergone very rapid changes in the last ten years, and there is no general agreement yet on an ultimate classification schema.

The following taxonomy of medically important funguslike bacteria and true fungi is compiled from Ainsworth (1973) and Alexopoulos and Mims (1979). McGinnis (1980) and others have changed the subdivisions to divisions and the subclasses to classes, but it is rather a moot academic point to clinical mycologists. Organisms in parentheses represent the asexual (ana-

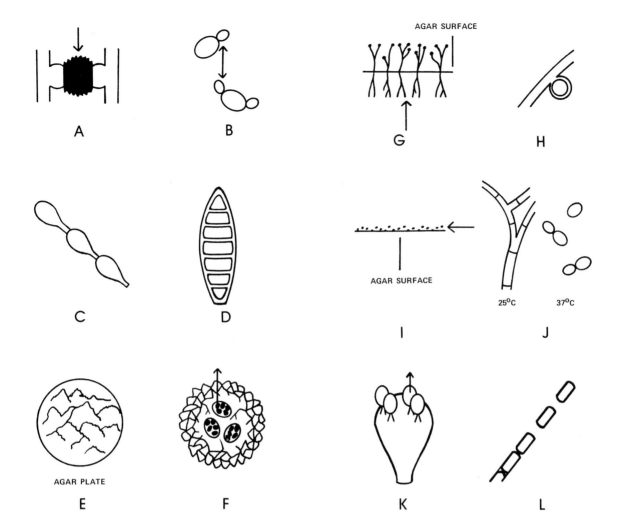

morph) names, while those without parentheses indicate the sexual **(teleomorph)** names. Some species of a genus may have known sexual stages, while other species of the genus do not. Thus, the genus is placed under both the known sexual classification and the asexual one. Some asexual fungi may exhibit two or three different sexual appearances and thus may possess two or three different sexual names. The reverse is also true: some sexual organisms may possess two or three different asexual names. **See Chart 1-2 on pages 20-21 at end of module.**

Key to Identification of Clinically Important Fungi

See Charts 1-3 to 1-13 on pages 22-39 at end of module.

Types of Mycoses Based on Body Site

Mycoses, fungal diseases, may be classified according to the tissue or body site invaded.

Superficial mycoses affect only the outermost layers of skin and hair. Little or no pathology is evidenced, and the patients are mainly worried about cosmetic effects. Some superficial mycoses are otomycosis, black and white piedra, pityriasis versicolor, and tinea nigra.

Cutaneous mycoses involve destruction of the keratin of skin, hair, and nails. There is rarely invasion of deeper body tissues. Cutaneous mycoses are caused primarily by the dermatophytes *(Trichophyton, Microsporum,* and *Epidermophyton)* and by *Candida.*

Subcutaneous mycoses involve the skin, muscle, and connective tissue immediately below the skin. Deeper tissue involvement is rare. Some subcutaneous mycoses are chromoblastomycosis, mycetoma, and sporotrichosis.

Systemic mycoses involve the deep tissues and organs of the body. In disseminated forms of these diseases, subcutaneous and cutaneous areas may also be invaded. Some systemic mycoses are blastomycosis, paracoccidioidomycosis, histoplasmosis, and coccidioidomycosis.

Study Questions— Supplemental Rationale

1. A patient is seen by his physician for a hard, nonmoving nodule below the skin on his right index finger. There are no other symptoms. Circle the letter of the correct answer:

   The infection that this patient is most likely presenting is:

   A. Superficial

   B. Cutaneous

   C. Subcutaneous

   D. Systemic

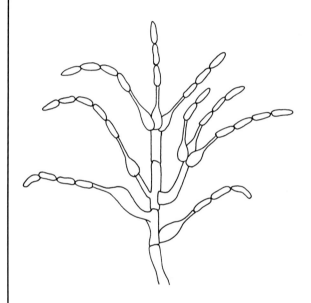

FIGURE 1-40. Study question demonstration.

2. In the laboratory, you have isolated a rapid growing, powdery, olive-tan fungal colony. After setting up a slide culture (Module 2), you see only the light-colored microscopic structures in Figure 1-40. Using Charts 1-3 to 1-13, this fungus is _____ sp.

3. In the blanks, write the letter of the correct answer below.

   The taxonomic subdivision Zygomycotina is distinct in that the hyphae are usually _____ . The typical asexual reproductive structures are _____ , while the sexual stage is characterized by the formation of _____ .

   A. Septate

   B. Basidiospores

   C. Zygospores

   D. Aseptate

   E. Ascospores

   F. Arthroconidia

   G. Sporangiospores

STOP HERE UNTIL YOU HAVE COMPLETED THE ANSWERS.

Look up the answers in the back of the book. If you missed more than one, go back and repeat the Supplemental Rationale section. Correctly complete any missed questions.

CHART 1-1. Conidiogenesis*

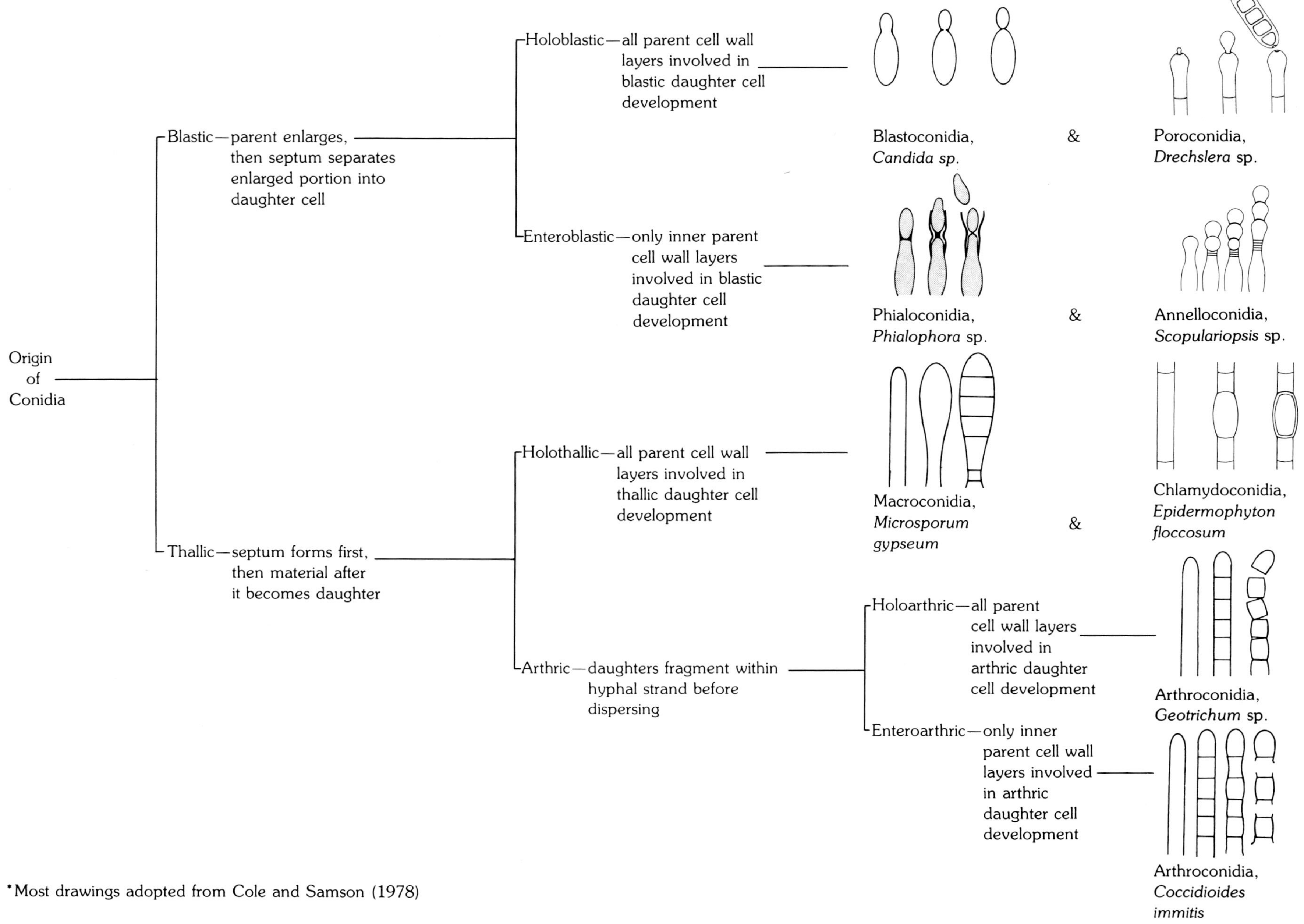

Origin of Conidia

Blastic—parent enlarges, then septum separates enlarged portion into daughter cell

- **Holoblastic**—all parent cell wall layers involved in blastic daughter cell development

  Blastoconidia, *Candida sp.*

  &

  Poroconidia, *Drechslera sp.*

- **Enteroblastic**—only inner parent cell wall layers involved in blastic daughter cell development

  Phialoconidia, *Phialophora sp.*

  &

  Annelloconidia, *Scopulariopsis sp.*

Thallic—septum forms first, then material after it becomes daughter

- **Holothallic**—all parent cell wall layers involved in thallic daughter cell development

  Macroconidia, *Microsporum gypseum*

  &

  Chlamydoconidia, *Epidermophyton floccosum*

- **Arthric**—daughters fragment within hyphal strand before dispersing

  - **Holoarthric**—all parent cell wall layers involved in arthric daughter cell development

    Arthroconidia, *Geotrichum sp.*

  - **Enteroarthric**—only inner parent cell wall layers involved in arthric daughter cell development

    Arthroconidia, *Coccidioides immitis*

*Most drawings adopted from Cole and Samson (1978)

CHART 1-2. Taxonomic Classification of Clinically Important Fungi and Funguslike Bacteria

True Fungi:

REPRESENTATIVE GENERA	ASEXUAL REPRODUCTION	SEXUAL REPRODUCTION	HYPHAE
Kingdom Myceteae (Fungi)			
Division Amastigomycota			
Subdivision Zygomycotina			
Class Zygomycetes	Sporangiospores, sometimes chlamydoconidia or budding	Zygospores	6-10 μm in diameter, usually aseptate, except at bases of reproductive structures or across damaged areas
Order Mucorales			
Family Mucoraceae—*Absidia, Mucor, Rhizopus, Circinella*			
Family Cunninghamellaceae—*Cunninghamella*			
Family Syncephalastraceae—*Syncephalastrum*			
Family Mortierellaceae—*Mortierella*			
Subdivision Ascomycotina			
Class Ascomycetes	Fission, fragmentation, chlamydoconidia, conidia	Ascospores	3-4 μm in diameter, septate
Subclass Hemiascomycetidae			
Order Endomycetales			
Family Endomycetaceae—*Endomyces (Geotrichum)*			
Family Saccharomycetaceae—*Saccharomyces*			
Subclass Plectomycetidae			
Order Onygenales			
Family Gymnoascaceae—*Arthroderma (Trichophyton), Nannizzia (Microsporum), Ajellomyces (Blastomyces, Histoplasma)*			
Order Eurotiales			
Family Eurotiaceae—*Talaromyces, Eupenicillium (Penicillium); Eurotium, Sartorya, Emericella (Aspergillus); Byssochlamys (Paecilomyces)*			
Subclass Loculoascomycetidae			
Order Myriangiales			
Family Saccardinulaceae—*Piedraia*			
Subdivision Basidiomycotina			
Class Basidiomycetes	Budding, arthroconidia, conidia, oidia, mycelial fragmentation	Basidiospores	3-4 μm in diameter, septate
Subclass Teliomycetidae			
Order Ustilaginales			
Family Ustilaginaceae—*Filobasidium, Filobasidiella (Cryptococcus); Rhodosporidium (Rhodotorula)*			
Subdivision Deuteromycotina			
Form—Class Deuteromycetes	Conidia	None or not yet discovered	3-4 μm in diameter, septate
Form—Subclass Blastomycetidae			
Form—Order Sporobolomycetales—*(Sporobolomyces)*			
Form—Order Cryptococcales—*(Rhodotorula), (Cryptococcus), (Candida), (Trichosporon), (Malassezia)*			

CHART 1-2. Continued

REPRESENTATIVE GENERA	ASEXUAL REPRODUCTION	SEXUAL REPRODUCTION	HYPHAE
Form—Subclass Coelomycetidae			
Form—Order Sphaeropsidales			
Form—Family Sphaeropsidaceae—(Phoma), (Sphaeropsis)			
Form—Subclass Hyphomycetidae			
Form—Order Moniliales			
Form—Family Moniliaceae—(Aspergillus), (Penicillium), (Botrytis), (Verticillium), (Trichoderma), (Paracoccidioides), (Sporothrix), (Geotrichum), (Coccidioides), (Microsporum), (Trichophyton), (Epidermophyton)			
Form—Family Dematiaceae—(Alternaria), (Curvularia), (Drechslera), (Cladosporium), (Phialophora), (Fonsecaea), (Exophiala), (Wangiella)			
Form—Family Tuberculariaceae-(Volutella), (Fusarium)			
Funguslike Bacteria:			
Kingdom Monera (Bacteria)			
Subdivision Schizomycotina			
Order Actinomycetales			0.5–1.0 μm in diameter
Family Mycobacteriaceae			
Family Actinomycetaceae—Actinomyces, Nocardia			
Family Streptomycetaceae—Streptomyces			

CHART 1-3. Key to Identification of Some Clinically Important Fungi*

Ascocarps and/or asci present . . . . Subdivision Ascomycotina

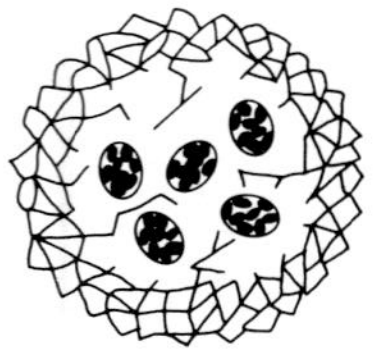

isolate on **potato dextrose agar** 2 wks at 30°C

Sporangia or zygospores present . . . . Subdivision Zygomycotina: See Chart 1-4.

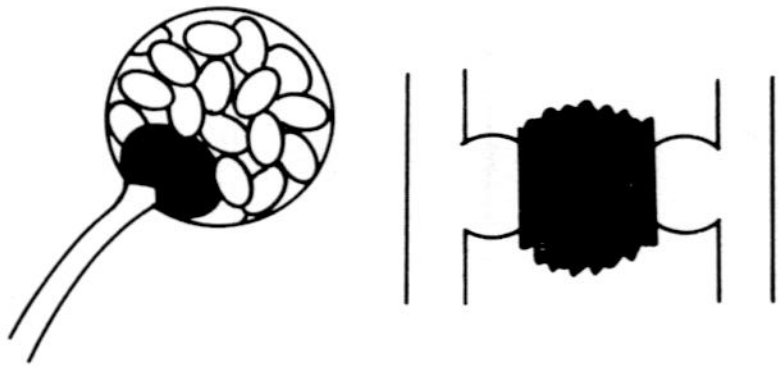

Ascocarps and/or asci absent

Yeasts with or without pseudohyphae; true hyphae absent or rudimentary . . . . Subdivision Deuteromycotina, Form—Subclass Blastomycetidae: See Chart 1-5.

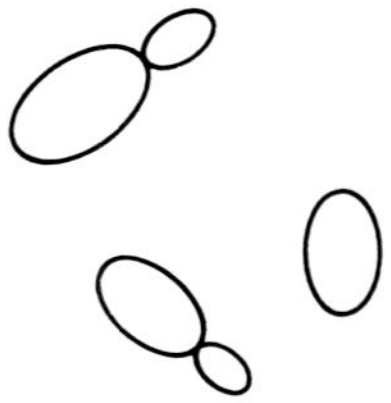

Sporangia or zygospores absent

Pycnidia (asexual sacs containing conidia) or **acervuli** (thick hyphal mats supporting bunches of conidiophores) present . . . . Subdivision Deuteromycotina, Form—Subclass Coelomycetidae

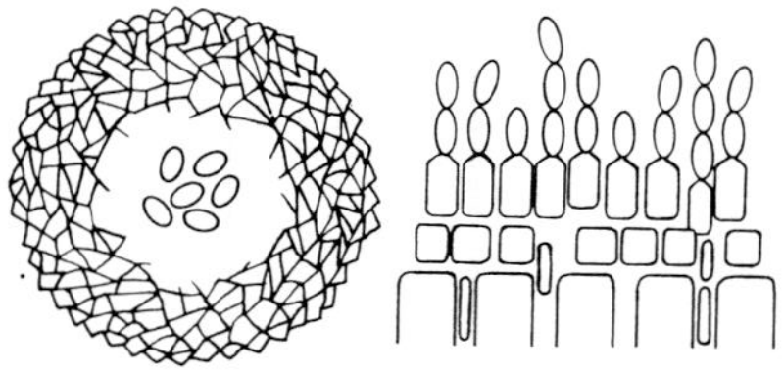

Yeasts typically absent, hyphae well developed

Pycnidia or acervuli absent . . . . Subdivision Deuteromycotina, Form—Subclass Hyphomycetidae: See Chart 1-6.

*Modified from McGinnis (1980). The Subdivision Basidiomycotina is not included here, since so few of these organisms are clinically important.

22

CHART 1-4. Key to Identification of Clinically Important Zygomycotina*

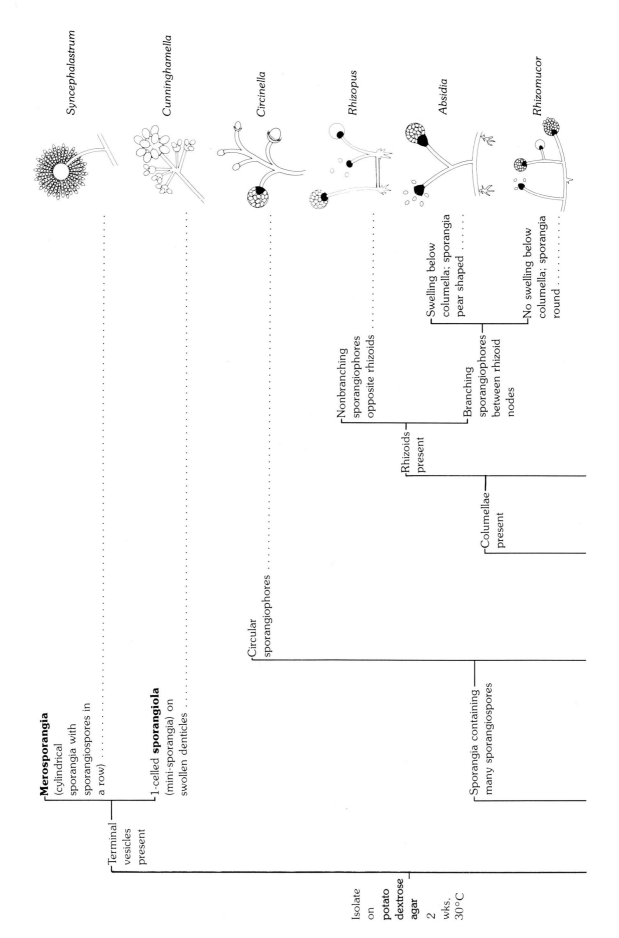

Syncephalastrum

Cunninghamella

Circinella

Rhizopus

Absidia

Rhizomucor

Merosporangia (cylindrical sporangia with sporangiospores in a row) . . . . . .

1-celled **sporangiola** (mini-sporangia) on swollen denticles . . . .

Terminal vesicles present

Circular sporangiophores . . . .

Nonbranching sporangiophores opposite rhizoids

Branching sporangiophores between rhizoid nodes

Swelling below columella; sporangia pear shaped . . . .

No swelling below columella; sporangia round . . . .

Rhizoids present

Columellae present

Sporangia containing many sporangiospores

Isolate on **potato dextrose agar** 2 wks, 30°C

CHART 1-4. Continued

Terminal vesicles absent

Sporangiophores not circular

Rhizoids absent; branching sporangiophores . . . . *Mucor*

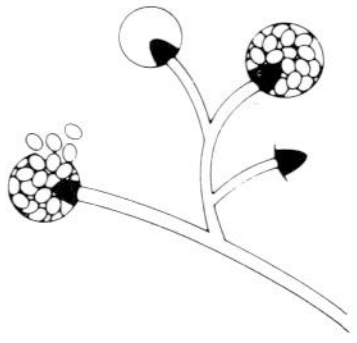

Columellae absent; tapering sporangiophores . . . . *Mortierella*

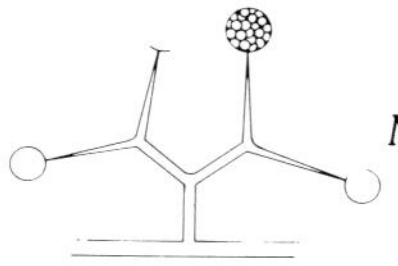

Sporangia absent; hyphae sparse; 1-celled conidia forcibly discharged

Zygospores with 2 beaklike appendages . . . . *Basidiobolus*

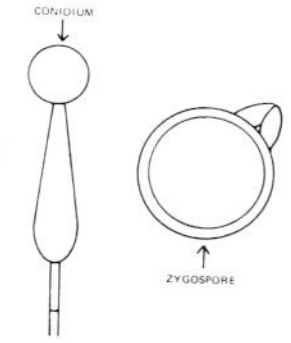

Zygospores when present, without appendages . . . . *Conidiobolus*

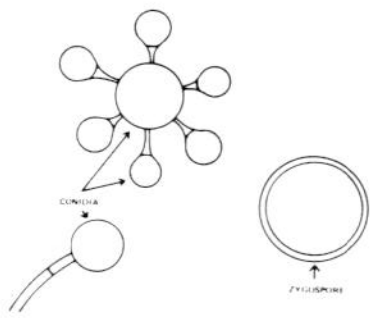

*Modified from McGinnis (1980).

CHART 1-5. Key to Identification of Clinically Important Blastomycetidae*

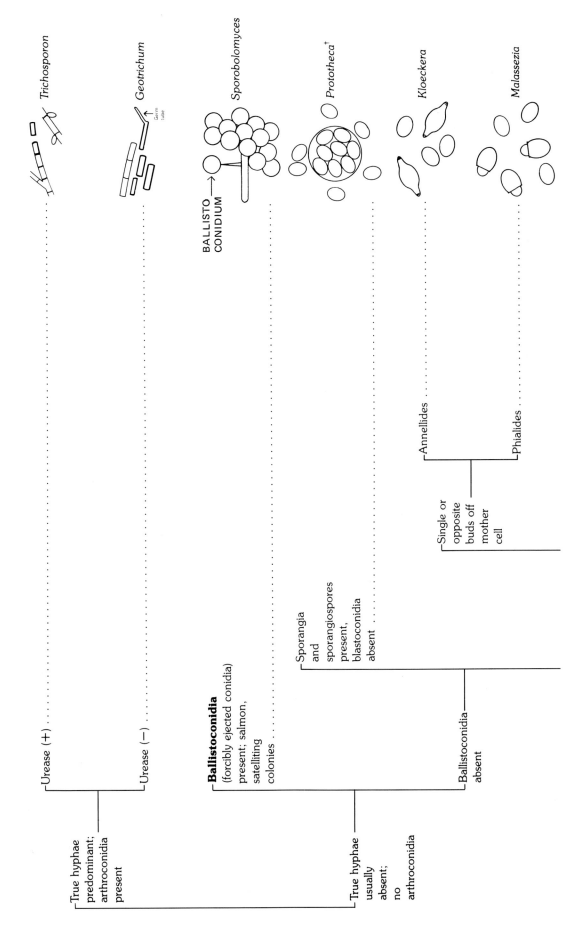

CHART 1-5. Continued

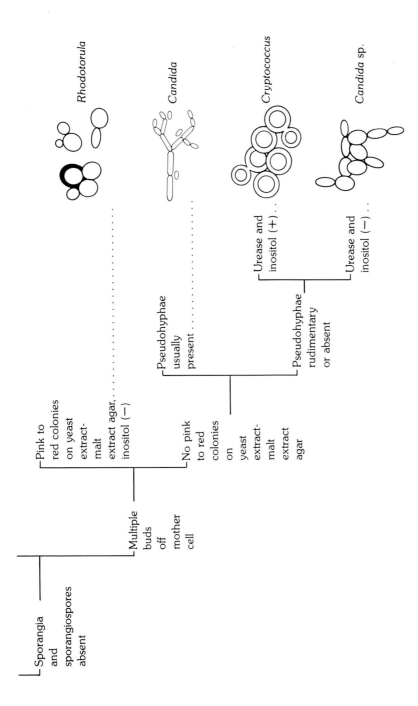

Sporangia and sporangiospores absent

Multiple buds off mother cell

Pink to red colonies on yeast extract-malt extract agar, inositol (−) . . . . *Rhodotorula*

No pink to red colonies on yeast extract-malt extract agar

Pseudohyphae usually present . . . . *Candida*

Pseudohyphae rudimentary or absent

Urease and inositol (+) . . . *Cryptococcus*

Urease and inositol (−) . . . *Candida sp.*

*Modified from McGinnis (1980)
†Alga commonly mistaken for a yeast

26

CHART 1-6. Key to Identification of Clinically Important Hyphomycetidae*

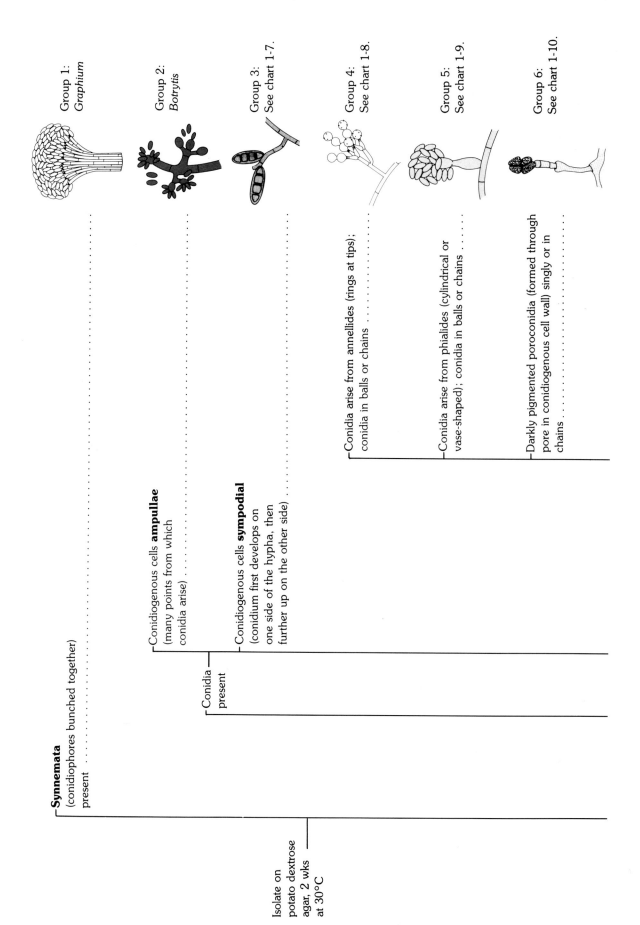

Isolate on
potato dextrose
agar, 2 wks
at 30°C

Synnemata
(conidiophores bunched together)
present . . . .
    Group 1:
    Graphium

Conidiogenous cells **ampullae**
(many points from which
conidia arise) . . . .
    Group 2:
    Botrytis

Conidia
present

Conidiogenous cells **sympodial**
(conidium first develops on
one side of the hypha, then
further up on the other side) . . . .
    Group 3:
    See chart 1-7.

Conidia arise from annellides (rings at tips);
conidia in balls or chains . . . .
    Group 4:
    See chart 1-8.

Conidia arise from phialides (cylindrical or
vase-shaped); conidia in balls or chains . . . .
    Group 5:
    See chart 1-9.

Darkly pigmented poroconidia (formed through
pore in conidiogenous cell wall) singly or in
chains . . . .
    Group 6:
    See chart 1-10.

CHART 1-6. Continued

Synnemata absent

Conidiogenous cells neither ampullae nor sympodial

Arthroconidia (formed by hyphal fragmentation) in chains . . . .

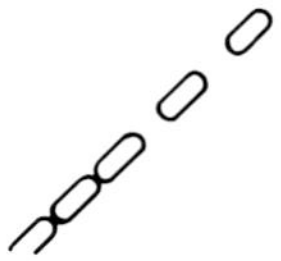

Group 7:
See chart 1-11.

Single conidia arising as terminal swollen cells, usually with an **annular frill** (skirtlike remnant at conidial base) . . . .

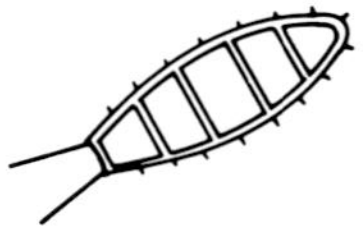

Group 8:
See chart 1-12.

Single or chained conidia "blown out" and constricted at their bases; no annular frill . . . . .

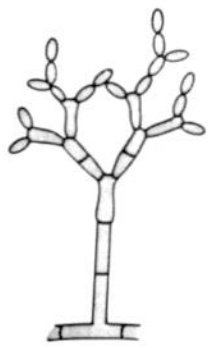

Group 9:
See chart 1-13.

Conidia absent . . . .

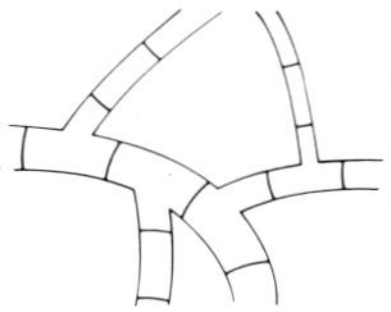

Group 10:
Mycelia
Sterilia

28

*Modified from McGinnis (1980)

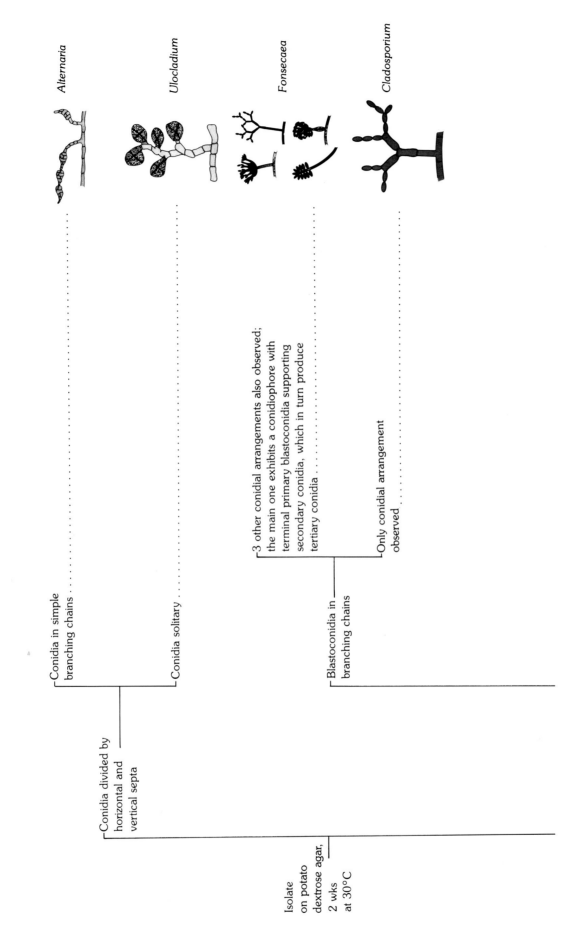

CHART 1-7. Key To Identification of Group 3 Hyphomycetidae*

Isolate on potato dextrose agar, 2 wks at 30°C

Conidia divided by horizontal and vertical septa

Conidia in simple branching chains .... *Alternaria*

Conidia solitary .... *Ulocladium*

Blastoconidia in branching chains

3 other conidial arrangements also observed; the main one exhibits a conidiophore with terminal primary blastoconidia supporting secondary conidia, which in turn produce tertiary conidia .... *Fonsecaea*

Only conidial arrangement observed .... *Cladosporium*

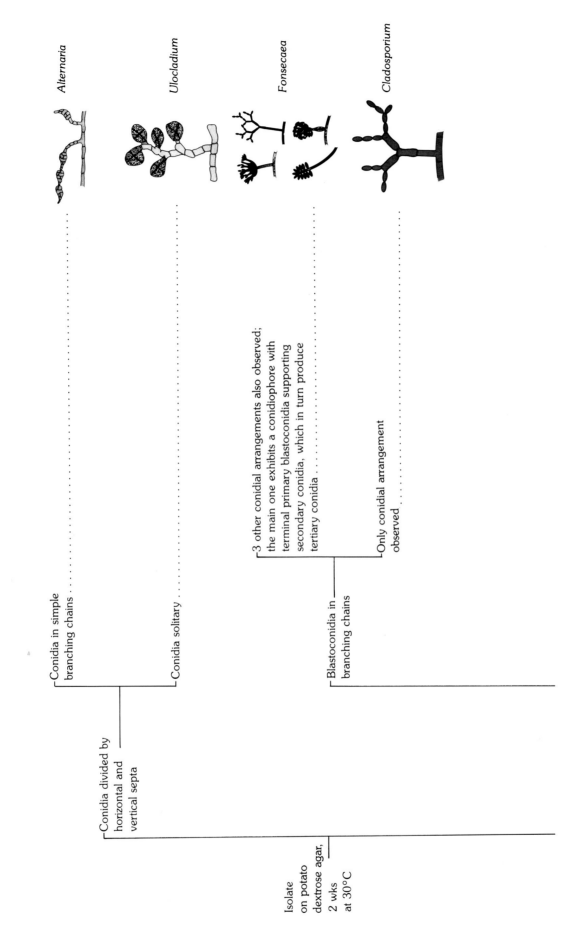

CHART 1-7. Continued

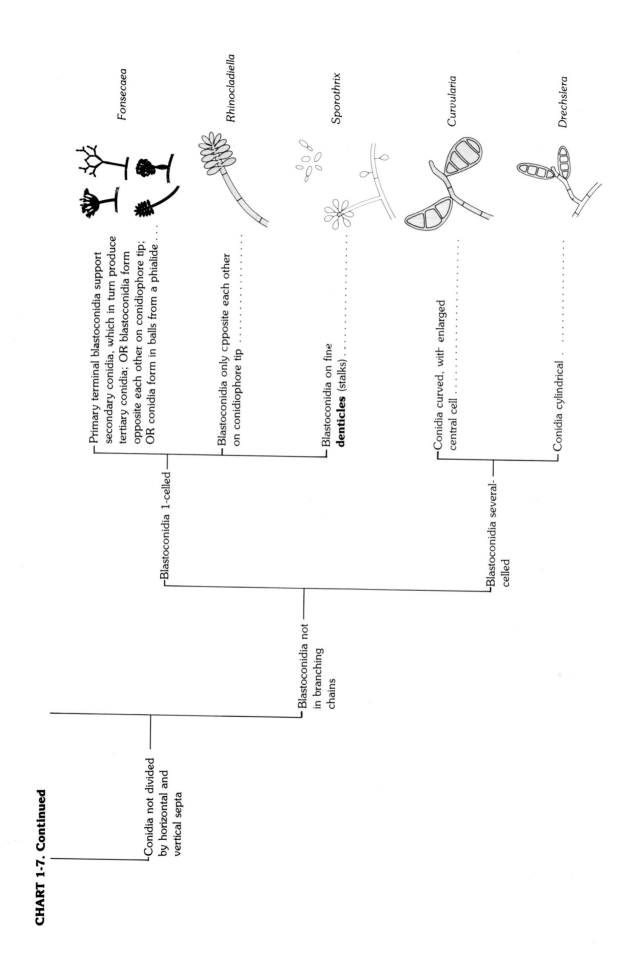

Conidia not divided by horizontal and vertical septa

Blastoconidia not in branching chains

Blastoconidia 1-celled

Primary terminal blastoconidia support secondary conidia, which in turn produce tertiary conidia; OR blastoconidia form opposite each other on conidiophore tip; OR conidia form in balls from a phialide . . . . . *Fonsecaea*

Blastoconidia only opposite each other on conidiophore tip . . . . *Rhinocladiella*

Blastoconidia on fine **denticles** (stalks) . . . . *Sporothrix*

Blastoconidia several-celled

Conidia curved, with enlarged central cell . . . . *Curvularia*

Conidia cylindrical . . . . *Drechslera*

*Modified from McGinnis (1980)

CHART 1-8. Key to Identification of Group 4 Hyphomycetidae*

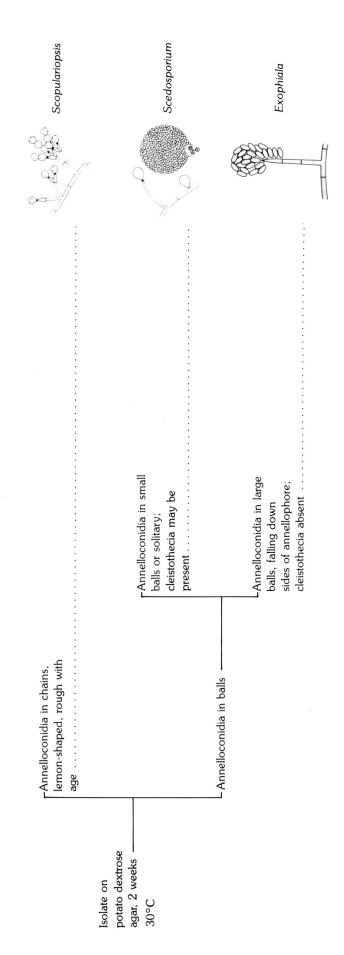

Isolate on
potato dextrose
agar, 2 weeks
30°C

Annelloconidia in chains,
lemon-shaped, rough with
age . . . . *Scopulariopsis*

Annelloconidia in balls

Annelloconidia in small
balls or solitary;
cleistothecia may be
present . . . . *Scedosporium*

Annelloconidia in large
balls, falling down
sides of annellophore;
cleistothecia absent . . . . *Exophiala*

*Modified from McGinnis (1980)

CHART 1-9. Key to Identification of Group 5 Hyphomycetidae*

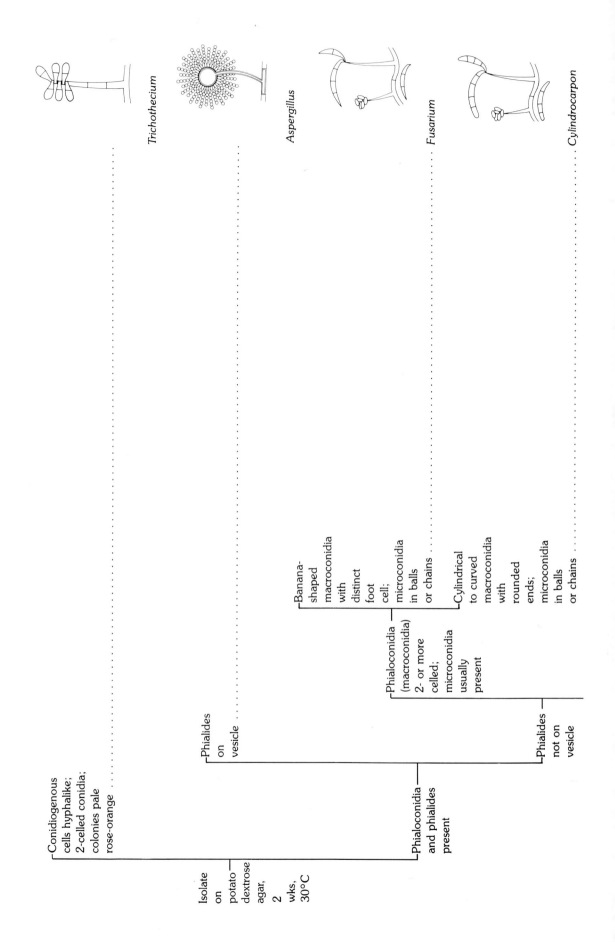

Isolate on potato dextrose agar, 2 wks, 30°C

Conidiogenous cells hyphalike; 2-celled conidia; colonies pale rose-orange .... *Trichothecium*

Phialoconidia and phialides present

Phialides on vesicle .... *Aspergillus*

Phialides not on vesicle

Phialoconidia (macroconidia) 2- or more celled; microconidia usually present

Banana-shaped macroconidia with distinct foot cell; microconidia in balls or chains .... *Fusarium*

Cylindrical to curved macroconidia with rounded ends; microconidia in balls or chains .... *Cylindrocarpon*

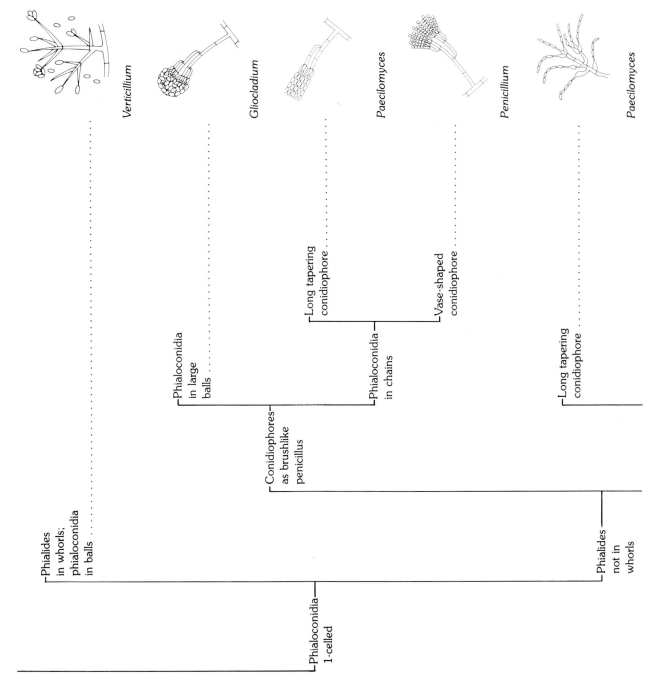

Verticillium

Gliocladium

Paecilomyces

Penicillium

Paecilomyces

Long tapering
conidiophore

Vase-shaped
conidiophore

Long tapering
conidiophore

Phialoconidia
in large
balls

Phialoconidia
in chains

Conidiophores
as brushlike
penicillus

Phialides
in whorls;
phialoconidia
in balls

Phialides
not in
whorls

Phialoconidia
1-celled

CHART 1-9. Continued

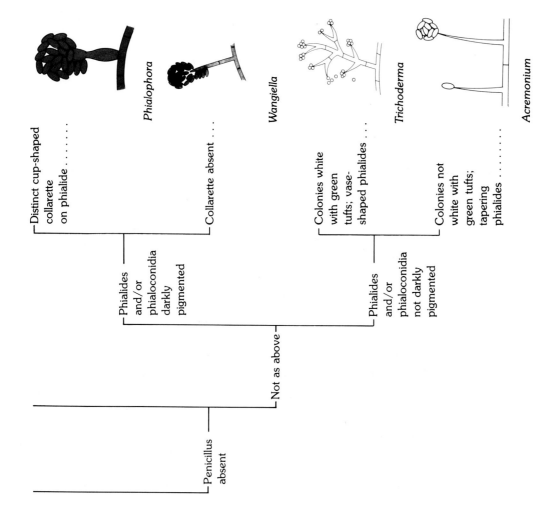

CHART 1-9. Continued

*Modified from McGinnis (1980)

Distinct cup-shaped
collarette
on phialide . . . .

Phialophora

Collarette absent . . .

Wangiella

Colonies white
with green
tufts; vase-
shaped phialides . . . .

Trichoderma

Colonies not
white with
green tufts;
tapering
phialides . . . .

Acremonium

Phialides
and/or
phialoconidia
darkly
pigmented

Phialides
and/or
phialoconidia
not darkly
pigmented

Not as above

Penicillus
absent

CHART 1-10. Key to Identification of Group 6 Hyphomycetidae*

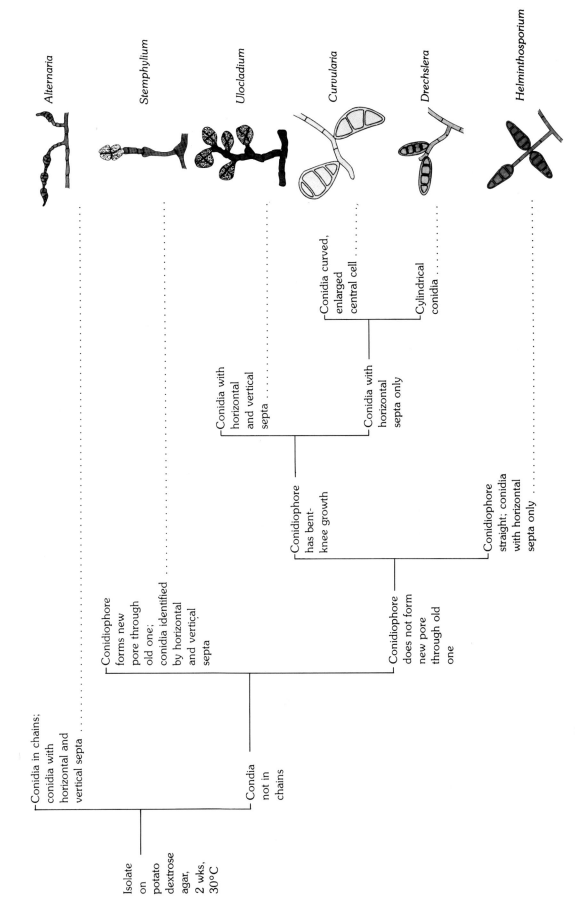

Alternaria

Stemphylium

Ulocladium

Curvularia

Drechslera

Helminthosporium

Conidia in chains; conidia with horizontal and vertical septa . . . .

Conidiophore forms new pore through old one; conidia identified by horizontal and vertical septa . . . .

Conidia with horizontal and vertical septa . . . .

Conidia curved, enlarged central cell . . . .

Cylindrical conidia . . . .

Conidiophore has bent-knee growth

Conidia with horizontal septa only

Conidiophore straight; conidia with horizontal septa only . . . .

Condia not in chains

Conidiophore does not form new pore through old one

Isolate on potato dextrose agar, 2 wks, 30°C

*Modified from McGinnis (1980)

CHART 1-11. Key to Identification of Group 7 Hyphomycetidae*

Isolate on potato dextrose agar, 2 wks, 30°C

Empty (disjunctor) cells between arthroconidia

Spherules and endospores at 37° in tissue or special media . . . . *Coccidioides*

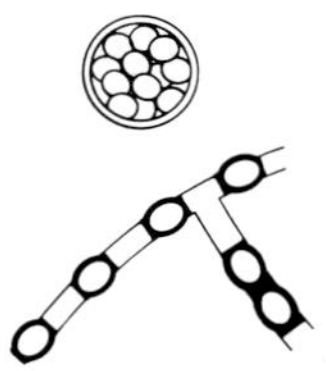

No spherules or endospores . . . . *Malbranchea*

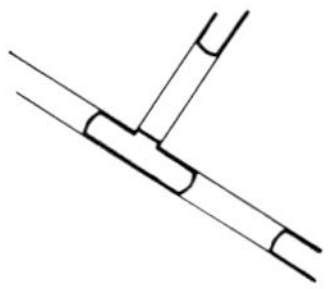

Disjunctor cells absent . . . . *Geotrichum*

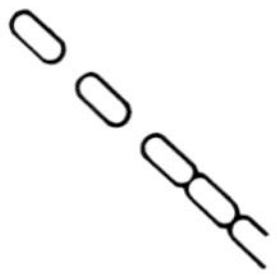

*Modified from McGinnis (1980)

CHART 1-12. Key to Identification of Group 8 Hyphomycetidae*

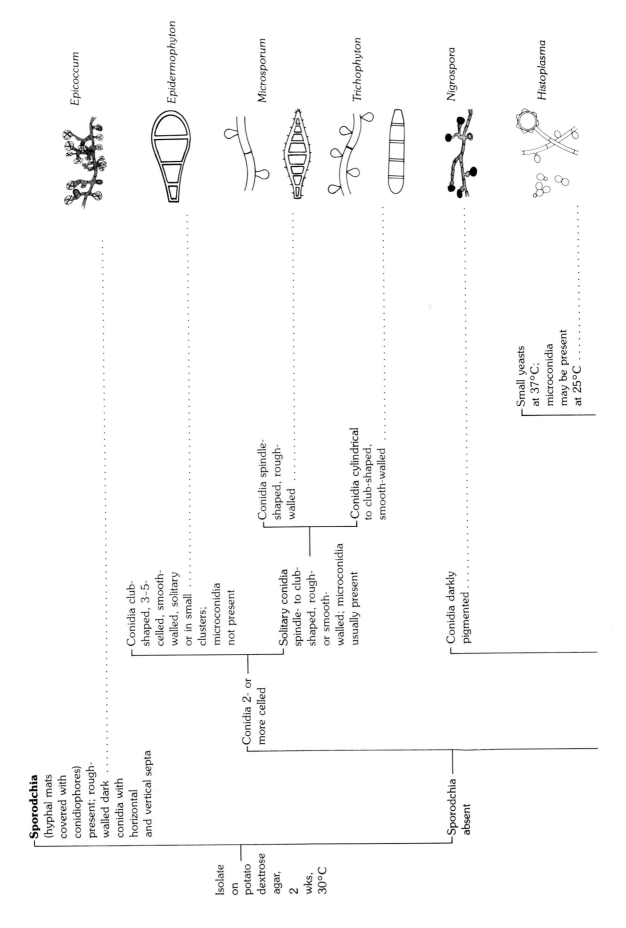

Epicoccum

Epidermophyton

Microsporum

Trichophyton

Nigrospora

Histoplasma

Small yeasts at 37°C; microconidia may be present at 25°C

Conidia spindle-shaped, rough-walled

Conidia cylindrical to club-shaped, smooth-walled

Conidia club-shaped, 3-5-celled, smooth-walled, solitary or in small clusters; microconidia not present

Solitary conidia spindle- to club-shaped, rough-or smooth-walled; microconidia usually present

Conidia darkly pigmented

Sporodchia (hyphal mats covered with conidiophores) present; rough-walled dark conidia with horizontal and vertical septa

Conidia 2- or more celled

Sporodchia absent

Isolate on potato dextrose agar, 2 wks, 30°C

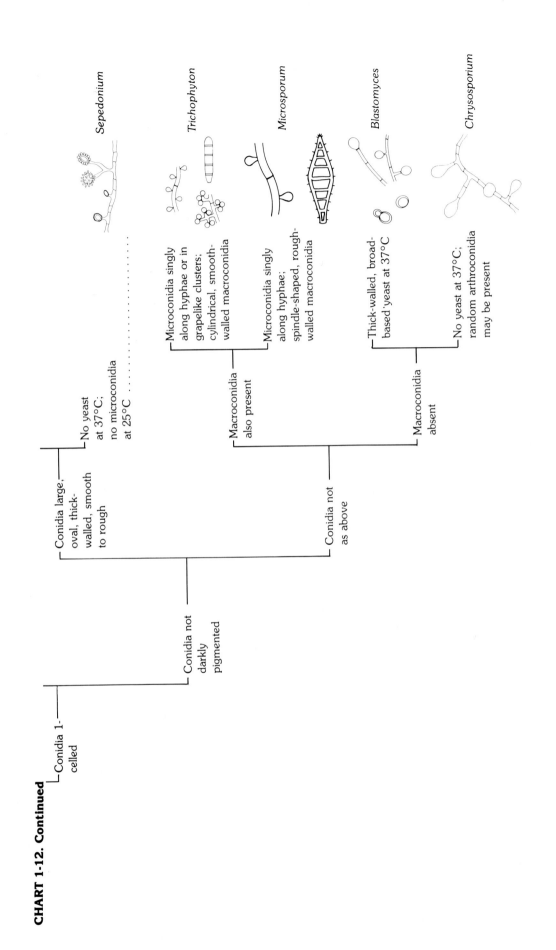

CHART 1-12. Continued

Conidia 1-celled

Conidia not darkly pigmented

Conidia large, oval, thick-walled, smooth to rough

Conidia not as above

No yeast at 37°C; no microconidia at 25°C .... *Sepedonium*

Macroconidia also present

Microconidia singly along hyphae or in grapelike clusters; cylindrical, smooth-walled macroconidia *Trichophyton*

Microconidia singly along hyphae; spindle-shaped, rough-walled macroconidia *Microsporum*

Macroconidia absent

Thick-walled, broad-based yeast at 37°C *Blastomyces*

No yeast at 37°C; random arthroconidia may be present *Chrysosporium*

•Modified from McGinnis (1980)

CHART 1-13. Key to Identification of Group 9 Hyphomycetidae*

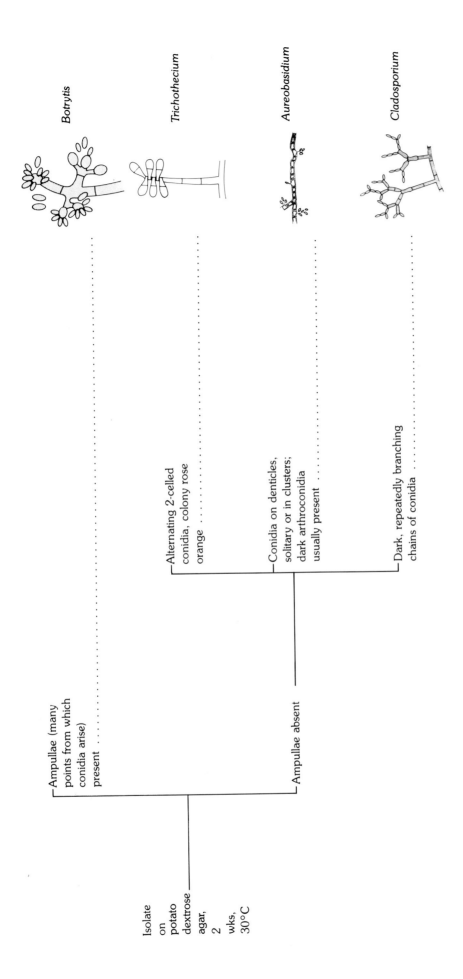

Isolate on potato dextrose agar, 2 wks, 30°C

Ampullae (many points from which conidia arise) present .... *Botrytis*

Ampullae absent

Alternating 2-celled conidia, colony rose orange .... *Trichothecium*

Conidia on denticles, solitary or in clusters; dark arthroconidia usually present .... *Aureobasidium*

Dark, repeatedly branching chains of conidia .... *Cladosporium*

*Modified from McGinnis (1980)

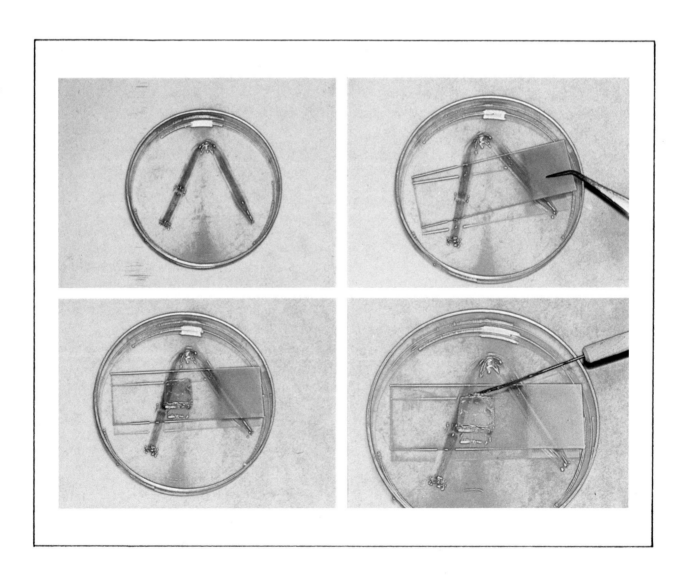

MODULE 2
LABORATORY PROCEDURES FOR FUNGAL CULTURE AND ISOLATION

PREREQUISITES. The learner must possess a good background knowledge in clinical microbiology and must have finished Module 1, Basics of Mycology.

BEHAVIORAL OBJECTIVES. Upon completion of this module, the learner should be able to:

1. List at least four general rules for good fungal specimen collection.

2. Correctly collect and process a fungal specimen from a given body source.

3. List at least two fungi which may be found at a given body site.

4. Explain why respiratory and urine specimens are collected in the morning, and why 24-hour collections should be avoided.

5. State two reasons why direct examination of every specimen for mycology is essential.

6. Discuss the types of specimen direct examinations, including the principle, procedure, and appearance of fungi in each.

7. Compile a rationale for use of the following primary isolation media:
   Sabouraud dextrose agar
   Sabouraud dextrose agar with cycloheximide and chloramphenicol
   Brain heart infusion agar with blood
   Brain heart infusion agar with blood, cycloheximide, and chloramphenicol

   Include which medium is best for isolating a given organism and which combination of media is best for maximal fungal recovery, and justify your reasons.

8. Comment on the optimal incubation temperature(s) for primary fungal cultures and justify the reasons.

9. Define rapid, intermediate, and slow growth rates, as discussed in this module.

10. Compare and contrast the advantages and disadvantages of the tease mount, slide culture, and coverslip sandwich techniques for fungal examination.

11. Synthesize a fungal identification scheme, using the general criteria below:

Specimen source
Fungal growth rate
Colonial appearance
General fungal microscopic morphology (mold, yeast, funguslike bacterium, dimorphic organism)
Specific fungal microscopic morphology (reproductive structures and so forth)

12. List two purposes for animal inoculation in mycology.

13. Discuss the pitfalls of skin tests for fungal infections.

14. Describe the principle of the following serologic tests used in mycology:

Immunodiffusion
Tube agglutination
Latex agglutination (indirect LA and indirect reverse LA)
Complement fixation
Indirect and direct fluorescent antibody
Counterimmunoelectrophoresis

List which detect circulating antibodies and which identify fungal antigens. Be sure to include what reaction comprises positive and negative test results.

CONTENT OUTLINE

I. Introduction
II. Obtaining and processing the specimen
  A. General considerations
    1. Collected from area affected
    2. Sterile technique in collecting specimen
    3. Adequate specimen
    4. Specimen delivered and processed quickly
    5. Specimen adequately labelled
  B. Specific fungal specimen sources:
    1. Blood, bone marrow
    2. Cerebrospinal fluid
    3. Cutaneous: hair, nails, skin
    4. Respiratory: bronchial washings, sputa, throats, transtracheal aspirates
    5. Tissue, biopsies
    6. Urine
    7. Vaginal, uterine cervix
    8. Wounds, subcutaneous lesions, mucocutaneous lesions
  C. Study questions
III. Direct examination of the specimen
  A. Saline wet preparation
  B. Lactophenol cotton blue wet mount
  C. Potassium hydroxide preparation
  D. Gram stain
  E. Acid-fast stain
  F. India ink preparation

FOLLOW-UP ACTIVITIES

1. Students may perform direct mounts of patient specimens or fungus cultures and observe them under the microscope.

2. Students may inoculate a specific fungus onto each of the media described in this module, then compare colonial morphology, microscopic morphology, and amount of fungal growth on each medium.

3. Students may inoculate *Geotrichum candidum* onto two tubes of Sabouraud dextrose agar, incubate one tube at room temperature (25°C) and the other tube at 37°C, then compare the two tubes for fungal growth.

4. Students may observe positive and negative reactions of the various serologic tests listed in the Supplemental Rationale section.

REFERENCES

BENEKE, ES AND ROGERS, AL: *Medical Mycology Manual*, ed 4. Burgess Publishing Co., Minneapolis, 1980.

BOTTONE, EJ: *Cryptococcus neoformans: Pitfalls in diagnosis through evaluation of gram-stained smears of purulent exudates.* J Clin Microbiol 12:790, 1980.

DOLAND, CT: *Evaluation of various media for growth of selected pathogenic fungi and Nocardia asteroides.* Am J Clin Pathol 58:339, 1972.

GORMAN, JW: *Sabhi: A new culture medium for pathogenic fungi.* Am J Med Tech 33:151, 1967.

HALEY, LD AND CALLAWAY, CS: *Laboratory Methods in Medical Mycology*, ed 4. U.S. Department of Health, Education, and Welfare, Washington, DC, 1978.

KAUFMAN, L: *Serodiagnosis of fungal diseases.* In ROSE, NR AND FRIEDMAN, H (EDS): *Manual of Clinical Immunology*, ed 2. American Society for Microbiology, Washington, DC, 1980.

KONEMAN, EW, ROBERTS, GD, AND WRIGHT, SF: *Practical Laboratory Mycology*, ed 2. Williams & Wilkins, Baltimore, 1978.

KOZINN, PJ, ET AL: *Efficiency of serologic tests in the diagnosis of systemic candidiasis.* Am J Clin Pathol 70:893, 1978.

KURUP, VP AND FINK, JN: *Evaluation of methods to detect antibodies against Aspergillus fumigatus.* Am J Clin Pathol 69:414, 1978.

MACCANI, JE: *Detection of cryptococcal polysaccharide using counterimmunoelectrophoresis.* Am J Clin Pathol 68:39, 1977.

MACKENZIE, DWR AND PHILPOT, CM: *Counterimmunoelectrophoresis as a routine mycoserological procedure.* Mycopathologia 57:1, 1975.

MANN, JL: *Autofluorescence of fungi: An aid to detection in tissue sections.* Am J Clin Pathol 79:587, 1983.

MCDONOUGH, ES, ET AL: *Growth of dimorphic human pathogenic fungi on media containing cycloheximide and chloramphenicol.* Mycopathol Mycol Appl 13:113, 1960.

MCGINNIS, MR: *Laboratory Handbook of Medical Mycology.* Academic Press, New York, 1980.

MITCHELL, JL AND BRITT, EM: *A coverslip culture technique for preparing permanent fungus mounts.* Mycopathologia 76:23, 1981.

PALMER, DF, ET AL: *Serodiagnosis of Mycotic Diseases.* Charles C Thomas, Springfield, Ill, 1977.

RINALDI, MG: *Use of potato flakes agar in clinical mycology.* J Clin Microbiol 15:1159, 1982.

TAPLIN, D, ET AL: *Isolation and recognition of dermatophytes on a new medium (DTM).* Arch Derm 99:203, 1969.

WOLF, PL, RUSSELL, B, AND SHIMODA, A: *Practical Clinical Microbiology and Mycology: Techniques and Interpretations.* John Wiley & Sons, New York, 1975.

INTRODUCTION

Fungal culture and isolation is a boundless subject area. Almost every month, someone publishes a new fungal medium or procedure. Therefore, only the most widely accepted and used media, stains, and procedures will be discussed.

This module will progress in the same order of events as occurs in the clinical situation.

OBTAINING AND PROCESSING THE SPECIMEN

General Considerations

There are several general rules for good fungal specimen collection.

1. Make sure the specimen is collected from the area most likely to be affected. For example, when a hair infection is suspected, choose hair specimens that look broken and scaly, since these will be the ones most likely to contain organisms. For a sputum specimen, instruct the patient to produce material from a deep cough, not just spit up saliva.

2. Use sterile technique in collecting the specimen. Any fungus in the specimen may contaminate your hands and possibly cause an infection. Use only flamed and cooled forceps and sterile swabs and specimen containers.

3. The specimen must be adequate. Often the physician will send down one swab to be used on bacteriology, tuberculosis, and fungal media. By the time the swab is rolled over multiple media, any organisms present might be removed and the fungal culture could be falsely negative. If several cultures are requested, ask for additional swab specimens for use in mycology.

4. The specimen must be delivered promptly to the laboratory and the laboratory must quickly process the specimen. Slow-growing, **pathogenic** (disease-producing) fungi are rapidly overgrown by bacteria and fungal contaminants. If the specimen must sit before processing, refrigerate it. Besides keeping fungi alive and bacterial/fungal contaminant colony counts down, refrigeration prevents yeasts like *Candida albicans* from multiplying and therefore increasing their significance in the specimen. If the specimen must be mailed, add 50,000 units of penicillin AND 100,000 μg of streptomycin, or alternatively, add 0.2 mg of chloramphenicol to each milliliter of material.

5. The specimen must be adequately labelled, including what disease the physician suspects. For certain fungus diseases, a special protocol is followed. For example, if actinomycosis is suspected, the specimen must be maintained, processed, and cultured under an-

aerobic conditions, or the causative (**etiologic**) organism will die. It must be remembered that the final laboratory results are only as good as the specimen that the laboratory has to work with.

Specific Fungal Specimen Sources

See Chart 2-1 (**on pages 68-70 at end of module**) for fungal organisms that may be found in various specimens.

BLOOD AND BONE MARROW

These specimens are collected in the same aseptic manner as for bacteriology. Ten milliliters of blood or any quantity of bone marrow is obtained, one drop is placed on a slide and smeared to a feathered edge, and the rest of the specimen is put into a biphasic bottle containing brain heart infusion (BHI) agar and 100 ml BHI broth. Bactec* blood culture bottles work well also. The slide is dried, Wright stained, and examined for fungal elements, especially intracellular yeast forms of *Histoplasma capsulatum*. The biphasic culture bottle is kept vented and is tilted daily to allow broth to flow over the

---

*Johnston Laboratories, 383 Hillen Road, P.O. Box 20086, Towson, Maryland 21204

agar surface. It is then carefully checked daily for growth. Note that fungi will not turn the broth very cloudy; therefore, it is imperative to frequently Gram stain the bottle contents.

If feasible, the membrane filter technique (see gray box) should be used to concentrate and culture specimens of blood and cerebrospinal fluid. Not only are more fungi recovered by this method, but growth is noticed within 18 to 24 hours, as opposed to 3 to 4 days for conventional techniques.

An excellent new commercial system for quicker and better recovery of fungi from blood is the isolator.*

CEREBROSPINAL FLUID

Cerebrospinal fluid is aseptically collected as for bacteriology. The specimen is centrifuged, one drop of sediment is placed on a slide, a coverslip is added, and the mount is microscopically examined for fungal elements. More sediment direct mounts, particularly the India ink preparation and Wright stain, may be indicated, depending on the agent suspected. The remaining sediment is inoculated to Sabouraud dextrose agar (SDA) and brain heart infusion agar with blood (BHIAB). If *Actinomyces* is suspected, inoculate a BHIAB anaerobically.

---

*E.I. DuPont Co., Concord Plaza, Wilmington, DE 19898

MEMBRANE FILTER TECHNIQUE FOR PROCESSING BLOOD AND CEREBROSPINAL FLUID SPECIMENS

Collection

Blood: Aseptically collect 8.5 ml of blood into a sterile yellow-topped Vacutainer (containing 1.7 ml of SPS), and mix well. Place the tube in a 37°C incubator and process within one hour.

CSF: The physician aseptically collects at least 3 ml of CSF. Centrifuge the specimen at 2000 rpm for 15 minutes and, placing a sterile Pasteur pipette through the supernatant, remove some of the sediment to make direct preps. Vortex the specimen.

Reagent Preparation

0.2 percent Triton X-100 solution:

Triton X-100 (octylphenoxy polyethoxyethanol)	1.0 ml
Distilled water	500 ml

   1. Mix reagents and autoclave at 15 psi for 15 minutes. Cool.

0.08 percent sodium carbonate:

Sodium carbonate	0.4 gm
Distilled water	500.0 ml

   1. Mix reagents and autoclave at 15 psi for 15 minutes. Cool.

Procedure

1. Either place a 0.45 mm membrane into a permanent filter apparatus or use a Falcon disposable filter No. 7102.
2. BEFORE turning on the vacuum, pour 50 ml of sterile 0.2 percent Triton X-100 solution into the funnel.
3. Transfer 4.0 ml of blood from the yellow-topped tube or all of the CSF into the funnel of Triton X-100 solution and swirl gently to mix.

Box continues on next page.

4. **Add 50 ml of sterile 0.08 percent sodium carbonate to the funnel, mix, and allow the mixture to sit for 2 to 3 minutes to complete the lysing action on the red blood cells.**
5. **Turn on the vacuum and, after the funnel contents have been filtered, wash the membrane with 50 ml of sterile water.**
6. **Turn off the vacuum and remove the membrane, top (inoculated) side up, to a Sabouraud dextrose agar plate or brain heart infusion agar with blood plate. Place the plate in a plastic bag to maintain moisture, incubate at 30°C, and examine daily for growth.**

CUTANEOUS: HAIR, NAILS, AND SKIN

Hair is plucked out by the roots with sterile forceps. Many fungi that infect hair will fluoresce with a Wood's lamp (366 nm). Hairs that fluoresce should be chosen for the specimen. If none of the hairs fluoresce, choose ones that are broken and scaly. Place the specimen in a sterile Petri dish for processing.

Nails are cleaned with 70 percent alcohol. With a sterile blade, scrape away and then dispose of the outer layers of nail. Scrape bits of the inner infected nail into a sterile Petri dish.

Skin is first cleaned with 70 percent alcohol to remove surface contaminants. If ringworm is present, scrape the outer portions of the red ring with a sterile blade. If there is no ring, scrape areas that look most infected. Place the scrapings in a sterile Petri dish for processing.

In the laboratory, large skin and nail scrapings are cut into tiny sections. A small portion of soft skin or hair is mixed with potassium hydroxide, while nail or hard skin is put into potassium hydroxide-dimethyl sulfoxide. For both mounts, a coverslip is added and examined for fungal elements. The rest of the specimen is inoculated onto SDA and SDA with cycloheximide and chloramphenicol (C & C). If systemic pathogens with cutaneous manifestations are suspected, also inoculate BHIAB-C & C. If *Malassezia furfur* is a consideration, set up an SDA tube layered with olive oil.

RESPIRATORY: BRONCHIAL WASHINGS, SPUTA, THROATS, TRANSTRACHEAL ASPIRATES

Usually the respiratory tract becomes infected with organisms that have been inhaled. Many mycoses exhibit a pulmonary origin and then spread to other parts of the body.

Bronchial washings are obtained by threading a tube down the patient's throat to his bronchi, injecting a little sterile saline to pick up organisms in the lungs, and aspirating up the material. Since the tube passes down the throat, bronchial washings are usually contaminated with throat flora. As with sputum, this procedure should be performed upon rising in the morning, before eating.

Sputa should be collected upon rising in the morning. Overnight incubation and multiplication of fungi in the lungs will increase the chance of isolating fungi on culture. A 24-hour collection is discouraged because it becomes easily overgrown with bacterial and fungal contaminants. The patient should not eat before donating the specimen, as food left in the mouth may contain fungi that will grow on the patient's culture. The patient should brush his teeth, rinse out his mouth with water, then produce material from a deep cough. This specimen is put in a sterile container and sent immediately to the laboratory. Since sputum is coughed up through the throat, it will be contaminated with throat flora.

Throat specimens are obtained by rolling two sterile swabs individually over the affected area. This should be performed prior to eating. The swabs are kept moist with 0.5 ml sterile saline until they are processed in the laboratory. If culturing for *Candida*, the organisms will not stick well to the swab. Therefore, scrape off material with a sterile tongue depressor, put the depressor in a sterile tube, and send it immediately to the laboratory.

Transtracheal aspirates are obtained by putting a tube through a slit in the trachea (neck) down to the bronchi and aspirating lung secretions. This procedure should be performed in the morning, when lung secretions have accumulated. Since this technique bypasses the throat, no throat flora contamination should be seen.

If actinomycosis is suspected, bronchial washings or transtracheal aspirates are sent to the lab as soon as possible for processing and anaerobic culturing, with explicit instructions to culture for *Actinomyces*. Respiratory swab specimens are immediately placed in an anaerobic transport container. If a syringe is used to obtain the specimen, be sure to seal the needle with a cork.

Once in the laboratory, bronchial washings, sputa, and transtracheal aspirates are directly examined for bits of blood, pus, or necrotic material, and these are plated on to SDA and BHIAB-C & C. If *Actinomyces* is suspected, a BHIAB is inoculated before the other fungal media, then gassed to give anaerobiasis. Do not set up sputums and throats for *Actinomyces*, as there is too much normal anaerobic flora.

If the specimen is tenacious or also to be used for TB culture, it is treated with an equal quantity of plain N-acetyl-L-cysteine (NALC) solution and vortexed to liquefy the mucus and equally distribute the organisms. Do not use specimens that have been treated with sodium hydroxide, which is routinely used for processing mycobacteria, as this chemical destroys many fungi. The NALC treated specimen is poured into a sterile 50 ml centrifuge tube, brought up to the 50 ml mark with 0.07 M phosphate buffer (pH 6.8–7.1), and mixed. If the specimen is to be used for TB culture, divide it into two tubes. Centrifuge both tubes at 2100 rpm for 15 minutes, and decant the supernatants. If *Nocardia* or *Actinomyces* is suspected, place some of the sediment from the mycology tube onto 7H10 agar or prereduced anaerobic brain heart infusion agar with blood, respectively. Add enough chloramphenicol to the mycology tube to give a final concentration of 0.1 mg per ml. Inoculate 0.1 ml of the sediment onto SDA and BHIAB-C & C. For the mycobacteriology tube, add 2 ml of 1.0 percent NaOH to the sediment, incubate 15 minutes, bring the volume up to the 50 ml mark with buffer, centrifuge as before, decant the supernatant, and inoculate the sediment to appropriate media.

A drop of concentrated sediment for fungus is put on a slide, a coverslip is added, and the specimen observed under the microscope for budding yeasts, hyphae, spherules, or funguslike bacteria **(see Chart 2-2 on pages 72–75 at end of module).** Also various stains can be used as described in the section on direct examination of the specimen.

For the two throat swabs, roll one across a slide, stain, and examine for fungal elements. Roll the other swab across SDA and SDA-C & C. For the tongue depressor, aseptically remove some of the material to a slide for staining and inoculate the remaining specimen onto SDA and SDA-C & C.

TISSUE, BIOPSIES

These specimens are obtained by the physician and should include both normal tissue and the center and edge of the lesion. They are kept moist with sterile saline until ready for processing. Tissues are aseptically teased apart in a sterile Petri dish and searched for granules and areas of pus or necrosis. Use these areas as your specimen. If granules are present, proceed as described under wounds, subcutaneous lesions, and mucocutaneous lesions. If areas of pus or necrosis are evident, inoculate these directly onto SDA, SDA-C & C, and anaerobic BHIAB, also smearing some on slides for a potassium hydroxide prep and stained preparations. If there are no granules or areas of pus or necrosis, mince the rest of the tissue with a sterile scalpel and grind it in a tissue homogenizer. Inoculate the homogenized material onto the same media mentioned above and make direct smears. As with other specimens, if *Actinomyces* is suspected, keep the tissue as anaerobic as possible during processing.

URINE

Urine should be collected after overnight incubation in the bladder. A clean catch or catheterized specimen is best, as this minimizes the presence of genital flora. Twenty-four-hour urine specimens are discouraged because of overgrowth with contaminants. Urine should not be collected from a bedpan, as the pan may also contain contaminants. The urine specimen is placed in a sterile container and sent immediately to the laboratory.

In the laboratory, some of the urine is centrifuged and a direct mount for fungal exam made with one drop of the sediment.

Stains may also be performed as indicated. If fungi are observed, a preliminary report is sent to the physician.

Usually urine is inoculated for bacteriology (calibrated loop, uncentrifuged urine, blood agar plate) and if fungi grow, they are quantitated and identified. Lately, the efficacy of quantitating fungi has been questioned. Classically, for a clean catch urine, over 100,000 fungal colonies of one kind per milliliter of urine were significant of infection; 10,000 to 100,000 were suspect; and under 10,000 or three different fungal/bacterial organisms present on the culture were representative of probable genital contamination. Now significance is based more on clinical grounds, and identification is at the discretion of the individual physician. With urine obtained from a suprapubic puncture, any fungal colonies are significant and should be identified.

If an uncommon organism is suspected, the chance of recovery is increased if the urine is centrifuged and the sediment inoculated to SDA and SDA-C & C. This procedure cannot be used to quantitate organisms; any fungi that grow are identified.

VAGINAL, UTERINE CERVIX

These sites normally may contain yeasts. Usually the specimen is obtained to determine if these yeast flora, in particular *Candida albicans*, have overgrown their normal quantities to produce an infection. The affected area is rolled over with two sterile swabs, the swabs put in transport media,* for example, Stuart's or Amie's, and refrigerated until they are processed in the laboratory. Refrigeration slows multiplication of yeasts.

In the laboratory, one swab is rolled over a slide and the slide is stained for fungal elements. The other swab

---

*With the exception of *Candida albicans*, which survives well in most transport media, few data are available on the survival of other fungi. If an organism other than *C. albicans* is suspected, insert the swab into Sabouraud broth for transport.

is rolled over SDA and SDA-C & C. Any fungi that grow are semiquantitated (many, moderate, few) and identified.

WOUNDS, SUBCUTANEOUS LESIONS, MUCOCUTANEOUS LESIONS

In a wound, for example, a burn, the damaged tissue is very susceptible to infection and becomes easily colonized with opportunistic contaminants and yeasts. Also deep, ulcerated, and crusted subcutaneous and mucocutaneous lesions may be elicited by some fungi. Scrapings of the crusted portions and from the deep center and edge of active lesions are taken with a sterile scalpel. Remove the scrapings to 1 ml of sterile saline for transport. In addition to scrapings, material may be aspirated from deep cysts or abscesses in the tissue by needle and syringe. If there are any variously colored granules or tiny black dots, these are collected by laying sterile saline-wetted gauze on top of the lesion and pulling off the gauze. The granules should be trapped in the gauze mesh.

All specimens are kept in anaerobic containers in case *Actinomyces* is the causative agent. In the laboratory, a potassium hydroxide preparation is made with some of the scrapings and aspirate, and the mount is searched for fungal elements. The color of the granules is noted, since this may provide a clue as to the causative organism. Some of the granules are gently teased apart in a drop of sterile water or they are stained. They are observed microscopically for bacteria, funguslike bacteria, or hyphae interspersed with swollen chlamydosporelike cells. Some granules may contain a cementlike matrix or center of necrotic debris.

A potassium hydroxide-dimethyl sulfoxide prep (see section on direct examination of the specimen) is made with some of the black dots; they are observed for thick-walled, dark brown bodies (**sclerotic bodies**) which may be divided into two or four cells.

Concurrent with the direct mounts, the rest of the skin scrapings, aspirated material, and black dots are inoculated to SDA, SDA-C & C, and anaerobic BHIAB. The granules are washed several times in sterile saline to remove contamination before culturing, then crushed and placed on the media listed above. Be sure to first plate the brain heart infusion agar with blood, and immediately gas it to maintain anaerobiasis.

STUDY QUESTIONS

1. **List three general rules for good collection of fungal specimens.**

2. **Circle true or false:**

   T F With a sputum culture, one would expect to observe growth of throat organisms.

3. **Why is a urine specimen obtained upon rising in the morning?**

4. **Circle the letter of the correct answer:**

   The fungal organism most commonly found in vaginal infections is:

   A. *Cryptococcus neoformans*

   B. *Coccidioides immitis*

   C. *Candida glabrata*

   D. *Candida albicans*

   E. *Geotrichum candidum*

5. **Circle true or false:**

   T F Do not disinfect skin or nail areas with alcohol before taking scrapings, as the disinfectant will kill any pathogenic fungi you want to recover.

6. **Why are more organisms recovered more quickly with the membrane filtration technique for blood and cerebrospinal fluid cultures than with conventional methods?**

7. Circle true or false:

   T F Sputum specimens may be placed in plain N-acetyl-L-cysteine solution for concurrent fungal and TB processing.

8. Circle true or false:

   T F Granules from subcutaneous lesions only represent necrotic material and therefore should be disregarded.

STOP HERE UNTIL YOU HAVE COMPLETED THE ANSWERS.

Look up the answers in the back of the book. If you missed more than two, go back and review the sections on general considerations and specific sources of fungal specimens. Correctly complete any missed questions before proceeding further.

DIRECT EXAMINATION OF THE SPECIMEN

It is most important that each specimen be examined microscopically before, or concurrent with, culturing. A direct examination allows you to send out an immediate preliminary report to the physician, telling him whether a fungus, and even possibly which genus, was seen. With a positive direct examination result, you may also inoculate special media to quickly isolate and specifically identify the organism.

In the patient with an acute disease, direct examination results can possibly save his life. If a fungus was observed, the physician can immediately begin treatment. Some pathogenic fungi require a long incubation period (three to four weeks) for growth. By this time the patient may have died, and isolation and identification of the causative fungal agent becomes academic.

On the other hand, if a fungus was not observed on a direct mount, the physician can avoid using antifungal drugs, which are generally toxic and require a long period of treatment. Also, the physician may start thinking about other possible disease agents, for example, tuberculosis.

It is obvious that to be of any use to the physician and patient you must be very careful and very thorough with the direct examination. Many times this may require performing more than one type of direct mount. Each will be discussed separately.

Saline Wet Mount

See gray box. Fungal elements that may be observed are budding yeasts, hyphae and pseudohyphae, conidia, thin branching filaments resembling bacteria (funguslike bacteria), granules, or *Coccidioides immitis* spherules. Chart 2-2 **(on pages 72-75 at end of module)** summarizes wet preparation findings.

SALINE WET MOUNT

Reagent Preparation
  Saline:
    Sodium chloride   0.85 gm
    Distilled water   100 ml
      1. Dissolve the sodium chloride in water and mix well.
Procedure
    1. Place one drop of specimen on a glass slide and add one drop of saline.
    2. Put on a coverslip and observe under low and high power on the microscope, using low light. Organisms will appear refractile, or shiny, and slightly green. Be sure to differentiate any yeast cells from bubbles or red blood cells: yeasts will contain inclusions, while the others will not.

Lactophenol Cotton Blue (LPCB) Wet Mount (Fig. 2-1)

See gray box. The phenol in the stain will kill any organisms, while the lactic acid preserves fungal structures. Cotton blue stains the chitin in fungal cell walls. The same structures may be seen as with the saline wet mount; however, the LPCB preparation can be made permanent.

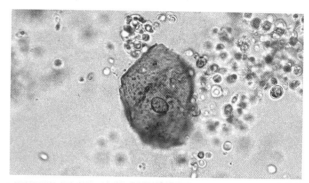

FIGURE 2-1. Lactophenol cotton blue (LPCB) wet mount, yeasts and epithelial cell, ×450.

LACTOPHENOL COTTON BLUE (LPCB) WET MOUNT

Reagent Preparation
LPCB: commercially available (Marion Scientific)*

Phenol, concentrated	20 ml
Lactic acid	20 ml
Glycerol	40 ml
Cotton blue (China blue) (National Aniline Division)†	0.05 gm
Distilled water	20 ml

1. Dissolve cotton blue in distilled water, then add the rest of the ingredients. Mix well.

Procedure
1. Place one drop of specimen on a slide, and add one drop of LPCB. Some specimens, for example, pleural fluid, will precipitate with this stain.
2. Mix well and add a coverslip. Observe under the microscope for fungal elements; see Chart 2-2 at end of module.
3. For a permanent preparation, rim the coverslip with clear nail polish or Permount.

---

*Marion Scientific, 9233 Ward Parkway, Kansas City, Missouri 64114
†Cotton blue is a carcinogen, so handle with care. Trypan blue or aniline blue may be used instead. Lactophenol aniline blue is commercially available from Remel, 12076 Santa Fe Drive, Lenexa, Kansas 66215.

Potassium Hydroxide (KOH) Preparation (Fig. 2-2)

If the specimen is skin, hair, or nail, the background cellular material may mask fungal elements. Potassium hydroxide will dissolve the keratin in these specimens, thus making any fungi more visible (gray box).* If there is a lot of cellular material in sputum or vaginal secretions, a KOH mount may be prepared to dissolve the background, thus making any yeasts more visible. However, a saline mount must be additionally done to quantitate epithelial cells and white blood cells and to note presence of *Trichomonas*.

For nail and very hard skin scrapings or for sclerotic bodies of chromoblastomycosis, potassium hydroxide-dimethyl sulfoxide may be used instead (gray box).

KOH-DMSO is not recommended for hair or thin scrapings, as it may distort them.

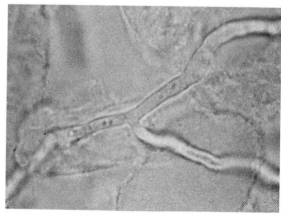

FIGURE 2-2. Potassium hydroxide (KOH) preparation, hyphae in scrapings. (Courtesy of Dr. Robert Kenney, William Beaumont Medical Center, El Paso, Texas.

---

*Calcofluor white-KOH (pg. 53) is more sensitive than plain KOH for detecting fungi.

POTASSIUM HYDROXIDE (KOH) PREPARATION

Reagent Preparation
10 percent potassium hydroxide: commercially available (Marion Scientific)

Potassium hydroxide	10 gm
Glycerol	20 ml
Distilled water	80 ml

1. Dissolve the potassium hydroxide in water, then add glycerol. Glycerol prevents crystalization of the reagent and allows KOH preparations to be maintained for two days before drying up.

Procedure
1. Thinly smear some of the specimen on a glass slide.
2. Add one drop of 10 percent KOH, put on a coverslip, and gently heat by passing through a flame two or three times. Do not boil.
3. When the specimen has cleared (about 20 minutes), observe it under low and high power for any mycologic elements: hyphae, arthroconidia, and yeasts. On hair specimens, determine if the fungus is growing outside the hair shaft (ectothrix invasion) or inside the hair shaft (endothrix invasion). As with saline preparations, the organisms are not stained and thus they appear refractile. Low light is best for observing the fungi.

POTASSIUM HYDROXIDE-DIMETHYL SULFOXIDE (KOH-DMSO) PREPARATION

Reagent Preparation
KOH-DMSO:

Dimethyl sulfoxide, water solvent (Calbiochem Co., Los Angeles)	40 ml
Distilled water	60 ml
Potassium hydroxide (KOH)	10 gm

1. Using a safety pipette, add DMSO to distilled water.
2. Dissolve the KOH in solution and mix well.

Procedure
1. Place the specimen, ground in small pieces, on a glass slide. Add one drop of KOH-DMSO, and put on a coverslip. Do not heat the preparation.
2. The mount must be examined within 20 minutes. Look for the same structures as with the 10 percent KOH prep.

Gram Stain (Fig. 2-3)

Often, fungal presence is first noted on the routine specimen Gram stain performed for bacteriology. Fungi stain Gram positive, or blue. Any fungal forms may be observed, although yeasts and pseudohyphae are the most common.

Yeasts are two to three times larger than Gram-positive cocci and will usually be budding if they are causing an infection. On a vaginal or urethral Gram-stained smear, a nonbudding yeast may be mistaken for a tailless spermatozoon. One must also be aware that on respiratory or CSF specimens, the capsule around *Cryptococcus neoformans* prevents definitive staining of the yeast itself, and thus the organism can easily be

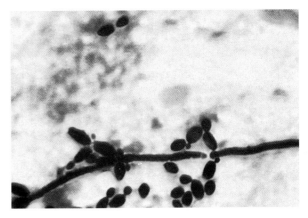

FIGURE 2-3. Gram stain, yeasts and pseudohyphae, ×1000.

completely overlooked. This point is especially important since the physician may not order histologic stains or fungus cultures, and the patient's disease would remain undiagnosed. On a Gram stain, *C. neoformans* appears either as a round, pale lavender cell with Gram-positive, granular inclusions, or as a Gram-negative fat body.

Hyphae are two to three times wider than Gram-positive rods, and often hyphae will not stain solidly inside, eliciting a granular appearance.

Acid-fast Stain

The funguslike bacteria *Nocardia* are partially acid fast, appearing red against a blue background (Color Plate 12), and may be mistaken for mycobacteria; however, *Nocardia* possess branching filaments as well as bacillary forms. The acid-fast stain for mycobacteria may overdecolorize *Nocardia*, giving false-negative results. Another smear should be made and stained with the modified Kinyoun acid-fast stain (see gray box) if *Nocardia* is suspected. These organisms remain viable through the sputum digestion process for tuberculosis and will also grow on TB media. The disease caused by these funguslike bacteria may resemble tuberculosis; hence, the diagnosis of nocardiosis must always be considered when working up a patient for TB. See the Supplemental Rationale section of Module 6 for a description of nocardiosis.

MODIFIED KINYOUN ACID-FAST STAIN

Reagent Preparation
  Kinyoun's carbolfuchsin: commercially available (Difco)

Basic fuchsin	4 gm
95 percent ethanol	20 ml
Phenol crystals	8 gm
Distilled water	100 ml

    1. Dissolve the basic fuchsin in ethanol.
    2. Carefully add phenol and water. Mix well.
  50 percent ethanol:

Concentrated (99–100 percent) ethyl alcohol	50 ml
Distilled water	50 ml

    1. Mix the above ingredients together.
  1 percent sulfuric acid:

Concentrated sulfuric acid	1 ml
Distilled water	99 ml

    1. Carefully add acid to water and mix well.
  Methylene blue: commercially available (Difco)

Methylene blue	2.5 gm
95 percent ethanol	100 ml

    1. Dissolve methylene blue in alcohol and mix well.
Procedure
  1. Make smears of the organism* and positive and negative controls. Heat fix.
  2. Flood the slides with Kinyoun's carbolfuchsin. Stain for 5 minutes.
  3. Wash with tap water.
  4. Flood the slides with 50 percent ethanol until all excess dye is removed. This step removes precipitated dye, eliminating a lot of background debris.
  5. Wash with tap water.
  6. Decolorize with 1 percent sulfuric acid for 3 minutes.[†]
  7. Wash with tap water.
  8. Counterstain with methylene blue for 1 minute.
  9. Wash with tap water and allow the slides to air dry. *Nocardia* stains red, while other bacteria and fungi are blue. If this procedure is used for yeast ascospore production, asci stain red, while blastoconidia are blue.

Nocardia should be taken from cultures on 7H10 or 7H11 agar, as these media enhance acid fastness.
[†]Acid alcohol for staining mycobacteria may be used for decolorization instead. Acid alcohol is flooded on the slides for 5 seconds and washed off. This method gives variable results and is thus not recommended.

India Ink Preparation (Fig. 2-4)

This procedure is employed to observe capsules around yeasts, especially *Cryptococcus neoformans* in cerebrospinal fluid sediment (see gray box). Unfortunately, all bacterial and fungal organisms, encapsulated or not, will stand out distinctly against the black India ink background, because the ink will not penetrate the cell wall or capsule. Therefore, be careful to search for capsules only. Some bacteria, for example *Klebsiella*, possess capsules that may be mistaken for yeasts. However, bacteria are one fourth the size of yeasts, and bacteria will not be budding. Some laboratories use a positive India ink preparation as definitive evidence for the presence of *Cryptococcus neoformans*. It must be emphasized that other *Cryptococcus* species, as well as *Rhodotorula, Candida (Torulopsis), Sporobolomyces, Trichosporon beigelii,* and *Prototheca stagnora* (an alga that may be confused with *Cryptococcus*) may be encapsulated. The laboratory must perform other studies,

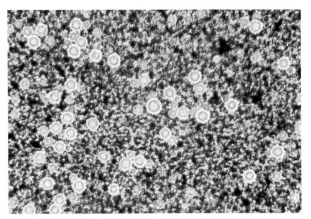

FIGURE 2-4. India ink preparation, *Cryptococcus neoformans*, ×1000.

such as dark brown pigment production on caffeic acid agar or specific carbohydrate assimilation reactions, before calling an organism *Cryptococcus neoformans*. See Module 5 for further information on *Cryptococcus*.

INDIA INK PREPARATION

Reagent Preparation
   India ink or nigrosin
Procedure
   1. **On a slide, mix a *tiny* drop of India ink or nigrosin*† with one drop of specimen sediment, add a coverslip, and let the mount sit 10 minutes to allow yeast cells to settle into one plane of focus.**
   2. **Observe the preparation under the microscope, with the condenser adjusted for maximum light, for capsules around budding yeasts.**

---

*Marion Scientific, 9233 Ward Parkway, Kansas City, Missouri 64114
†I prefer nigrosin over India ink, because nigrosin provides a homogenized background, which facilitates the search for capsules.

Other Stains

Stains for fungal detection may be done in laboratory sections other than microbiology. The technologists in histology perform the Gomori methenamine silver (GMS) stain, in which fungi and actinomycetes appear black against a green background (Color Plate 13), and the periodic acid-Schiff (PAS) stain, in which fungal elements, but not actinomycetes, look magenta against a light pink or green background (Color Plate 64). They can also perform Mayer's mucicarmine stain when *Cryptococcus* is suspected. The capsules of these organisms appear red against a yellow background, while other similar-appearing fungi do not take up the red stain. The hematoxylin and eosin (H&E) stain is the workhorse of pathologists: the background is pink, with tissue nuclei and fungal elements staining purple. An added advantage to the H&E preparation is that stained sections may be placed directly under a fluorescent microscope, where fungi such as *Blastomyces, Cryptococcus, Candida, Aspergillus, Coccidioides, Paracoccidioides,* and occasionally *Histoplasma* will brightly autofluoresce while tissue and background material remain dark. See Mann (1983) for further details.

The hematology technologists perform the Wright stain on blood and bone marrow smears to look for purple pseudoencapsulated yeast forms of *Histoplasma capsulatum* inside polymorphonuclear cells and monocytes.

A new technique for direct mounts or histologic sections utilizes Calcofluor white-KOH or Calcofluor white-Evans blue. The prep is observed under a fluorescent microscope, and is very sensitive for detecting fungal structures. It is far preferred to the plain KOH prep. See Hageage, George and Harrington, Brian "Use of Calcofluor white in Clinical Mycology," Laboratory Medicine 15:109, 1984.

Study Questions

1. Why is it important to perform a direct mount examination on every specimen? Give two reasons.

Matching: Place the letter of the answer in Column B in front of the words in Column A.

Column A		Column B
2. _____ KOH preparation		A. *Nocardia*
3. _____ Acid-fast stain		B. *Histoplasma capsulatum*
		C. Fungi stain magenta
4. _____ India ink preparation		D. Hair
		E. Hard nail scrapings
5. _____ Wright stain		F. *Cryptococcus neoformans*
6. _____ Gram stain		G. Fungi stain blue
7. _____ KOH-DMSO preparation		

8. Circle true or false:

   T   F   With the India ink preparation, only encapsulated organisms are visible against the black background.

9. Circle the letter of the correct answer.

   _____ is the most useful mounting fluid for nail scrapings.
   A. Lactophenol cotton blue
   B. Potassium hydroxide-dimethyl sulfoxide
   C. Acetic acid
   D. Saline
   E. Potassium hydroxide

10. Circle true or false:

    T   F   With positive lactophenol cotton blue mounts, the specimen may then be removed from under the coverslip and cultured.

STOP HERE UNTIL YOU HAVE COMPLETED THE ANSWERS.

Look up the answers in the back of the book. If you missed more than one, go back and review the section on direct examinations. Correctly complete any missed questions before proceeding further.

CULTURING THE SPECIMEN

Primary Fungal Media

Once a direct mount has been examined, specific fungal media are inoculated to initially isolate any organisms (primary media). Tubed media are preferred over plates, as the former will not dry out over the long incubation period, and also the chance for fungal reproductive structures to become airborne and contaminate the room and people is decreased. Never use plates when *Coccidioides immitis* is suspected; this fungus is extremely infectious and aerosols may be inhaled. Always work under a microbiologic hood, wear gloves, auto-clave specimens and inoculated media when finished, and disinfect the work area daily. See individual sections on specimen collection and processing, plus Chart 2-1 **(on pages 68-70 at end of module),** for media to be inoculated for various specimens.

SABOURAUD DEXTROSE AGAR (SDA)

This general medium has an acid pH of 5.6 and is nutritionally poor (see gray box). These conditions inhibit growth of many bacteria but allow fungal contaminants and pathogenic fungi to grow, with the exception of *Histoplasma capsulatum* and some strains of *Nocardia asteroides.*

SABOURAUD DEXTROSE AGAR (SDA)

Medium Preparation: commercially available (Difco, BBL)

Dextrose	40 gm
Neopeptone (Difco)	10 gm
Agar	15 gm
Distilled water	1 liter

1. Mix together the above ingredients and heat to dissolve.
2. Tube in 15 ml aliquots and autoclave at 15 psi for 10 minutes. Slant so there is a one-inch butt, cool, and refrigerate.

Procedure

1. Bring the tube to room temperature. Swab the entire surface of the agar slant. Pieces of specimen are pushed slightly into the agar. If media with antibiotics are also to be inoculated, be sure to swab plain Sabouraud dextrose agar and brain heart infusion agar with blood first so there is no antibiotic carryover.
2. Incubate with the cap loose, at 30°C for one month before discarding as negative.

SABOURAUD DEXTROSE AGAR WITH CYCLOHEXIMIDE AND CHLORAMPHENICOL (SDA-C&C)

See gray box. Cycloheximide and chloramphenicol are antibiotics that inhibit bacterial and most fungal contaminant organisms, thus allowing pathogens a better chance to flourish. However, many pathogens are also inhibited **(see Chart 2-3 on page 76 at end of module).** Since many disease-causing organisms will not grow on SDA-C&C, this medium is usually reserved for skin, hair, and nail specimens, in which only dermatophytes *(Trichophyton, Epidermophyton,* and *Microsporum)* or *Candida albicans* are suspected.

SABOURAUD DEXTROSE AGAR WITH CYCLOHEXIMIDE AND CHLORAMPHENICOL (SDA-C&C)

Medium Preparation: commercially available (Mycosel—BBL; Mycobiotic—Difco)

Dextrose	40 gm
Neopeptone (Difco)	10 gm
Agar	15 gm
Distilled water	1 liter
Cycloheximide (Upjohn)	500 mg
Acetone	10 ml

Box continues on next page.

---

1. Mix together the first four ingredients and bring to a boil.
2. Dissolve cycloheximide in acetone; dissolve chloramphenicol in alcohol. Add both to hot medium and mix well.
3. Tube in 15 ml aliquots, autoclave at 15 psi for 10 minutes, and slant so there is a one-inch butt. Cool and refrigerate.

Procedure
1. Bring the medium to room temperature. Swab the entire surface of the agar slant.
2. Incubate with the cap loose at 30°C for one month before discarding as negative.

These organisms are not sensitive to C&C and therefore will proliferate.

Dermatophyte test medium (DTM)* may be used in place of SDA-C&C for cutaneous specimens. DTM contains a phenol red indicator; when dermatophytes grow, they change the color from yellow to red, although a few fungi other than dermatophytes can accomplish this also. If Sabouraud dextrose agar with antibiotics is used for specimens other than skin, hair, and nails, a plain Sabouraud dextrose agar should additionally be inoculated so that all organisms (except *Histoplasma capsulatum* and some *Nocardia asteroides*) will be recovered.

---

*Oricult, Medical Technology Corp., 71 Veronica Ave., P.O. Box 218, Somerset, NJ 08873.

BRAIN HEART INFUSION AGAR WITH BLOOD (BHIAB)

See gray box. Brain heart infusion agar is a very nutritious medium, and the addition of blood makes it more so. Aerobically, bacteria, fungal contaminants, and pathogens, including *Histoplasma capsulatum* and *Nocardia asteroides*, will flourish. Because there is growth of contaminants, plain brain heart infusion agar with blood is of limited usefulness. Its value aerobically is to isolate *Histoplasma* and *Nocardia* from normally sterile specimens and to convert purified dimorphic fungi from the mold to the yeast phase. Prereduced brain heart infusion agar with blood is incubated anaerobically when *Actinomyces* is suspected. Be sure to inoculate it before any other mycologic media, and immediately gas it to create anaerobic conditions (95 percent N_2, 5 percent CO_2).

BRAIN HEART INFUSION AGAR WITH BLOOD (BHIAB)

Medium Preparation: commercially available

Brain heart infusion	37 gm
Agar	20 gm
Distilled water	1 liter
Sheep blood, defibrinated, sterile	100 ml

1. Mix together the brain heart infusion, agar, and water. Autoclave at 15 psi for 15 minutes and cool to 50°C.
2. While swirling the flask, add the sheep blood, then immediately pour into plates or aseptically aliquot in tubes and slant. Cool completely and refrigerate. If medium is to be used for anaerobic actinomycetes, prereduce it in an anaerobic chamber before inoculating.

Procedure
1. Bring the medium to room temperature. If it is to be used for dimorphic mold conversion, follow instructions in Module 7.
2. If it is to be used for anaerobic actinomycetes, swab one third of the prereduced plate, then streak out for isolation. Granules from specimens are first washed several times with sterile saline, crushed, then smeared on one third of the agar plate, before streaking for isolation. Try to maintain anaerobic conditions from time of specimen collection through processing, to incubation. Set inoculated media in an anaerobic chamber at 37°C for 7 to 10 days before discarding as negative.

BRAIN HEART INFUSION AGAR WITH BLOOD, CYCLOHEXIMIDE, AND CHLORAMPHENICOL (BHIAB-C&C)

In the previous section it was stated that brain heart infusion agar with blood is nutritious, that is, it will support the growth of fastidious organisms such as *Histoplasma capsulatum* and *Nocardia asteroides*. The cycloheximide and chloramphenicol inhibit bacterial and fungal contaminants, plus some pathogens, including *Nocardia asteroides* **(see Chart 2-3 on page 76 at end of** **module),** so that the slower growing dimorphic pathogens have an opportunity to grow. Any specimen contaminated with bacterial and fungal contaminants that is also suspected of containing *Histoplasma* should be plated on brain heart infusion agar with blood, cycloheximide, and chloramphenicol (gray box). Note that only the mold phase will grow, as chloramphenicol inhibits the yeast phase of dimorphic organisms. Brain heart infusion agar with blood, cycloheximide, and chloramphenicol may also be used in place of SDA-C&C.

BRAIN HEART INFUSION AGAR WITH BLOOD, CYCLOHEXIMIDE, AND CHLORAMPHENICOL (BHIAB-C&C)

Medium Preparation

Brain heart infusion	37 gm
Agar	20 gm
Distilled water	1 liter
Cycloheximide (Upjohn)	500 mg
Acetone	10 ml
Chloramphenicol (Parke-Davis)	50 ml
95 percent alcohol	10 ml
Sheep blood, defibrinated, sterile	100 ml

1. Mix together the brain heart infusion, agar, and water. Bring to a boil.
2. Dissolve cycloheximide in acetone; dissolve chloramphenicol in alcohol. Add both to boiling media and mix well.
3. Autoclave at 15 psi for 15 minutes and cool to 50°C.
4. While swirling the flask, add the sheep blood, then immediately aseptically aliquot in tubes and slant. Cool completely and refrigerate.

Procedure

1. Bring medium to room temperature. Swab the entire surface of the slant.
2. Incubate at 30°C with the cap loose for one month (12 weeks if *Histoplasma* is suspected) before discarding as negative.

Incubation Temperature

Fungal cultures should be generally incubated at 30°C. Room temperature (25°C) is acceptable, although some organisms may multiply slower at this temperature. A 37°C incubation may actually inhibit some fungi. Since so few dimorphic fungi are recovered, it is preferable to first isolate them in the mold phase (room temperature or 30°C), then set up cultures at 37°C for conversion to the yeast phase. Anaerobic cultures for *Actinomyces* should always be incubated at 37°C.

Incubation Time

Some fungi mature within three to four days, while others may require three to four weeks. **(See Chart 2-4 on page 77 at end of module for incubation times of various organisms.)** Growth rates may vary, depending on conditions such as media used, temperature of incubation, or inhibitors in the patient's specimen. To decrease the risk of false-negative reports, keep all cultures at least one month before reporting final results and discarding media. Incubate cultures suspected of containing *Histoplasma capsulatum* for 12 weeks before discarding as negative. Maintaining a moist atmosphere helps keep inoculated media from drying out and enhances fungal growth.

Study Questions

For statements 1 to 5, place the letter of the correct answers in front of the statements. An answer may be used more than once, and each statement will be marked with the number of answers required.

A. Sabouraud dextrose agar
B. Sabouraud dextrose agar with cycloheximide and chloramphenicol
C. Brain heart infusion agar with blood
D. Brain heart infusion agar with blood, cycloheximide, and chloramphenicol

1. _____ Best media for isolation of *Histoplasma capsulatum* (2 answers).

2. _____ Media that are inoculated to obtain the most fungal contaminants and pathogens (2 answers).

3. _____ Best medium for isolation of dermatophytes (1 answer).

4. _____ Best medium for isolation of the anaerobe *Actinomyces.*

5. _____ Best medium for isolation of all strains of *Nocardia asteroides* (1 answer).

6. According to this module, what is an intermediate growth rate?

STOP HERE UNTIL YOU HAVE COMPLETED THE ANSWERS.

Look up the answers in the back of the book. If you missed more than two of them, go back and review the section on primary fungal media. Correctly complete any missed questions before proceeding further.

EXAMINING THE CULTURE

Once a mature colony has formed, observe it for macroscopic appearance. Module 1 contains descriptive terms of colonial morphology. Colonial appearance may help to identify a fungus. However, this morphology may vary greatly between fungal strains, times and temperatures of incubation, and culture media. For molds, the final identification is basically dependent on microscopic morphology, although there are a few useful biochemical tests. For yeasts and funguslike bacteria, biochemical tests are the primary basis for identification, with less emphasis on microscopic and macroscopic appearance. There are three often used procedures to microscopically examine a culture: the tease mount, slide culture, and coverslip sandwich techniques.

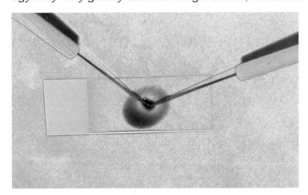

FIGURE 2-5. Teasing apart hyphae, tease mount.

Tease Mount Method

See gray box and Figure 2-5. The advantage of this method is that it can be performed and examined immediately after maturation of the fungal colony on the primary isolation plate. The disadvantage is that the rough action of teasing apart hyphae disturbs the juxtaposition of conidia so that oftentimes the structural morphology of the organism cannot be discerned.

TEASE MOUNT

Reagent Preparation
   Lactophenol Cotton Blue—see LPCB wet mount
Procedure
   1. Put one drop of LPCB stain on a glass slide.
   2. With a flamed and cooled stiff wire inoculating needle, pick up a small portion of the

fungal colony, cutting through the aerial and vegetative mycelium. Do not take the center or edge of the colony: the center is so old that hyphae may be sterile, while the edge is so young that reproductive structures may not yet have formed.

3. Place the fungal portion in the LPCB and, with a second needle, tease apart the hyphae so that they form a thin layer.
4. Put on a coverslip and press down hard to spread out the fungus. Examine under the microscope for reproductive structures.
5. For a permanent preparation, rim the edges of the coverslip with clear nail polish or Permount.

Slide Culture Method

See gray box and Figures 2-6 through 2-13. The advantage of this method is that the fungal elements are grown and maintained in their original juxtaposition, thus making it easier to morphologically identify the organism. Also there are two mounts obtained from one culture. The disadvantages of this method are that it requires some technical expertise to set up the slide culture, and there is a waiting period for incubation of the slide culture in addition to incubation on the primary isolation medium before identifying the fungus. Also, cottony fungi, for example, the Zygomycotina, grow past the edges of the coverslip before forming reproductive structures.

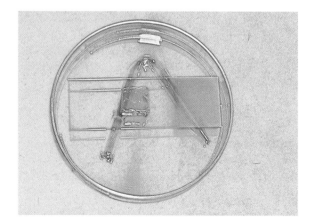

FIGURE 2-6. Glass rod in Petri dish, slide culture.

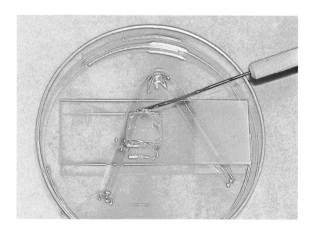

FIGURE 2-7. Glass slide over rod, slide culture.

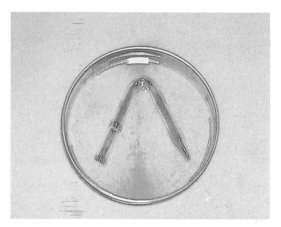

FIGURE 2-8. Agar block on slide, slide culture.

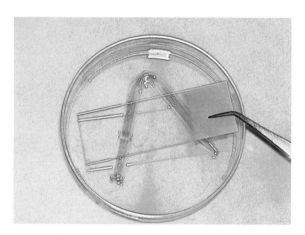

FIGURE 2-9. Inoculating agar block, slide culture.

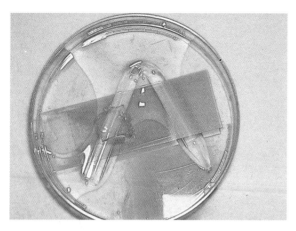

FIGURE 2-10. Flamed coverglass over agar and water in dish, slide culture.

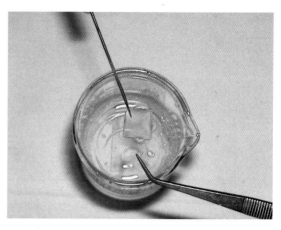

FIGURE 2-11. Agar block removed into disinfectant, slide culture.

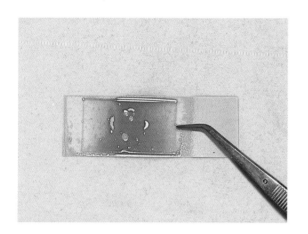

FIGURE 2-12. Coverslip put on slide with LPCB stain, slide culture.

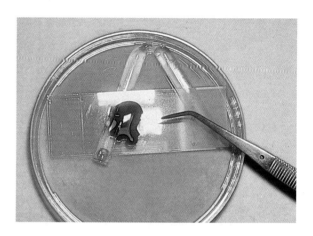

FIGURE 2-13. LPCB stain and coverslip put on slide from culture, slide culture.

SLIDE CULTURE METHOD

Medium Preparation

Potato dextrose agar (PDA): commercially available, but this recipe is easy and far superior*

Potato flakes, for example, Betty Crocker Potato Buds	20 gm
Glucose	10 gm
Agar	15 gm
Distilled water	1 liter

1. Mix together the above ingredients and autoclave at 15 psi for 15 minutes.
2. While frequently swirling the flask, pour plates of medium 4 mm thick. Cool and refrigerate.

Procedure

1. Bring medium to room temperature. Bind together the ends of two applicator sticks with rubber bands. Break the sticks almost all the way through the middle so they form a V-shape. Alternatively, bend a glass rod or broken off Pasteur pipette in a flame until it forms a V-shape, then cool. The sticks or glass rod serves as a platform on which to place the slide culture.

2. Place the sticks or rod in alcohol, dry, and put in the bottom of a sterile Petri dish.
3. Label a glass slide, dip in alcohol, flame dry, and set across the platform.
4. Place a 1-cm square block of potato dextrose agar (PDA) on the slide. This particular medium greatly enhances sporulation, although occasionally Sabouraud dextrose agar works better.
5. Using aseptic technique, inoculate a small piece of fungal colony from the primary isolation tube to one side of the agar block. When obtaining the inoculum, be sure to cut into the colony to get the vegetative as well as aerial growth. Do not take inoculum from the center or edge of the colony. Repeat this procedure for each side of the agar block.
6. Dip a glass coverslip (22 × 40 mm is recommended) in alcohol, flame, and place over the inoculated agar block. Press down lightly to ensure good contact between the agar and coverslip.
7. For moisture, pour about 5 ml of sterile distilled water into the bottom of the Petri dish. Cover the dish and set at room temperature to incubate. If all the water evaporates with time, add more.
8. The fungus will first grow on the sides of the agar, then out onto the slide and coverslip. Periodically examine the slide culture under a microscope. Look for fungal maturation, that is, characteristic reproductive structures.
9. When maturation is evident, remove the coverslip from the slide culture. Usually the agar block will come off with the coverslip; with a teasing needle, gently loosen the suction between agar and coverslip and decant the agar into disinfectant. Place the coverslip on a clean slide with one drop of LPCB.
10. If still remaining, remove the agar block from the bottom slide on the slide culture and drop into disinfectant. Put a drop of LPCB on this bottom slide and add a clean coverslip. Do not tamp down the coverslips, as this may jar conidia loose from the hyphae.
11. Gently heat the two LPCB preparations to release any trapped air bubbles and concentrate dye in the hyphae and reproductive structures. Observe the LPCB mounts under a microscope.
12. For permanent preparations, rim the coverslip edges with clear nail polish or Permount.

*Rinaldi, MG: *Use of potato flakes agar in clinical mycology.* J Clin Microbiol 15:1159, 1982.

Coverslip Sandwich Technique

See gray box and Figures 2-14 through 2-18. Several advantages of this technique are that more than two preparations may be made; each can be removed from the agar at different intervals; the set up is easier than for the slide culture; and the juxtaposition of reproductive structures to hyphae is almost as good as the slide culture method. The disadvantages are that the coverslip easily breaks while trying to insert it into the agar or taking it out, cottony fungi grow past the edges of the coverslip before forming reproductive structures, and there is a waiting period for incubation on the potato dextrose agar plate in addition to incubation on the primary isolation medium. Be cognizant that fungal elements formed on the coverslip beneath the agar are vegetative; only the aerial structures should be observed for mycologic identification.

COVERSLIP SANDWICH TECHNIQUE

Medium Preparation
    Potato dextrose agar (PDA): see Slide Culture Method
Procedure
1. Bring PDA to room temperature. Streak small bits of fungal colony from the primary isolation medium onto the PDA surface. Be sure to take vegetative as well as aerial mycelium when obtaining the inoculum. Also, do not take fungus from the center or edge of the colony.
2. Dip a 22 × 22 mm glass coverslip in alcohol, dry, and insert it into the agar at a 45-degree angle, over the fungal streaks. Repeat Step 2 with more glass coverslips.
3. Cover the plate and incubate at room temperature. At first the fungus will grow on the agar, then eventually up both sides of each coverslip.
4. When you think maturation is evident, gently remove one coverslip with forceps and place it on a slide containing a drop of LPCB. Add two to three drops more LPCB on top of the coverslip and put on a larger coverslip (24 × 40 mm works well). The 22 × 22 mm glass coverslip is now sandwiched between the larger one and the slide.
5. Observe under the microscope. Because there is fungal growth on both sides of the small coverslip, two different planes of focus are required to thoroughly examine the preparation.
6. If reproductive structures are present, remove the other glass coverslips from the PDA and mount them as in Step 4. If reproductive structures are not yet observed, reincubate the PDA plate and remove each glass coverslip when maturation occurs.
7. For permanent preparations, rim the large coverslips with clear nail polish or Permount.

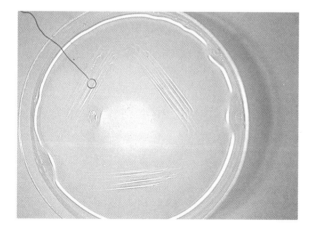

FIGURE 2-14. Streaks of fungus on potato dextrose agar (PDA), coverslip sandwich.

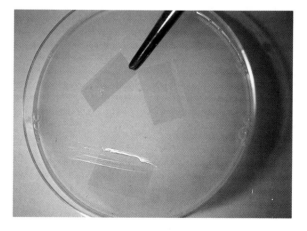

FIGURE 2-15. Coverslips inserted into streaks at 45-degree angle, coverslip sandwich.

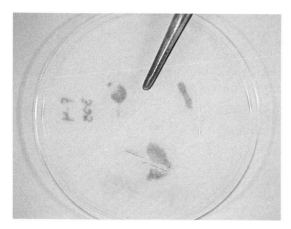

FIGURE 2-16. Coverslip removed when colony is mature, coverslip sandwich.

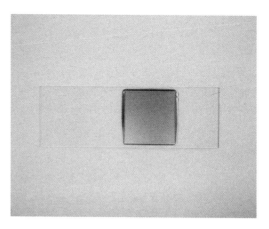

FIGURE 2-17. Coverslip on slide with LPCB stain, coverslip sandwich.

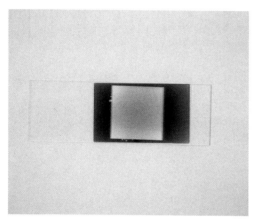

FIGURE 2-18. Second coverslip and LPCB stain over first coverslip, coverslip sandwich.

PROCEEDING TO SPECIFIC MODULES

Now that you know the specimen site, rate of growth, colonial morphology, and microscopic morphology, you may turn to specific modules for further differentiation of organisms. Also, Charts 1-3 to 1-13 at the end of Module 1 may aid in identification.

Growth Rate	Microscopic	Module Number and Title
Rapid	Mold	3 Common Fungal Contaminants
Intermediate-slow	Mold	4 Superficial and Dermatophytic Fungi
Rapid	Yeast	5 Yeasts
Intermediate-slow	Mold, dimorphic fungus, fungus-like bacterium	6 Organisms Causing Subcutaneous Mycoses
Intermediate-slow	Dimorphic fungus	7 Organisms Causing Systemic Mycoses

FINAL EXAM

1. Why should you not accept 24-hour collections on respiratory specimens?

2. Fill in the blanks: Two fungi that may be found in cerebrospinal fluid are _____ and _____ .

3. Circle true or false:

   T F Fungal growth can be easily detected in blood culture bottles, because the medium quickly becomes turbid.

4. Circle the correct answer: Lactophenol cotton blue stains the chitin/keratin in fungal cell walls.

5. One role of the mycology laboratory is to isolate fungi as quickly as possible, while keeping down costs. In your opinion, what is the best general incubation temperature for primary fungal cultures? Justify your answer.

6. List the advantages and disadvantages of the following:

   A. Tease Mount

   B. Slide Culture

   C. Coverslip Sandwich

7. How do specimen site, colonial morphology, and general microscopic morphology (i.e., mold, yeast, dimorphic fungus, or funguslike bacteria) aid in identification?

STOP HERE UNTIL YOU HAVE COMPLETED THE ANSWERS.

Look up the answers in the back of the book. If you missed more than one of them, go back and repeat this module. Correctly complete any missed questions before proceeding.

SUPPLEMENTAL RATIONALE

Animal Inoculation

Animal inoculation is beyond the scope of most clinical laboratories. It requires an animal room, and the procedures take more time than is helpful to the patient. Thus, animal work is reserved for reference laboratories and research purposes.

Sometimes when a fungus fails to grow from a specimen, the specimen can be inoculated into susceptible animals, in which the organism will multiply and produce disease. The animal is then sacrificed, infected tissues sectioned and stained, and fungal elements observed.

Animal inoculation is used for converting dimorphic fungi from the mold phase to the yeast phase. This is especially useful for *Coccidioides immitis*, in which the yeast phase is not easily cultivated in vitro. Animals are inoculated and allowed time to develop the disease. Sections of infected tissues are stained and observed for the yeast forms characteristic of various dimorphic organisms.

Animals may also be used to establish the pathogenicity of fungi. Animals are injected with a pure culture preparation of the fungal isolate and observed for symptoms of overt disease. If there are no symptoms, sections are stained to see if the organism proliferated in the tissues and produced subclinical disease.

See Beneke and Rogers (1980) for details of these procedures.

Seromycology

Serologic procedures are gaining importance in the diagnosis and treatment of mycologic disease. Some of the more important methods follow.

SKIN TESTS

An extract of the antigen (known fungus) is injected into the patient's skin. After 24 to 48 hours, the site is observed for **erythema** (redness) and swelling, and measured for **induration** (hardness). This reaction is caused by a delayed hypersensitivity in patients who have been previously exposed to the antigen. Skin tests are usually performed in patients suspected of having histoplasmosis, blastomycosis, or coccidioidomycosis. Since there is cross reactivity between these three antigens, all three are injected at the same time but at different sites. More than one site may give hardness and redness; however, the one with induration of 5 mm or more in diameter is the organism the patient was previously exposed to.

Since the skin will test positive years after the patient came in contact with the antigen, the skin test is of limited use in diagnosis of present active infection. Also the skin test may be negative in the acute stage of infection (no immunologic response synthesized yet), in patients who are immunosuppressed, or in patients who have overwhelming fungal infection. Do not administer a skin test before taking blood for other serologic studies. Injected skin test antigen will stimulate antibody production, which may give a false-positive reaction in serologic procedures.

DETECTING CIRCULATING ANTIBODIES IN SERA FROM PATIENTS

These are the most widely used serologic tests. Ideally, one should test paired sera, one serum taken while the patient is in the early, acute phase of the illness, and one serum taken at least four weeks later, in the convalescent phase. A fourfold increase in antibody titer is indicative of active infection. **(See Chart 2-5 on pages 78-80 and Chart 2-7 on page 83 at end of module.)** Also see Kaufman (1980) for test procedure sensitivity and specificity of the various serologic methods. Note that, although serologic reagents are commercially available, they are not always standardized.

Immunodiffusion (ID)

Punch two holes, or wells, in an agarose gel plate or purchase a commercially prepared plate. Fill one well with the patient's serum (which contains unknown antibody), and fill the other well with a known fungal extract (antigen). Allow time for the antigen and antibody to diffuse out from the wells into the agarose. If the antibody is specific against that particular antigen, a visible band of precipitate will form in the gel where the antigen and antibody meet. If the antibody is not against that antigen, no precipitate will be formed.

Tube Agglutination (TA)

A known killed whole fungus, not an extract, is the antigen. It is mixed with the patient's serum (containing unknown antibody) in a tube. After sufficient time, if the antibody is specific against that fungal antigen, it will clump to form a visible agglutinate. If the antibody is not specific against that antigen, there is no agglutination.

Indirect Latex Agglutination (ILA)

An extract of a known fungus (antigen) is bound to inert latex particles. The patient's serum (with unknown antibody) is added. If the antibody is specific against the antigen, the antigen-coated latex particles will agglutinate. If the antibody is not against that antigen, no agglutination will occur.

Complement Fixation (CF)

Complement is capable of binding to fungal antigen-antibody complexes or to red blood cell antigen-antibody complexes. When complement binds to the latter, it will lyse the red blood cells. An extract of a known fungus (antigen) is mixed with the patient's serum (containing unknown antibody) and complement and allowed to react. Red blood cells coated with anti-red blood cell antibody are added. If the antibody in the patient's serum is specific against the fungal antigen, complement will bind to this fungal antigen-antifungal antibody complex and not to the red blood cell-anti-red blood cell antibody complex. Therefore, the red blood cells will not be lysed. A positive test is no lysis. If the antibody in the patient's serum is not directed against that fungal antigen, no fungal antigen-antifungal antibody complex will form. This means complement is now available to bind to the red blood cell-anti-red blood cell antibody complex, which then lyses the red blood cells. Lysis is a negative test.

Indirect Fluorescent Antibody (IFA)

Known killed whole fungal cells (antigen) are attached to a glass slide. The slide is covered with the patient's serum (containing unknown antibody) and allowed to react. The slide is washed and covered with fluorescent labelled anti-human antibody and allowed to react. The slide is washed, dried, and observed under the fluorescent microscope. If the patient's antibody is specific against the fungal cell antigen, it will attach to the cells and not be washed away. Fluorescent labelled anti-human antibody attaches to the antibody now on the fungal cells so that the cells fluoresce. If the patient's antibody is not directed against the fungal cell antigen, the antibody is all washed away. The fluorescent labelled anti-human antibody has nothing to attach to, so it is also washed away, and the fungal cells will not fluoresce.

Counterimmunoelectrophoresis (CIE)

Counterimmunoelectrophoresis combines electrophoresis and immunodiffusion. Agarose is layered on a slide, then two wells are punched out of the solidified gel. An extract of a known fungus (antigen) is placed in one well, while the patient's serum (containing unknown antibody) is placed in the other. An electric field is applied with the negative pole on the antigen side and the positive pole on the antibody side. With time, the negatively charged antigen molecules migrate toward the positive pole, and the antibody molecules migrate toward the negative pole. Where antigen meets its specific antibody, a line of precipitate is formed. If the antibody is not specific for the antigen, the molecules continue to migrate past each other without forming a line of precipitate. The rate of antigen and antibody movement depends on many things: charge, size, and shape of the molecules, type of support media, pH and ionic strength of the buffer, strength of the electric field, and the incubation temperature of the test.

DETECTING FUNGAL ANTIGENS IN SPECIMENS OR CULTURES FROM PATIENTS

Serologic techniques for identifying fungi are becoming increasingly popular. They are very useful for quickly identifying the slow-growing dimorphic fungi that will not readily convert to the diagnostic yeast phase. Rapidly determining the presence of specific fungal antigens in cerebrospinal fluid is also very important, since this is an emergency situation and treatment must immediately begin. **See Chart 2-6 on pages 81-82 and Chart 2-7 on page 83.** See Kaufman (1980) for test procedure and sensitivity and specificity of the various serologic methods. Serologic reagents, though commercially available, are not always standardized.

Immunodiffusion (ID)

The principle and procedure are the same as for the immunodiffusion to detect fungal antibodies, except known antiserum (antibody) and unknown antigen (extract of the patient's specimen or culture) are used in the agarose wells. If the known antibody is specific for the unknown antigen, a visible band of precipitate will form in the gel where the antibody and antigen meet. If the known antibody is not specific for the unknown antigen, no band of precipitate will form.

Indirect Reverse Latex Agglutination (IRLA)

Inert latex particles coated with known fungal antiserum (antibody) are mixed with an extract of the patient's specimen or culture (containing unknown antigen) and allowed to react. If the known fungal antibody is specific for the unknown antigen, the antibody coated latex particles will agglutinate. If the fungal antibody is not specific for the unknown fungal antigen, no agglutination will occur.

Direct Fluorescent Antibody (DFA)

Tissue sections or smears of patient specimen or culture (containing unknown cellular fungal antigen) are fixed to a glass slide. Fluorescent labelled known fungal antiserum (antibody) is applied to the slide and allowed to react, and the excess is washed off. After the slide is dried, it is observed under the fluorescent microscope. If the fluorescent labelled antibody is specific for the unknown fungal antigen, the fungal cells will fluoresce, giving a positive test. If the fluorescent labelled antibody is not specific for the unknown fungal antigen, the antibody is washed away, and the cells do not fluoresce.

Study Questions—Supplemental Rationale

1. Circle true or false:

   T   F   Fungi that do not convert to the yeast phase in the laboratory may do so when inoculated into animals.

2. All of the following are true concerning skin tests for blastomycosis, histoplasmosis, and coccidioidomycosis *except:*

   A. Since all three antigens cross-react, the one that produces 5 mm or more of hardness is the positive test.

   B. Give the skin tests before taking blood for serology.

   C. Overwhelming fungal infection may produce a negative skin test to the corresponding antigen.

   D. Skin tests remain positive years after the active infection.

   E. Immunologically suppressed patients may not give a positive skin test, even in active infection.

3. Circle the correct answer:

   With the complement fixation procedure, lysis indicates a positive/negative result.

4. Matching. Place the letter of the correct answer from Column B in front of the words in Column A:

Column A	Column B
___Band of precipitate between matching Ag* and Ab[†]	A. Indirect fluorescent Ab
___Uses red blood cells	B. Counterimmunoelectrophoresis
___Fluorescent labelled known fungal Ab	C. Indirect latex agglutination
___Combines diffusion and electric field	D. Immunodiffusion
___Uses Ag coated latex particles	E. Indirect reverse latex agglutination
	F. Direct fluorescent Ab
	G. Complement fixation

*Ag=Antigen
[†]Ab=Antibody

STOP HERE UNTIL YOU HAVE COMPLETED THE ANSWERS.

Look up the answers in the back of the book. If you missed more than two of them, go back and review the Supplemental Rationale section. Correctly complete any missed questions.

CHART 2-1. Fungi That May Be Isolated From Various Specimens and Suggested Primary Isolation Media

SPECIMEN	NORMAL FUNGAL FLORA	ABNORMAL FUNGI	PRIMARY ISOLATION MEDIA
Blood, bone marrow	None	Any growth of *Candida* sp. *Histoplasma capsulatum* *Cryptococcus neoformans* other organisms that have become systemic *Blastomyces dermatitidis*	Brain heart infusion broth
Cerebrospinal fluid	None	Any growth of *Coccidioides immitis* *Histoplasma capsulatum* *Actinomyces* *Nocardia* *Candida* sp. *Cryptococcus neoformans* contaminants repeatedly isolated	Sabouraud dextrose agar Brain heart infusion agar with blood Anaerobic brain heart infusion agar with blood
Hair	Possibly a few contaminants	Common: Any growth of *Trichophyton* *Microsporum* Uncommon: Any growth of *Piedraia hortai* *Trichosporon beigelii*	Sabouraud dextrose agar Sabouraud dextrose agar with cycloheximide and chloramphenicol
Mucocutaneous scrapings	None	Any growth of *Candida* sp. *Paracoccidioides brasiliensis* Microscopic observation of *Rhinosporidium seeberi*	Sabouraud dextrose agar Sabouraud dextrose agar with cycloheximide and chloramphenicol
Nail scrapings	None	Any growth of *Candida* sp. *Trichophyton* *Epidermophyton* *Aspergillus* *Scopulariopsis*	Sabouraud dextrose agar Sabouraud dextrose agar with cycloheximide and chloramphenicol
Skin scrapings	Possibly a few contaminants Possibly a few yeast (*Candida*)	Common: Moderate-heavy growth of *Candida* sp. Any growth of *Trichophyton* *Microsporum* *Epidermophyton* Uncommon: Any growth of contaminants repeatedly isolated *Cryptococcus* *Malassezia furfur* *Exophiala werneckii*	Sabouraud dextrose agar Sabouraud dextrose agar with cycloheximide and chloramphenicol Brain heart infusion agar with blood, cycloheximide, and chloramphenicol Sabouraud dextrose agar layered with olive oil

CHART 2-1. Continued

SPECIMEN	NORMAL FUNGAL FLORA	ABNORMAL FUNGI	PRIMARY ISOLATION MEDIA
Sputum, bronchial washings	Few yeast (Candida) Few contaminants	Blastomyces dermatitidis Paracoccidioides brasiliensis Coccidioides immitis Histoplasma capsulatum agents of chromoblastomycosis (Fonsecaea, Phialophora, Cladosporium) agents of mycetoma (Scedosporium, Exophiala, Nocardia, Streptomyces, Actinomyces) Common: Moderate-heavy growth of Candida sp. esp. C. albicans & glabrata Moderate-heavy growth of contaminants repeatedly isolated (esp. Aspergillus, Rhizopus, Mucor, Penicillium, Geotrichum) Uncommon: Any growth of Nocardia Actinomyces Cryptococcus neoformans Blastomyces dermatitidis Paracoccidioides brasiliensis Coccidioides immitis Histoplasma capsulatum Sporothrix schenckii	Sabouraud dextrose agar Brain heart infusion agar with blood, cycloheximide, and chloramphenicol Anaerobic brain heart infusion agar with blood (bronchial washings, transtracheal aspirates)
Subcutaneous lesions and abscesses	None	Moderate-heavy growth of Saccharomyces Any growth of Candida sp. contaminants repeatedly isolated agents of chromoblastomycosis (Fonsecaea, Phialophora, Cladosporium) agents of mycetoma (Scedosporium, Exophiala, Nocardia, Streptomyces, Actinomyces) Sporothrix schenckii Coccidioides immitis Blastomyces dermatitidis Cryptococcus neoformans Histoplasma capsulatum Wangiella	Sabouraud dextrose agar Sabouraud dextrose agar with cycloheximide and chloramphenicol Anaerobic brain heart infusion agar with blood
Throat	Few yeast (Candida) Few contaminants	Common: Moderate-heavy growth of Candida albicans Uncommon: Moderate-heavy growth of Geotrichum candidum Saccharomyces cerevisiae	Sabouraud dextrose agar Sabouraud dextrose agar with cycloheximide and chloramphenicol

CHART 2-1. Continued

SPECIMEN	NORMAL FUNGAL FLORA	ABNORMAL FUNGI	PRIMARY ISOLATION MEDIA
Tissue, biopsy material	None	Any growth of *Paracoccidioides brasiliensis* (lymph nodes) agents of zygomycosis (*Rhizopus, Mucor, Absidia, Mortierella, Cunninghamella*) repeatedly isolated agents of mycetoma (*Scedosporium, Nocardia, Streptomyces, Actinomyces*) Microscopic observation of *Rhinosporidium seeberi*	Sabouraud dextrose agar Sabouraud dextrose agar with cycloheximide and chloramphenicol Anaerobic brain heart infusion agar with blood
Transtracheal aspirate	None	Same as for sputum, bronchial washings	Same as for sputum, bronchial washings
Urine	None from catheterized specimen	*Common:* Over 100,000 colonies/ml of *Candida* sp., esp. *C. albicans & glabrata* *Uncommon:* Any growth of *Blastomyces dermatitidis* *Coccidioides immitis* *Histoplasma capsulatum* *Cryptococcus neoformans*	Sabouraud dextrose agar Sabouraud dextrose agar with cycloheximide and chloramphenicol
Vaginal, uterine cervix	Few-moderate number of yeast colonies (*Candida*)	*Common:* Heavy growth of *Candida albicans or glabrata* *Uncommon:* Heavy growth of *Geotrichum candidum*	Sabouraud dextrose agar Sabouraud dextrose agar with cycloheximide and chloramphenicol
Wound	None	Any growth of *Candida* sp. contaminants repeatedly isolated other opportunistic pathogens	Sabouraud dextrose agar Sabouraud dextrose agar with cycloheximide and chloramphenicol

CHART 2-2. Structures and Associated Organisms Commonly Seen in Specimen Direct Examinations*

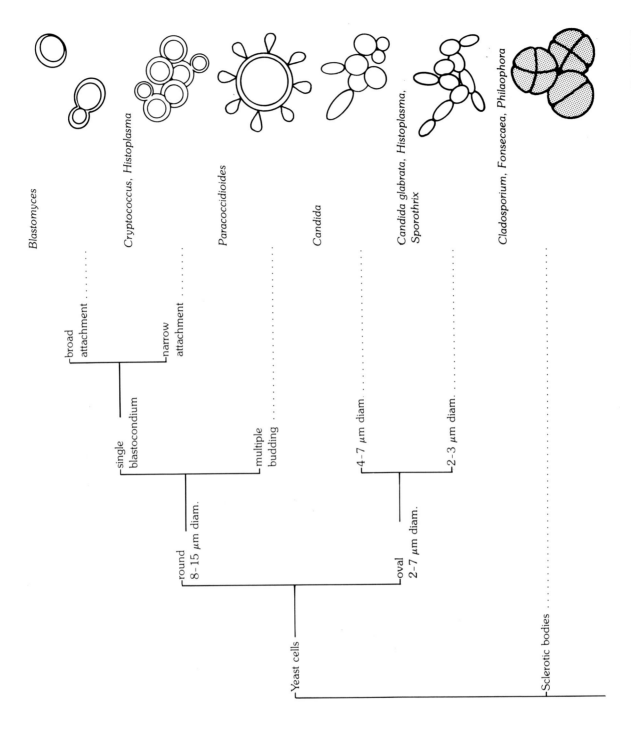

Yeast cells — round 8–15 µm diam. — single blastocondium — broad attachment .... *Blastomyces*

narrow attachment .... *Cryptococcus, Histoplasma*

multiple budding .... *Paracoccidioides*

oval 2–7 µm diam. — 4–7 µm diam. .... *Candida*

2–3 µm diam. .... *Candida glabrata, Histoplasma, Sporothrix*

Sclerotic bodies .... *Cladosporium, Fonsecaea, Philaophora*

CHART 2-2. Structures and Associated Organisms Commonly Seen in Specimen Direct Examinations*

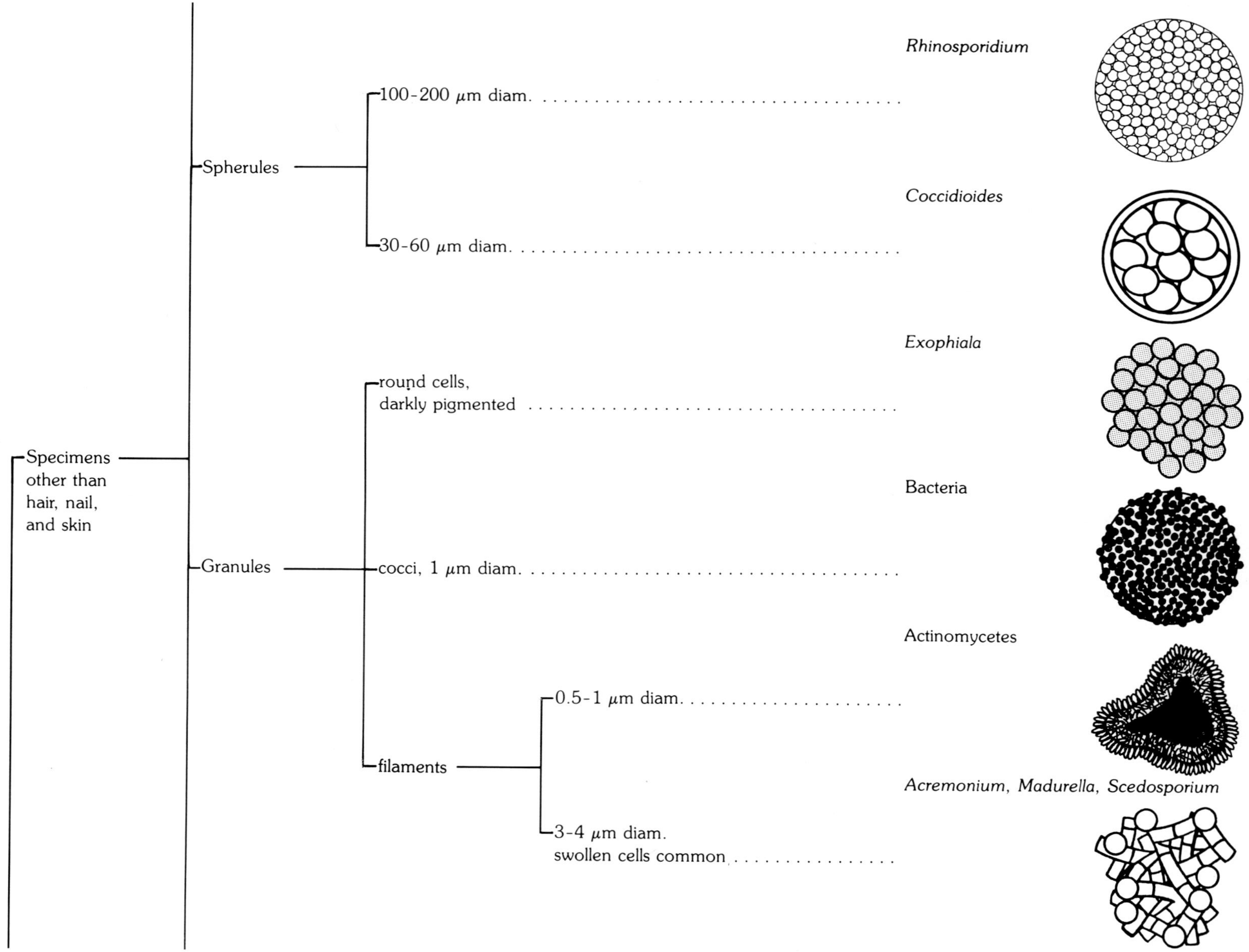

Specimens other than hair, nail, and skin

Spherules
- 100-200 μm diam. .... *Rhinosporidium*
- 30-60 μm diam. .... *Coccidioides*

Granules
- round cells, darkly pigmented .... *Exophiala*
- cocci, 1 μm diam. .... Bacteria
- filaments
  - 0.5-1 μm diam. .... Actinomycetes
  - 3-4 μm diam. swollen cells common .... *Acremonium, Madurella, Scedosporium*

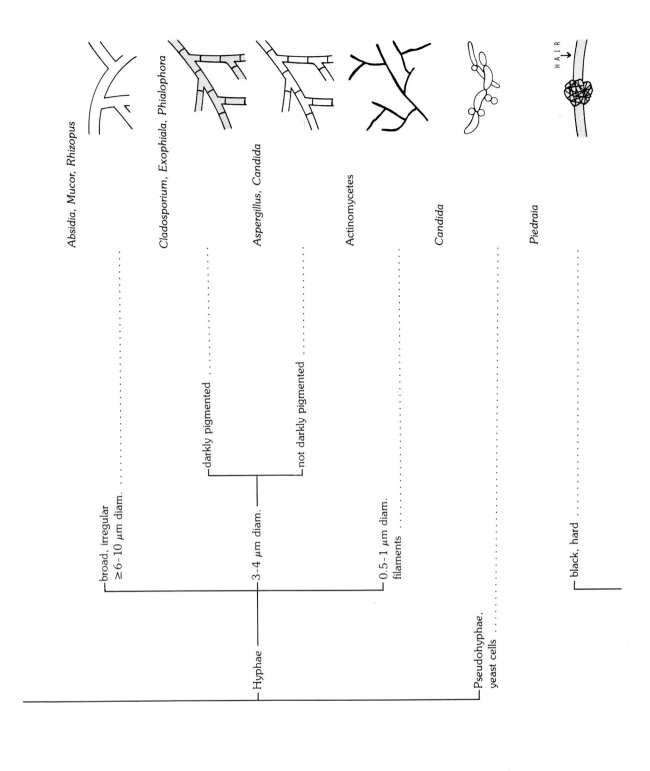

Absidia, Mucor, Rhizopus ....

Cladosporium, Exophiala, Phialophora ....

Aspergillus, Candida ....

Actinomycetes ....

Candida ....

Piedraia ....

darkly pigmented ....

not darkly pigmented ....

broad, irregular ≥ 6–10 μm diam. ....

3–4 μm diam.

0.5–1 μm diam. filaments ....

black, hard ....

Hyphae

Pseudohyphae, yeast cells ....

CHART 2-2. Continued

73

CHART 2-2. Structures and Associated Organisms Commonly Seen in Specimen Direct Examinations*

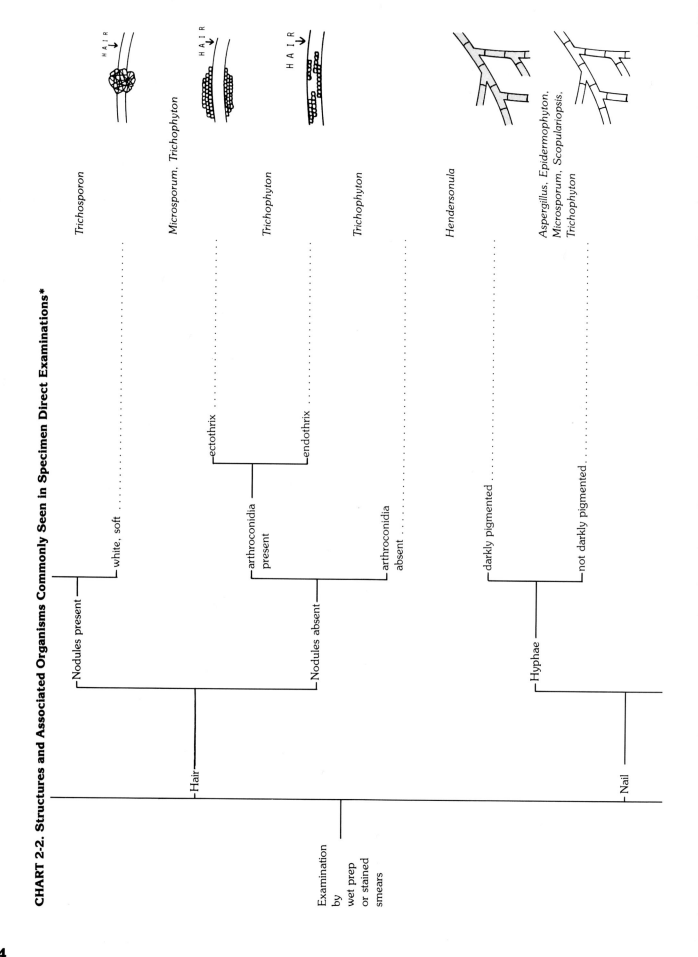

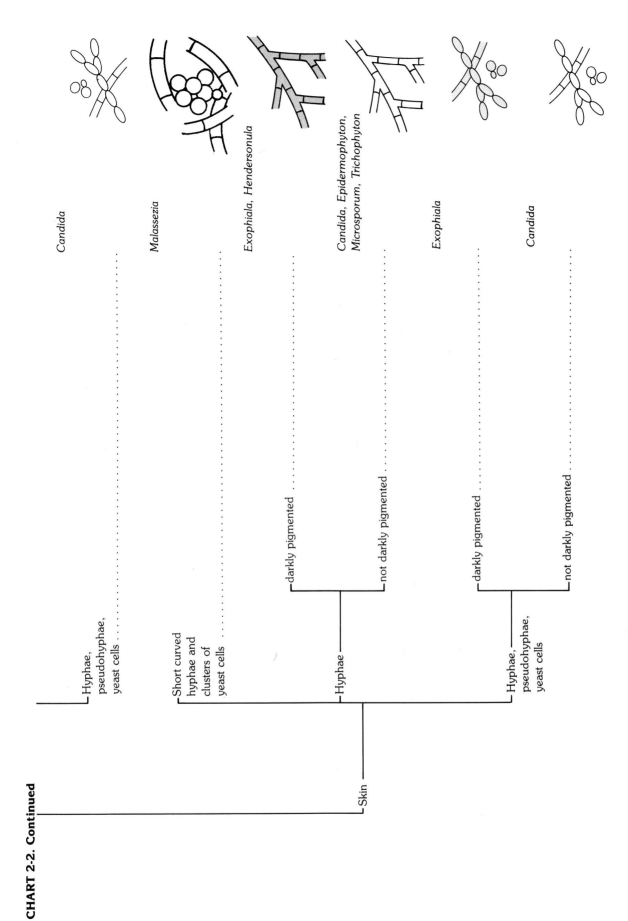

CHART 2-2. Continued

Skin

Hyphae, pseudohyphae, yeast cells . . . . *Candida*

Short curved hyphae and clusters of yeast cells . . . . *Malassezia*

Hyphae
- darkly pigmented . . . . *Exophiala, Hendersonula*
- not darkly pigmented . . . . *Candida, Epidermophyton, Microsporum, Trichophyton*

Hyphae, pseudohyphae, yeast cells
- darkly pigmented . . . . *Exophiala*
- not darkly pigmented . . . . *Candida*

•Modified from McGinnis (1980).

CHART 2-3. Pathogenic Fungi Inhibited by Cycloheximide and Chloramphenicol

CYCLOHEXIMIDE INHIBITS:	CHLORAMPHENICOL INHIBITS:
Cryptococcus neoformans	*Nocardia asteroides*[†]
Cryptococcus sp.	*Nocardia brasiliensis*
Candida parapsilosis	Other funguslike bacteria
Candida krusei	Yeast phases of dimorphic fungi*
Candida tropicalis	
Candida rugosa	
Candida glabrata	
Yeast phases of dimorphic fungi*	
Actinomyces sp.	
Nocardia sp.	
Streptomyces sp.	
Aspergillus fumigatus[†]	
Penicillium sp.	
Geotrichum sp.	
Scopulariopsis sp.	
Saccharomyces sp.	
Absidia sp.	
Mucor sp.	
Rhizopus sp.	

*Yeast phases are inhibited only at 37°C, not 25°C.
[†]Partially inhibited

CHART 2-4. Growth Rates of Various Fungi

GROWTH RATE	MOLDS	YEASTS	FUNGUSLIKE BACTERIA
Rapid growers (form mature colonies in 5 days or less)	Fungal contaminants: Absidia, Acremonium, Alternaria, Aspergillus, Aureobasidium, Chrysosporium, Cladosporium, Curvularia, Drechslera, Fusarium, Mucor, Nigrospora, Paecilomyces, Penicillium, Rhizopus, Scopulariopsis, Sepedonium, Syncephalastrum, Trichoderma Subcutaneous: Dimorphic—Sporothrix schenckii	Candida, Cryptococcus, Geotrichum, Rhodotorula, Saccharomyces, Trichosporon Subcutaneous: Dimorphic conversion—Sporothrix schenckii Systemic: Dimorphic conversion—Blastomyces dermatitidis	Actinomyces (anaerobic only), Nocardia, Streptomyces
Intermediate growers (form mature colonies in 6 to 10 days)	Dermatophytes: Epidermophyton floccosum, Microsporum canis, distortum, gypseum, nanum, vanbreuseghemii, Trichophyton ajelloi, mentagrophytes Subcutaneous: Pseudallescheria boydii Systemic: Dimorphic—Coccidioides immitis	Systemic: Dimorphic conversion—Histoplasma capsulatum	
Slow growers (form mature colonies in 11 to 21 days)	Dermatophytes: Microsporum audouinii, Trichophyton rubrum, schoenleinii, tonsurans, verrucosum, violaceum Subcutaneous: Cladosporium carrionii, Exophiala jeanselmei, Fonsecaea compacta, pedrosoi, Phialophora verrucosa Systemic: Dimorphic—Blastomyces dermatitidis, Histoplasma capsulatum, Paracoccidioides brasiliensis	Systemic: Dimorphic (primary growth)—Paracoccidioides brasiliensis	

CHART 2-5. Serologic Tests to Detect Patient's Antibodies

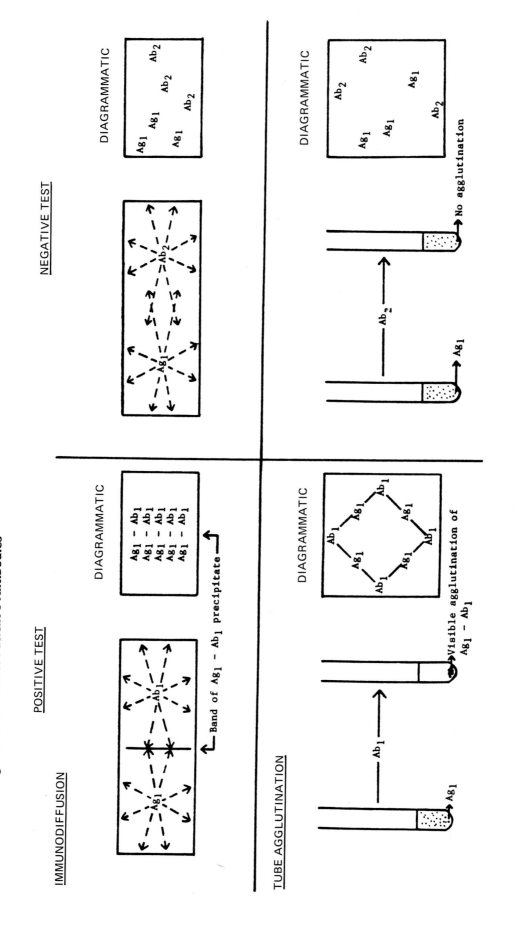

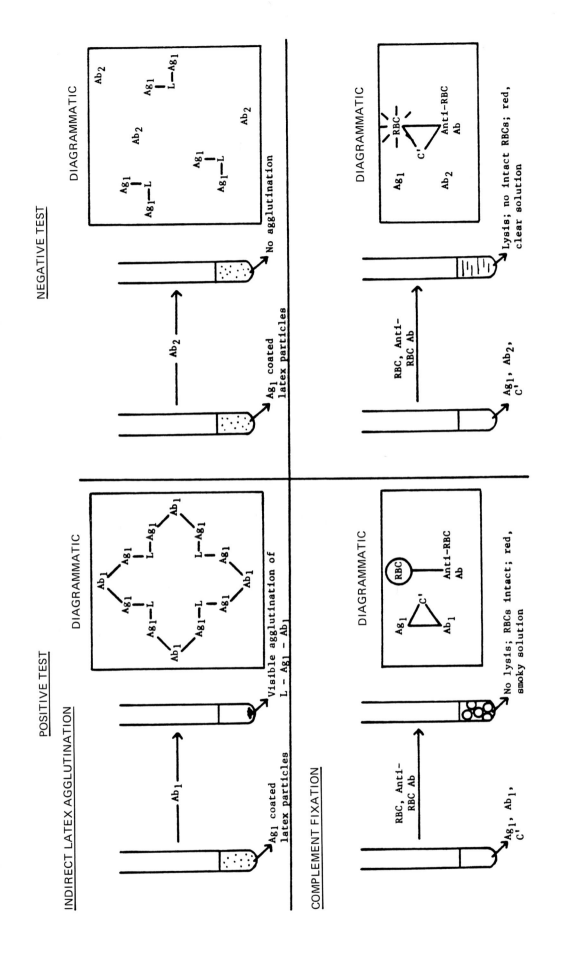

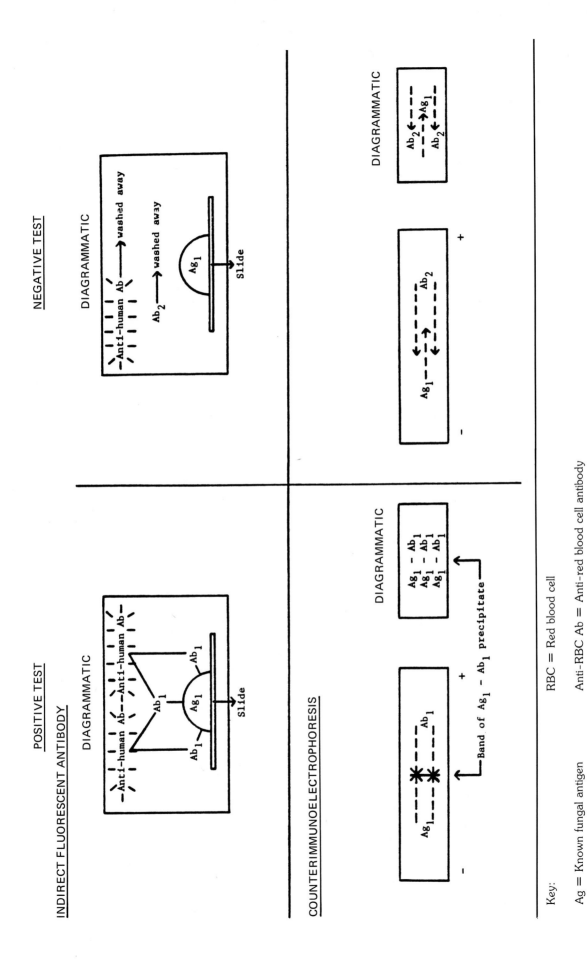

NEGATIVE TEST

DIAGRAMMATIC

POSITIVE TEST

INDIRECT FLUORESCENT ANTIBODY

DIAGRAMMATIC

COUNTERIMMUNOELECTROPHORESIS

DIAGRAMMATIC

DIAGRAMMATIC

Key:

Ag = Known fungal antigen

Ab = Patient's unknown antibody

L = Latex particle

RBC = Red blood cell

Anti-RBC Ab = Anti-red blood cell antibody

C' = Complement

Anti-human Ab = Anti-human antibody

CHART 2-6. Serologic Tests to Detect Fungal Antigens in Patient Specimens

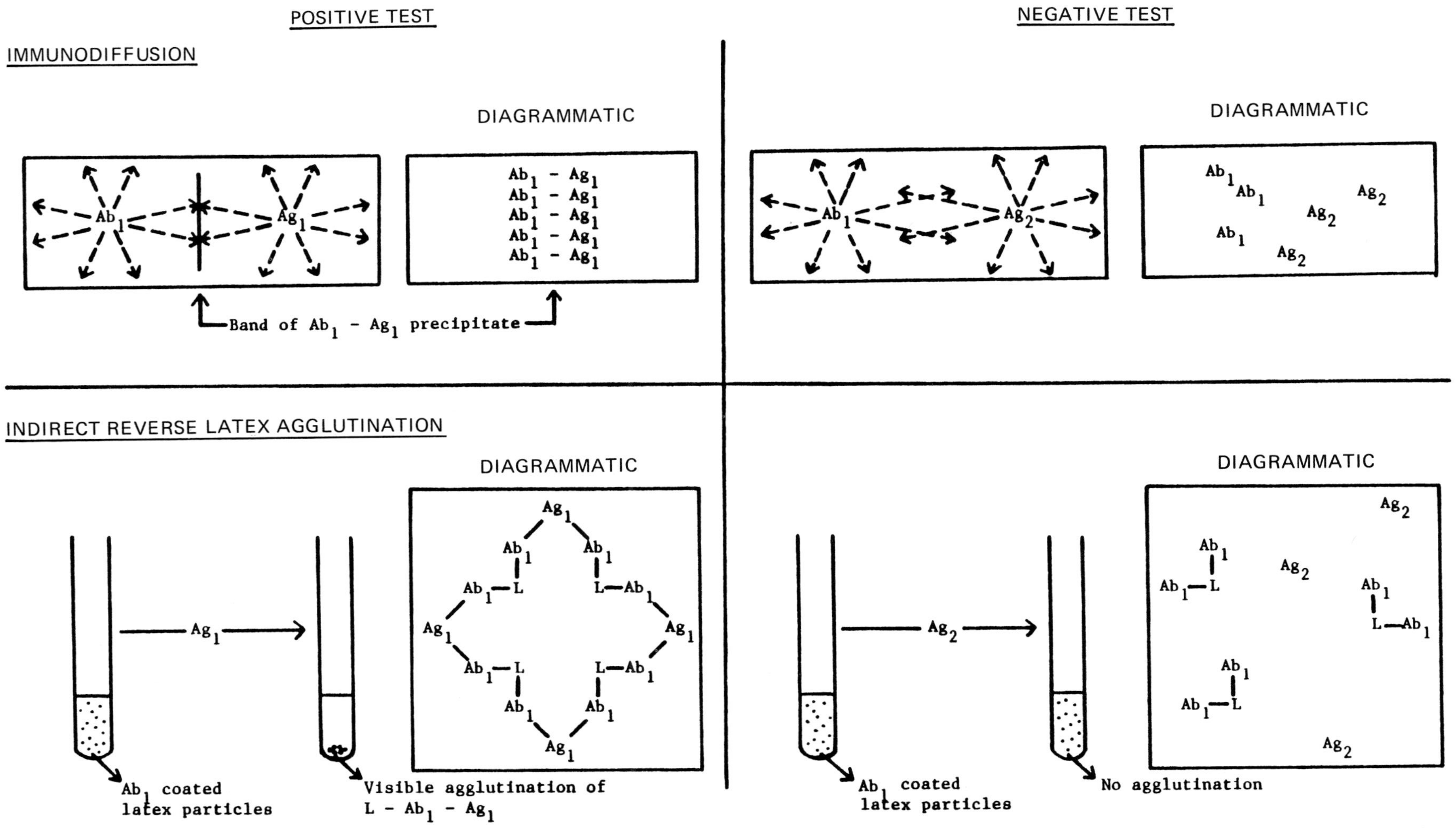

IMMUNODIFFUSION

POSITIVE TEST

DIAGRAMMATIC

Band of $Ab_1 - Ag_1$ precipitate

$Ab_1 - Ag_1$
$Ab_1 - Ag_1$
$Ab_1 - Ag_1$
$Ab_1 - Ag_1$
$Ab_1 - Ag_1$

NEGATIVE TEST

DIAGRAMMATIC

$Ab_1 Ab_1$ Ag_2
Ab_1 Ag_2
Ag_2

INDIRECT REVERSE LATEX AGGLUTINATION

DIAGRAMMATIC

Ab_1 coated latex particles Ag_1 Visible agglutination of $L - Ab_1 - Ag_1$

DIAGRAMMATIC

Ab_1 coated latex particles Ag_2 No agglutination

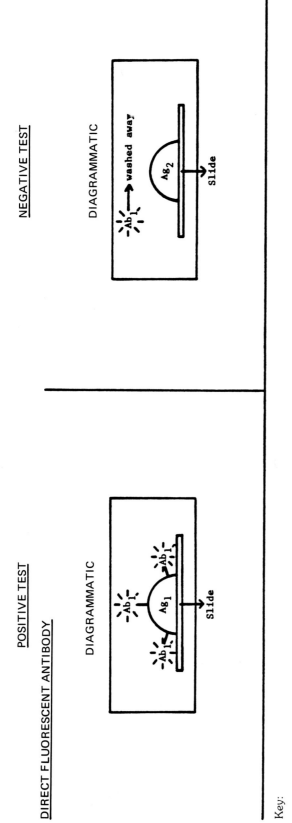

DIRECT FLUORESCENT ANTIBODY

POSITIVE TEST

DIAGRAMMATIC

NEGATIVE TEST

DIAGRAMMATIC

Key:

Ag = Patient's unknown fungal antigen

Ab = Known antibody

L = Latex particle

CHART 2-7. Serologic Tests to Diagnose Various Diseases

	HISTOPLASMOSIS	BLASTOMYCOSIS	COCCIDIOI-DOMYCOSIS	PARACOCCIDI-OIDOMYCOSIS	CRYPTO-COCCOSIS	INVASIVE ASPERGILLOSIS	SYSTEMIC CANDI-DOSIS
Tests to detect circulating fungal antibodies:							
Immunodiffusion	X	X	X	X		X	X
Tube agglutination					X		X
Latex agglutination	X		X				X
Complement fixation	X	X	X	X		X	
Indirect fluorescent antibody					X		
Counterimmunoelectrophoresis	X		X	X		X	X
Tests to detect fungal antigens:							
Immunodiffusion	X		X	X			
Latex agglutination					X		
Direct fluorescent antibody	X		X		X	X	X

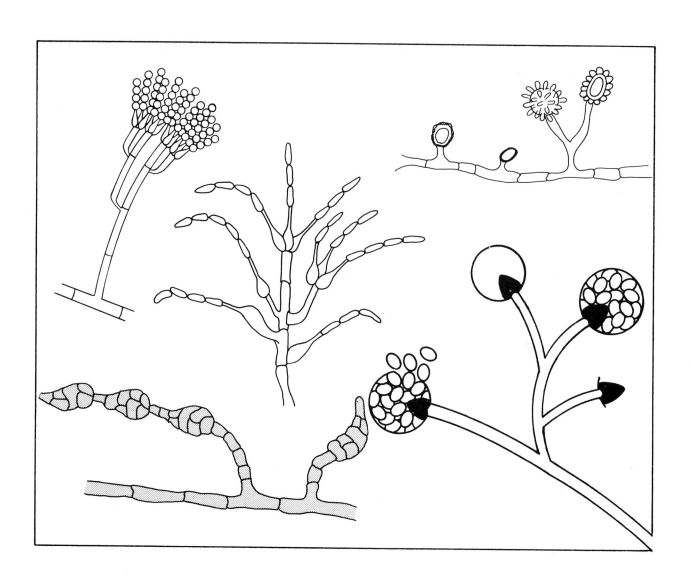

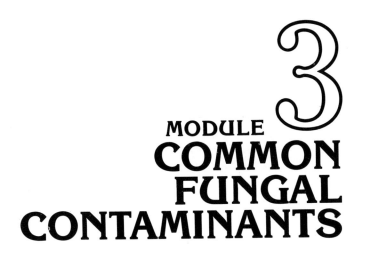

MODULE
COMMON FUNGAL CONTAMINANTS

PREREQUISITES. The learner must possess a good background knowledge in clinical microbiology and must have finished Module 1, Basics of Mycology, and Module 2, Laboratory Procedures for Fungal Culture and Isolation.

BEHAVIORAL OBJECTIVES. Upon completion of this module, the learner should be able to:

1. Define:

   Saprobe
   Opportunistic pathogen
   Hyaline
   Dematiaceous
   Penicillus

2. Discuss at least five common properties of fungal contaminants.

3. From fungal colonies and microscopic preparations, recognize the following:

   Absidia sp.
   Mucor sp.
   Rhizopus sp.
   Alternaria sp.
   Cladosporium sp.
   Aureobasidium sp.
   Curvularia sp.
   Epicoccum sp.
   Drechslera sp.
   Nigrospora sp.
   Acremonium sp.

Syncephalastrum sp.
Aspergillus sp., especially *A. fumigatus*
Chrysosporium sp.
Fusarium sp.
Gliocladium sp.
Penicillium sp.
Paecilomyces sp.
Scopulariopsis sp.
Sepedonium sp.
Ulocladium sp. .
Stemphylium sp.
Shield cells
Foot cells of *Aspergillus* and *Fusarium*

4. Given a fungal microscopic preparation, classify the organism as aseptate or septate, and if septate, categorize as hyaline or dematiaceous.

5. Compare and contrast the microscopic features of *Absidia* sp., *Mucor* sp., and *Rhizopus* sp.

6. Describe at least two ways to differentiate the similar-appearing dark molds *Epicoccum*, *Ulocladium*, and *Stemphylium*.

7. Contrast the poroconidial arrangement of *Curvularia*, *Drechslera*, and *Helminthosporium* sp.

8. Discuss ways to distinguish *Acremonium* from the subcutaneous pathogen *Sporothrix schenckii*.

9. Compare and contrast the contaminants *Chrysosporium* and *Sepedonium* with the subcutaneous disease producer *Scedosporium apiospermum* and the systemic pathogens *Histoplasma capsulatum* and *Blastomyces dermatitidis*.

10. List three microscopic differences between *Aspergillus* sp. and the similar-appearing organism, *Syncephalastrum* sp.

11. From microscopic mounts and cultural characteristics, differentiate *Aspergillus fumigatus* from other *Aspergillus* species.

12. Compare and contrast colonial and microscopic morphology of *Penicillium* sp., *Paecilomyces* sp., *Gliocladium* sp., and *Scopulariopsis* sp.

13. List two differences between *Fusarium* sp. and *Cylindrocarpon* sp.

14. Briefly elaborate on the symptoms for these contaminant-associated diseases:

Aspergillosis
Mycotic keratitis
Otomycosis
Penicilliosis
Zygomycosis

Include predisposing factors, basis for etiologic significance, and three causative agents for each.

CONTENT OUTLINE

I. Introduction
II. Common properties of fungal contaminants
  A. Rapid growing
  B. Saprobic and airborne
  C. Normally inhaled
  D. Opportunistic pathogens
  E. Laboratory diagnosis
III. Aseptate contaminants
  A. *Absidia* species
  B. *Mucor* species
  C. *Rhizopus* species
  D. Study questions
IV. Septate contaminants
  A. Dematiaceous contaminants
    1. *Alternaria* species
    2. *Aureobasidium* species
    3. *Cladosporium (Hormodendrum)* species
    4. *Curvularia* species
    5. *Drechslera* species
    6. *Epicoccum* species
    7. *Nigrospora* species
    8. Study questions
  B. Hyaline contaminants
    1. *Acremonium (Cephalosporium)* species
    2. *Aspergillus* species
    3. *Chrysosporium* species
    4. *Fusarium* species
    5. *Gliocladium* species
    6. *Paecilomyces* species
    7. *Penicillium* species
    8. *Scopulariopsis* species
    9. *Sepedonium* species
    10. Study questions
V. Final exam
VI. Supplemental Rationale
  A. Aspergillosis
  B. Mycotic keratitis
  C. Otomycosis
  D. Penicilliosis
  E. Zygomycosis
  F. Study questions

FOLLOW-UP ACTIVITIES

1. Students may identify unknown organisms by colonial and microscopic appearance.

2. Students may open up a sterile Sabouraud dextrose agar plate in a location of their choice (subway station, shower stall, or so forth) and expose the plate for five minutes. Incubate the plate at room temperature and observe which contaminants grow.

REFERENCES

BARNETT, HL AND HUNTER, BB: *Illustrated Genera of Imperfect Fungi*, ed 3. Burgess Publishing Co., Minneapolis, 1972.

BARRON, GL: *The Genera of Hyphomycetes from Soil.* Williams & Wilkins, Baltimore, 1968.

BENEKE, ES AND ROGERS, AL: *Medical Mycology Manual*, ed 4. Burgess Publishing Co., Minneapolis, 1980.

CHICK, EW, BALOWS, A, AND FURCOLOW, ML (EDS): *Opportunistic Fungal Infections. Proceedings of the Second International Conference.* Charles C Thomas, Springfield, Ill. 1975.

CONANT, NF, ET AL: *Manual of Clinical Mycology*, ed 3. WB Saunders, Philadelphia, 1971.

DELACRETAZ, J, GRIGORIU, D, AND DUCEL, G: *Color Atlas of Medical Mycology.* Hans Huber Publishers, Year Book Medical Publishers (distributor), Chicago, 1976.

EMMONS, CW, ET AL: *Medical Mycology*, ed 3. Lea & Febiger, Philadelphia, 1977.

KONEMAN, EW, ROBERTS, GD, AND WRIGHT, SF: *Practical Laboratory Mycology*, ed 2. Williams & Wilkins, Baltimore, 1978.

LOVELESS, MD, ET AL: *Mixed invasive infection with Alternaria species and Curvularia species.* Am J Clin Pathol 76:491, 1981.

McGINNIS, MR: *Laboratory Handbook of Medical Mycology.* Academic Press, New York, 1980.

NALESNIK, MA, ET AL: *Significance of Aspergillus species isolated from respiratory secretions in the diagnosis of invasive pulmonary aspergillosis.* J Clin Microbiol 11:370, 1980.

PANKE, TW, McMANUS, AT, AND SPEBAR, MJ: *Infection of a burn wound by Aspergillus niger.* Am J Clin Pathol 73:230, 1979.

RAPER, KB AND FENNELL, DF: *The Genus Aspergillus.* Williams & Wilkins, Baltimore, 1965.

ROGERS, AL (coordinator): *Identification of saprophytic fungi commonly encountered in a clinical environment.* 78th Annual Meeting of the American Society for Microbiology, Las Vegas, Nevada, American Society for Microbiology, Washington, DC, 1978.

ROGERS, AL: *Opportunistic and contaminating saprophytic fungi.* In LENNETTE, EH, ET AL (EDS): *Manual of Clinical Microbiology*, ed 3. American Society for Microbiology, Washington, DC, 1980.

WOLF, F: *Relation of various fungi to otomycosis.* Arch Otolaryngol 46:361, 1947.

INTRODUCTION

This module discusses some of the more common genera of fungal contaminants which the practicing medical mycologist may encounter. There are many more known contaminants, but it is beyond the scope of this module to present them all. (Refer to Barnett and Hunter (1972) for further information.) Contaminants will be seen very often in routine fungal cultures, and it is therefore important to be able to identify and differentiate them from the normally **pathogenic** fungi, which are presented in Modules 4 through 7.

COMMON PROPERTIES OF FUNGAL CONTAMINANTS

There are a number of generalizations that can be made regarding fungal contaminants.

Rapid Growing

Most are rapid growers, forming mature colonies in four or five days.

Saprobic and Airborne

They are **saprobic**, living on decaying organic matter in the soil, and sometimes become airborne.

Normally Inhaled

Since we constantly breathe in the conidia of fungal contaminants, routine cultures of sputum and other respiratory secretions may normally yield a few colonies of these organisms. Also, since the conidia are in the air, they may contaminate the skin as well as laboratory cultures.

Opportunistic Pathogens

Usually these organisms are nonpathogenic. However, they act as **opportunistic pathogens**. When the patient is debilitated in some way, as from illness or especially from immunosuppressive drugs, the common contaminants may multiply and cause disease, often with fatal consequences.

Laboratory Diagnosis

In order to isolate a contaminant, be sure to inoculate media free of antibiotics, since the drugs inhibit these fungi. Because they are so common in the environment, opportunistic pathogens must be repeatedly isolated in large numbers from cultured specimens of the patient to be considered the causative agent of a disease.

ASEPTATE CONTAMINANTS

All aseptate fungi, those that usually do not contain cross-walls, fall into the taxonomic subdivision Zygomycotina. A few of the more important Zygomycetes that act as opportunistic pathogens follow. Key identifying features are capitalized. Also Chart 1-4 (on pages 23-24) may be helpful.

Absidia Species
(Figs. 3-1 and 3-2)

Culture: On Sabouraud dextrose agar at room temperature, a woolly gray colony rapidly matures (Color Plate 14). The reverse side of the colony is colorless.

Microscopic: The mycelium is usually ASEPTATE, with BRANCHING SPORANGIOPHORES BETWEEN the **RHIZOID** nodes (rootlike hyphae) on the **STOLONS** (interconnecting runners). There is a slight swelling below the columella, and sporangia are PEAR SHAPED. When the sporangial wall dissolves, a collarette remains at the base of the columella.

Pathogenicity: *Absidia* may cause zygomycosis and mycotic keratitis. See the Supplemental Rationale section of this module for descriptions of these diseases.

Mucor Species
(Figs. 3-3 and 3-4)

Culture: On Sabouraud dextrose agar at room temperature, a white, fluffy mycelium quickly forms (Color Plate 15). It becomes gray to brown with age.

Microscopic: The mycelium is usually ASEPTATE. Single or BRANCHING SPORANGIOPHORES support round, spore-filled sporangia. Sometimes empty sporangial sacs may be seen or bare columellae with collarettes. The columella is variable in shape and light to pigmented in color. NO RHIZOIDS OR STOLONS are present.

Pathogenicity: *Mucor* may cause zygomycosis, **otomycosis** (ear infection), and allergies.

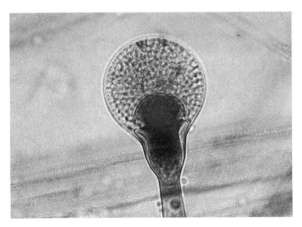

FIGURE 3-1. *Absidia* sp., lactophenol cotton blue (LPCB) stain, ×450.

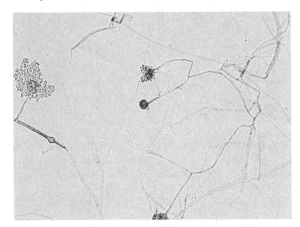

FIGURE 3-3. *Mucor* sp., LPCB stain, ×100.

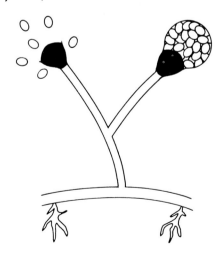

FIGURE 3-2. *Absidia* sp.

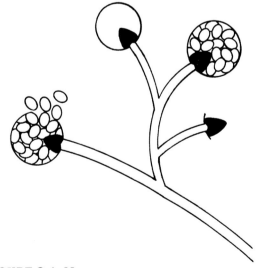

FIGURE 3-4. *Mucor* sp.

Rhizopus Species
(Figs. 3-5, 3-6, and 3-7)

Culture: On Sabouraud dextrose agar at room temperature, white, dense, cottony aerial hyphae rapidly form, which later become dotted with brown or black sporangia (Color Plate 3).

Microscopic: The hyphae are usually ASEPTATE. UNBRANCHED SPORANGIOPHORES arise OPPOSITE RHIZOIDS at the nodes, and each sporangiophore supports a round spore-filled sporangium with a flattened base. Sometimes the sporangia are completely black, or they may be empty. When the sporangial wall dissolves, a bare hemispherical columella without a collarette is observed. STOLONS connect the groups of rhizoids with each other.

Pathogenicity: *Rhizopus* causes zygomycosis and otomycosis.

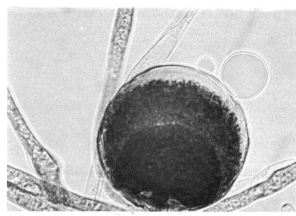

FIGURE 3-6. Sporangium, *Rhizopus* sp., LPCB stain, ×450.

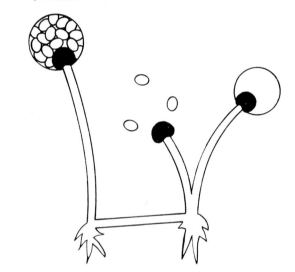

FIGURE 3-7. *Rhizopus* sp.

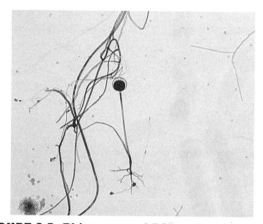

FIGURE 3-5. *Rhizopus* sp., LPCB stain, ×100.

Study Questions

1. **In your own words, describe at least five common properties that fungal contaminants possess.**

2. From Figure 3-8, fill in the blanks:

   A. _____

   B. _____

   C. _____

STOP HERE UNTIL YOU HAVE COMPLETED THE ANSWERS.

Look up the answers in the back of the book. If you missed more than two of them, go back and review the section on common properties of fungal contaminants and the section on aseptate contaminants. Correctly complete any missed study questions before proceeding further.

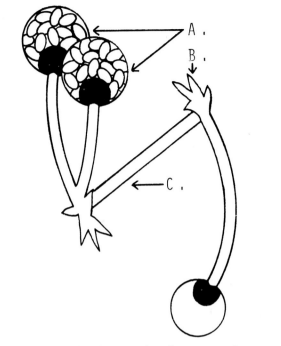

FIGURE 3-8. Study question demonstration.

SEPTATE CONTAMINANTS

Most contaminants contain cross-walls. Those of medical importance fall into the subdivision Deuteromycotina. The septate contaminants may be divided into those that are **dematiaceous** (dark-colored hyphae and/or conidia), and those that are **hyaline** (light-colored hyphae and conidia). **(See Chart 3-1 on page 107 at end of module.)** Organisms with dark hyphae on tease mounts also have dark green to black colonies, especially on the colony reverse. The colonial color aids in the initial identification. Hyaline organisms exhibit light-colored colonial aerial hyphae, but they may be covered over with brightly colored conidia; thus, a tease mount is required. In the following descriptions, key identifying features are capitalized.

Dematiaceous Contaminants

ALTERNARIA SPECIES (FIGS. 3-9 AND 3-10)

Culture: On Sabouraud dextrose agar at room temperature, the light gray, woolly colony rapidly matures to dark greenish black or brown, with a black reverse (Color Plate 16).

Microscopic: Reproductive structures and hyphae are DARK. The CHAINED POROCONIDIA, which contain HORIZONTAL and VERTICAL SEPTA, have

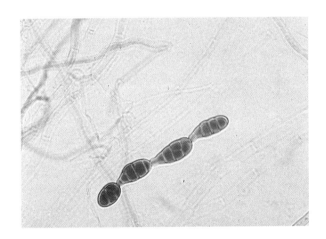

FIGURE 3-9. *Alternaria* sp., LPCB stain, ×450.

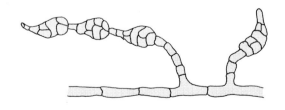

FIGURE 3-10. *Alternaria* sp.

club-shaped bases with tapered apices. If the poro-conidia are not in chains, they may be mistaken for the contaminant *Stemphylium* (see Fig. 3-22).

Pathogenicity: *Alternaria* has been reported in mycotic keratitis, skin infections, osteomyelitis, pulmonary disease, and nasal septum infection.

AUREOBASIDIUM SPECIES (FIGS. 3-11 AND 3-12)

Culture: On Sabouraud dextrose agar at room temperature, colonies are initially shiny white and yeastlike. With age, they become shiny black and leathery with a white fringe (BLACK YEAST) (Color Plate 17).

Microscopic: Light to DARK brown conidiophores are not differentiated from the hyphae. Short DENTI-CLES support HYALINE solitary or clustered CO-NIDIA, from which secondary blastoconidia may arise. With age, conidiophores become dark, one- to two-celled ARTHROCONIDIA.

Pathogenicity: *Aureobasidium* has been reported in a case of foot and leg lesions, in allergies, and in a case of cheloid blastomycosis.

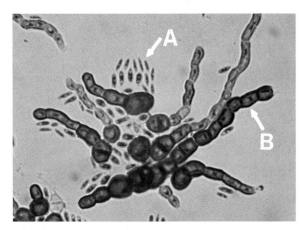

FIGURE 3-11. *Aureobasidium* sp., LPCB stain, ×450. Arrow A indicates hyaline blastoconidia; arrow B shows dark arthroconidia.

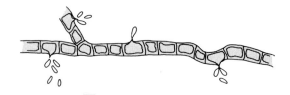

FIGURE 3-12. *Aureobasidium* sp.

CLADOSPORIUM (HORMODENDRUM) SPECIES (FIGS. 3-13 AND 3-14)

Culture: On Sabouraud dextrose agar at room temperature, the colony is moderately slow-growing for a contaminant, requiring seven days. It is powdery or velvety, heaped and folded, and dark gray-green with the reverse black (Color Plate 18).

Microscopic: The septate hyphae are DARK colored. Short CHAINS of dark one- to four-celled BLAS-TOCONIDIA with a distinct SCAR at each point of attachment are borne from REPEATEDLY FORKING, shield-shaped conidiogenous cells (SHIELD CELLS).

Other comments: In the past, contaminant strains of the genus were differentiated from pathogenic ones by the former's ability to hydrolyze nutrient gelatin. This test is not reliable and criteria such as growth rate, microscopic morphology, and clinical picture should be used instead.

Pathogenicity: *Cladosporium* may cause mycotic keratitis and allergies.

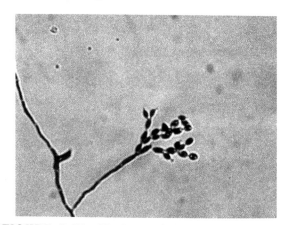

FIGURE 3-13. *Cladosporium* sp., LPCB stain, ×450.

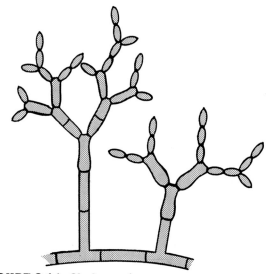

FIGURE 3-14. *Cladosporium* sp.

CURVULARIA SPECIES (FIGS. 3-15 AND 3-16)

Culture: On Sabouraud dextrose agar at room temperature, the colony is moderately rapid growing, cottony, and white, light pink, orange, or green, with a brown reverse (Color Plate 19).

Microscopic: The septate mycelium is DARK. Large, four- to five-celled, dark POROCONIDIA are borne on a BENT-KNEE type CONIDIOPHORE. The poroconidia are centrally distended owing to an OVER-ENLARGED CENTRAL CELL, and the ends are lighter than the middle.

Pathogenicity: *Curvularia* usually causes mycotic keratitis, but occasionally it may produce **mycetoma** (draining subcutaneous lesions on the extremities), endocarditis, pulmonary infection, allergies, and infection of the nasal septum.

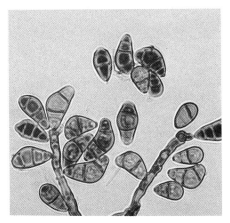

FIGURE 3-15. *Curvularia* sp., LPCB stain, ×450.

DRECHSLERA SPECIES (FIGS. 3-17 AND 3-18)

Culture: On Sabouraud dextrose agar at room temperature, the rapidly growing colony is velvety or woolly, at first appearing grayish-brown; later the center is matted and black, and the reverse is light or dark (Color Plate 20).

Microscopic: The septate hyphae are DARK. Numerous dark, CYLINDRICAL, four- or five-celled POROCONIDIA are usually in clusters. *Drechslera* resembles *Helminthosporium* sp. (Chart 1-10, page 35), but the former has a "BENT-KNEE" angle of the CONIDIOPHORE where the poroconidium attaches, while the latter does not.

Pathogenicity: *Drechslera* most frequently causes mycotic keratitis, while lesions of the nasal mucosa, meningitis, allergies, peritonitis, and **phaeohyphomycosis** (subcutaneous abscesses) have been reported.

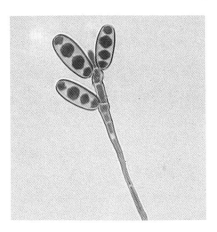

FIGURE 3-17. *Drechslera* sp., LPCB stain, ×450.

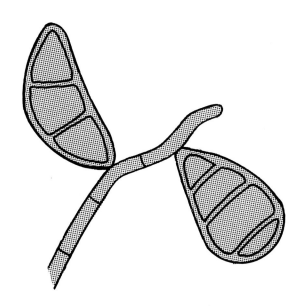

FIGURE 3-16. *Curvularia* sp.

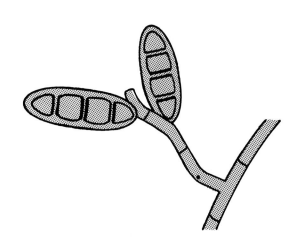

FIGURE 3-18. *Drechslera* sp.

EPICOCCUM SPECIES

Culture: On Sabouraud dextrose agar at room temperature, colonial rings of yellow, orange, and brown are seen, and pigments of the same color may diffuse into the agar (Color Plate 21).

Microscopic: Thick clusters of short conidiophores **(SPORODCHIA)** (Fig. 3-19) support terminal DARK round conidia with unconstricted HORIZONTAL and VERTICAL SEPTA. With age, the conidia become rough walled. *Epicoccum* (Fig. 3-20) superficially resembles the contaminants *Ulocladium* (Fig. 3-21) and *Stemphylium*. Figure 3-22 summarizes the differences.

Pathogenicity: *Epicoccum* has been associated with allergies.

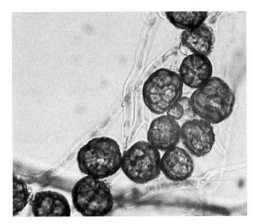

FIGURE 3-20. *Epicoccum* sp., LPCB stain, ×450.

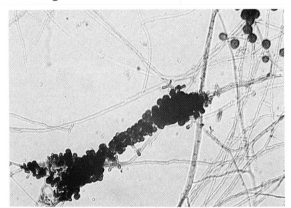

FIGURE 3-19. Sporodchia, *Epicoccum* **sp., LPCB stain, ×100.**

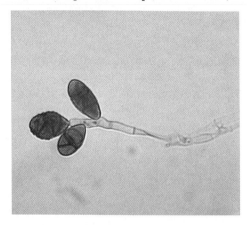

FIGURE 3-21. *Ulocladium* sp., LPCB stain, ×450.

1. Dark round conidia	Dark round to oval poroconidia	Dark oval poroconidia
2. Unconstricted horizontal and vertical septa in conidia	Unconstricted	Constricted
3. Sporodchia	No sporodchia: bent-knee type conidiophore	No sporodchia: new poroconidium produced through old scar
4. Orange colony, reverse brown	Gray to black colony, reverse black	Gray to black colony, reverse light gray

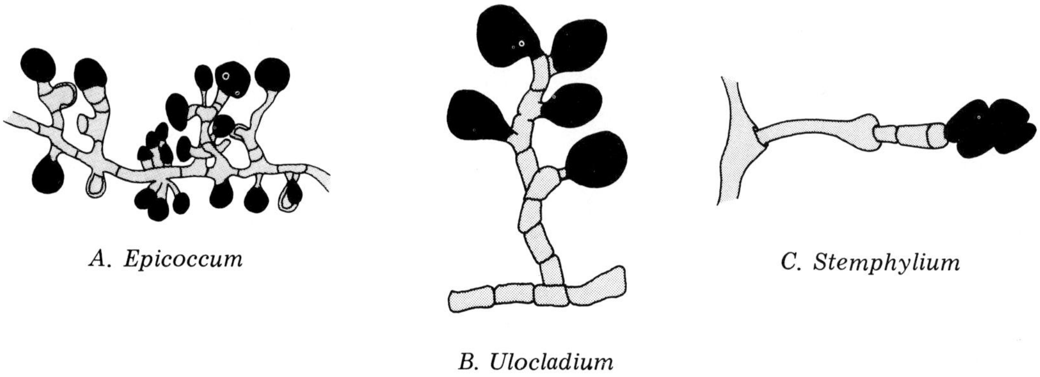

A. Epicoccum

B. Ulocladium

C. Stemphylium

FIGURE 3-22. Differentiation of *Epicoccum,* *Ulocladium,* **and** *Stemphylium.*

NIGROSPORA SPECIES (FIGS. 3-23 AND 3-24)

Culture: On Sabouraud dextrose agar at room temperature, a white, woolly colony with a black reverse rapidly fills the plate (Color Plate 22). With age, the aerial mycelium turns gray.

Microscopic: The hyphae are dark. SHORT, FAT CONIDIOPHORES support SINGLE, oval, smooth-walled, BLACK CONIDIA at the tips.

Pathogenicity: *Nigrospora* has been reported as a causative agent of mycotic keratitis.

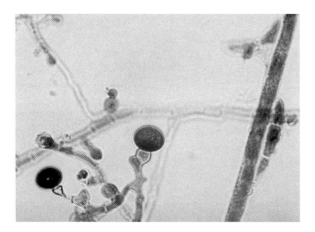

FIGURE 3-23. *Nigrospora* sp., LPCB stain, ×450.

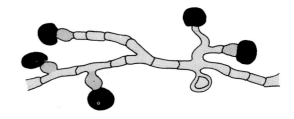

FIGURE 3-24. *Nigrospora* sp.

STUDY QUESTIONS

1. **Fill in the blank: If the conidia of *Alternaria* sp. are young and therefore not in chains, they may be mistaken for those of _____ .**

2. **Circle the correct answer(s).**
   Which of the following possess conidia with vertical and horizontal cross-walls?
   A. *Curvularia* sp.
   B. *Ulocladium* sp.
   C. *Aureobasidium* sp.
   D. *Epicoccum* sp.
   E. *Drechslera* sp.
   F. *Alternaria* sp.
   G. *Stemphylium* sp.

3. **Place the letter of the answer from Column B in front of the corresponding words in Column A. An answer may be used more than once.**

   Column A
   ___ Black yeast
   ___ Shield cells
   ___ Enlarged central cell
   ___ Arthroconidia
   ___ Single, one-celled, black conidia

   Column B
   A. *Nigrospora* sp.
   B. *Ulocladium* sp.
   C. *Aureobasidium* sp.
   D. *Drechslera* sp.
   E. *Cladosporium* sp.
   F. *Curvularia* sp.

STOP HERE UNTIL YOU HAVE COMPLETED THE ANSWERS.

Look up the answers in the back of the book. If you missed more than two, go back and repeat the section on dematiaceous contaminants. Correctly complete any missed questions before proceeding.

Hyaline Contaminants

ACREMONIUM (CEPHALOSPORIUM) SPECIES (FIGS. 3-25 AND 3-26)

Culture: On Sabouraud dextrose agar at room temperature, the colony is rapid growing. It is wrinkled, membranous, and white, gray, or rose, later becoming covered with loose aerial mycelium (Color Plate 23). The reverse is colorless, pale yellow, or pinkish.

Microscopic: The mycelium is septate. Unbranched TAPERING CONIDIOPHORES support closely packed BALLS of sickle- or elliptical-shaped CONIDIA. If the conidiophores are in whorls around the hyphae, *Acremonium* may resemble the contaminant Verticillium (see Chart 1-9, pages 32–34); however, *Verticillium* exhibits conidiophores in whorls. If the conidia are more loosely packed, *Acremonium* may resemble *Sporothrix schenckii* (covered in Module 6), but *Sporothrix* forms a yeast at 37°C, while *Acremonium* does not.

Pathogenicity: *Acremonium* may cause mycotic keratitis, rarely mycetoma, lesions of the hard palate, meningitis, arthritis and systemic disease.

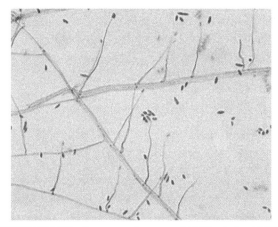

FIGURE 3-25. *Acremonium* sp., LPCB stain, ×450.

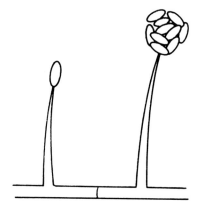

FIGURE 3-26. *Acremonium* sp.

ASPERGILLUS SPECIES (FIGS. 3-27 AND 3-28)

If possible, this genus should be speciated, especially *A. fumigatus.* **(See Chart 3-2 on page 108 at end of module.)**

Culture: On Sabouraud dextrose agar at room temperature, the rapid-growing colony is rugose and velvety. Various colors are due to dense production of conidia: blue, green, yellow, black, and white (Color Plates 8 and 24).

Microscopic: The mycelium is septate. Unbranched, rough or smooth conidiophores with a FOOT CELL at their base support a large VESICLE at their tip. The vesicle in turn supports short, flask-shaped PHIALIDES (old name: sterigmata) in a SINGLE OR DOUBLE ROW, which produce CHAINS of smooth or rough PHIALOCONIDIA. *Aspergillus* sp. must not be confused with the similar-appearing zygomycete, *Syncephalastrum* sp. (Fig. 3-29 and Color Plate 25), which is aseptate, possesses no phialides, and exhibits chains of spores in tubes **(merosporangia)** off the vesicle.

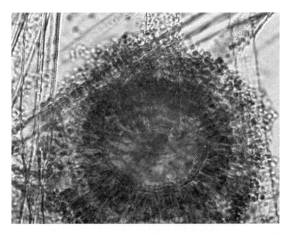

FIGURE 3-27. *Aspergillus* sp., LPCB stain, ×450.

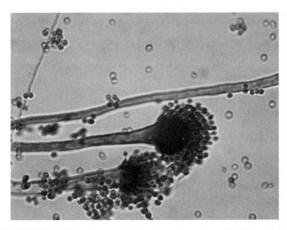

FIGURE 3-28. *Aspergillus fumigatus,* LPCB stain, ×450.

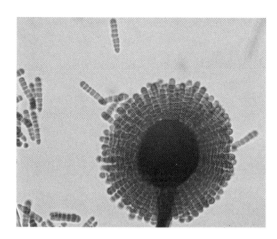

FIGURE 3-29. *Syncephalastrum* sp., LPCB stain, ×450.

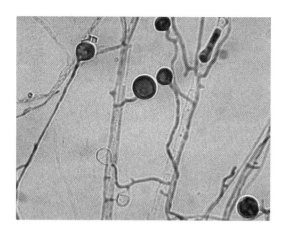

FIGURE 3-30. *Chrysosporium* sp., LPCB stain, ×450.

Other comments: *A. fumigatus* grows at 45°C, while most other *Aspergillus* species will not.

Pathogenicity: *A. fumigatus* is the most common opportunistic pathogen of the genus. It causes disseminated aspergillosis, pulmonary disease, and allergic bronchopulmonary disease (farmer's lung), as well as mycotic keratitis, otomycosis, and infection of the nasal sinuses.

CHRYSOSPORIUM SPECIES (FIGS. 3-30 AND 3-31)

Culture: On Sabouraud dextrose agar at room temperature, a heaped, velvety, buff-colored colony rapidly forms, with a white, yellow, or reddish-brown reverse (Color Plate 26).

Microscopic: SINGLE, round to club-shaped, smooth or rough CONIDIA perch on top of short conidiophores, which are poorly differentiated from the vegetative mycelium. Conidia also develop directly off the hyphae, and swollen arthroconidia may be present. *Chrysosporium* colonially and microscopically resembles the subcutaneous pathogen *Scedosporium apiospermum* (Module 6) and the mold phase of the systemic dimorphs *Blastomyces dermatitidis* and *Histoplasma capsulatum* (Module 7). However, *Chrysosporium* is a rapid grower, while *Scedosporium* is intermediate and *Blastomyces* and *Histoplasma* are slow. Unlike the dimorphs, *Chrysosporium* cannot be converted to a yeast phase at 37°C. *Scedosporium* also does not form a yeast phase but can be separated on the basis of clinical manifestations, annellides, and by the common presence of sexual stage cleistothecia.

Pathogenicity: *Chrysosporium* has rarely been reported as a pathogen.

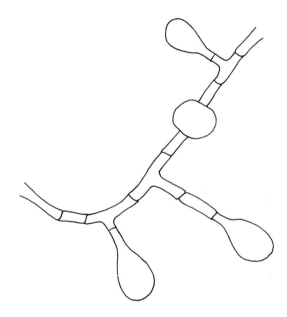

FIGURE 3-31. *Chrysosporium* sp.

FUSARIUM SPECIES (FIGS. 3-32 AND 3-33)

Culture: On Sabouraud dextrose agar at room temperature, the rapidly growing colony is white at first and woolly or cottony. Later it becomes LAVENDER, or sometimes yellow or orange, with a light reverse (Color Plate 27).

Microscopic: The mycelium is septate. Conidiophores are single or branching, occasionally producing whorls, and they terminate in tapering phialides. Microphialoconidia are one celled and occur in balls; if macrophialoconidia are not exhibited, *Fusarium* may be mistaken for *Acremonium*. Diagnostic MACRO-

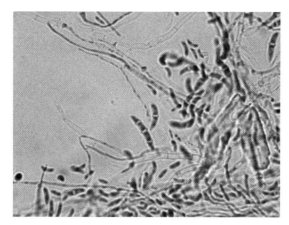

FIGURE 3-32. *Fusarium* sp., LPCB stain, ×450.

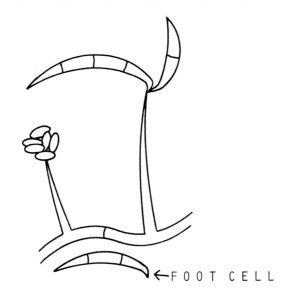

←FOOT CELL

FIGURE 3-33. *Fusarium* sp.

PHIALOCONIDIA are two to five celled, BANANA- or cylindrical-SHAPED, with a distinctive FOOT CELL at the point of attachment. The contaminant *Cylindrocarpon* (see Chart 1-9) produces similar-appearing macrophialoconidia; however, the ends are rounded, there are no foot cells, and one to ten septa may occur. Chlamydoconidia are common in *Fusarium*.

Pathogenicity: *Fusarium* is the most common cause of mycotic keratitis. It has also been isolated from skin lesions on burn patients, in **onychomycosis** (nail infection), otomycosis, varicose ulcers, mycetoma, osteomyelitis following trauma, and disseminated infection.

GLIOCLADIUM SPECIES (FIGS. 3-34 AND 3-35)

Culture: On Sabouraud dextrose agar at room temperature, the colony is initially white but it rapidly fills the plate with a green, furry growth mimicking a GREEN LAWN (Color Plate 28). Some strains may remain white or turn rose colored. The reverse is white. The contaminant *Trichoderma* (see Chart 1-9) is also initially white and later green; however, the color is usually more yellowish-green, and the growth is cottony.

Microscopic: Brushlike conidiophores (**PENICILLI**; singular, penicillus) bear flask-shaped PHIALIDES, which in turn produce terminal masses of hyaline to green PHIALOCONIDIA, held together in a LARGE BALL by a gelatinous matrix. Young penicilli with only one or two branches may be mistaken for *Trichoderma* and *Verticillium* (see Chart 1-9) which exhibit single or whorled phialides with terminal balls of phialoconidia. *Trichoderma* structures are smaller and more delicate than *Gliocladium*; also with careful searching, no penicilli should be found with either *Trichoderma* or *Verticillium*.

Pathogenicity: *Gliocladium* is not known to be a human pathogen.

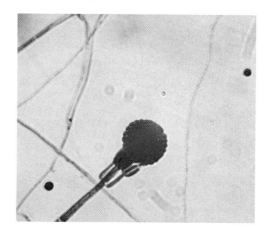

FIGURE 3-34. *Gliocladium* sp., LPCB stain, ×450.

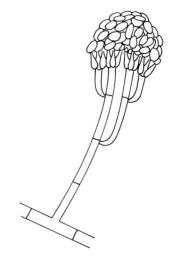

FIGURE 3-35. *Gliocladium* sp.

PAECILOMYCES SPECIES (FIGS. 3-36 AND 3-37)

Culture: On Sabouraud dextrose agar at room temperature, the powdery, velvety, or cottony mycelium very rapidly matures to an OLIVE TAN (Color Plate 29), although shades of violet or brown may be seen.

Microscopic: Single, whorled, or penicillus-type ELONGATED PHIALIDES bear CHAINS of smooth or rough, hyaline to pigmented oval CONIDIA. Microscopically, *Paecilomyces* maintains a close semblance to the contaminants *Penicillium* and *Verticillium* (see Chart 1-9), but the latter fungi do not exhibit elongated phialides.

Pathogenicity: *Paecilomyces* has been implicated in cases of penicilliosis, endophthalmitis, endocarditis, pleural effusion, and skin lesions.

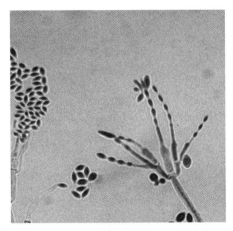

FIGURE 3-36. *Paecilomyces* sp., LPCB stain, ×450.

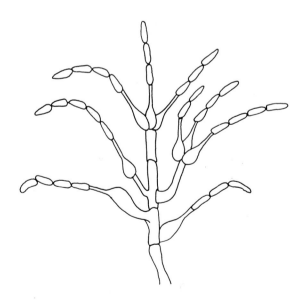

FIGURE 3-37. *Paecilomyces* sp.

PENICILLIUM SPECIES (FIGS. 3-38 AND 3-39)

Culture: On Sabouraud dextrose agar at room temperature, the rapid-growing colony is initially velvety and white, later becoming powdery and BLUE GREEN with a white periphery and colorless reverse (Color Plate 30).

Microscopic: The mycelium is septate. PENICILLI bear flask-shaped PHIALIDES, which in turn support CHAINS of round PHIALOCONIDIA. Conidiophores and phialoconidia may be hyaline to pigmented, and smooth to rough, depending on species.

Pathogenicity: *Penicillium* causes mycotic keratitis, penicilliosis, otomycosis, onychomycosis, and rarely, deep infection.

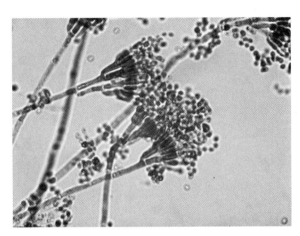

FIGURE 3-38. *Penicillium* sp., LPCB stain, ×450.

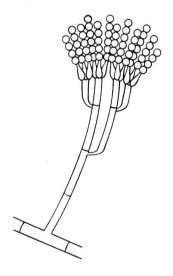

FIGURE 3-39. *Penicillium* sp.

SCOPULARIOPSIS SPECIES (FIGS. 3-40 AND 3-41)

Culture: On Sabouraud dextrose agar at room temperature, the rapid-growing colony is velvety, rugose, and white, later becoming light tan or brown, with a tan reverse (Color Plate 31).

Microscopic: The mycelium is septate. Single, unbranching, or PENICILLUS-type ANNELLOPHORES bear flask-shaped ANNELLIDES, which in turn support large LEMON-SHAPED ANNELLOCONIDIA in chains. With age, the conidia become **echinulate,** or SPINY.

Pathogenicity: *Scopulariopsis* causes mycotic keratitis, rarely bronchopulmonary disease (penicilliosis), otomycosis, and onychomycosis. It has been reported in an infection of the ankle and as the cause of an inguinal ulcer.

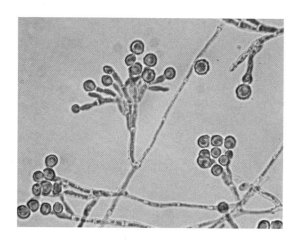

FIGURE 3-40. *Scopulariopsis* sp., LPCB stain, ×450.

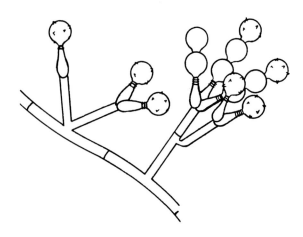

FIGURE 3-41. *Scopulariopsis* sp.

SEPEDONIUM SPECIES (FIGS. 3-42 AND 3-43)

Culture: On Sabouraud dextrose agar at room temperature, the waxy and white colony rapidly becomes velvety and lemon colored with a peripheral fringe, and white reverse (Color Plate 32).

Microscopic: SINGLE or clustered, THICK-WALLED, SMOOTH TO ROUGH (MACRO)CONIDIA form at the ends of simple or branched conidiophores which are not well differentiated from the vegetative mycelium. Formerly, it was thought that single, smooth, and thin-walled, elliptical (micro)conidia were also produced; now McGinnis (1980) and Rogers (1980) feel that these only represent young macroconidia. *Sepedonium* greatly imitates the systemic dimorph *Histoplasma capsulatum* (Module 7) which possesses macro- and microconidia, but the former does not convert to a yeast phase at 37°C.

Pathogenicity: *Sepedonium* is not known to be a human pathogen.

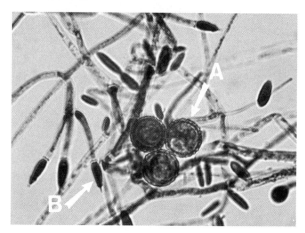

FIGURE 3-42. *Sepedonium* sp., LPCB stain, ×450. Arrow A indicates a macroconidium; Arrow B shows a previously named microconidium, now considered to be a young macroconidium.

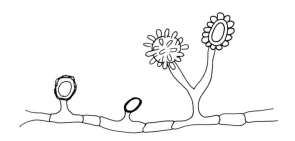

FIGURE 3-43. *Sepedonium* sp.

STUDY QUESTIONS

1. *Penicillium, Gliocladium, Paecilomyces,* and *Scopulariopsis* all possess a penicillus. Describe three ways in which they may be distinguished from each other.

2. *Aspergillus* and *Syncephalastrum* resemble each other microscopically. Put an A in front of each characteristic that pertains to *Aspergillus* sp., a B in front of those items that apply to *Syncephalastrum* sp., and a C where neither fungus is characterized.

    ___ Aseptate
    ___ Vesicles
    ___ Blastoconidia
    ___ Merosporangia
    ___ Foot cells
    ___ Phialides

3. Circle true or false:
    T F *Acremonium* exhibits repeatedly forking conidiophores with terminal balls of conidia.

4. The fungi listed in Column A below all possess single, one-celled, terminal conidia. The items in Column B may be used to differentiate them. Place the letter of the characteristic from Column B in front of the corresponding organism in Column A. More than one characteristic may be placed in front of each fungus.

    Column A
    ___ *Chrysosporium* sp.
    ___ *Sepedonium* sp.
    ___ *Scedosporium apiospermum*
    ___ *Blastomyces dermatitidis*
    ___ *Histoplasma capsulatum*

    Column B
    A. Dimorphic
    B. Rapid growing
    C. May possess microconidia
    D. Cleistothecia common
    E. Annellidic

STOP HERE UNTIL YOU HAVE COMPLETED THE QUESTIONS.

Look up the answers in the back of the book. If you missed more than two, go back and repeat the section on hyaline contaminants. Correctly complete any missed questions before proceeding.

FINAL EXAM

1. Circle the correct answer:
    Banana-shaped macrophialoconidia with foot cells are diagnostic of:
    A. *Cylindrocarpon* sp.
    B. *Nigrospora* sp.
    C. *Curvularia* sp.
    D. *Fusarium* sp.
    E. *Paecilomyces* sp.

2. Circle true or false:
    T F Dematiaceous organisms exhibit light-colored hyphae and/ or conidia.

3. In front of numbers 1. to 3., write the letter(s) of the fungus that represents each characteristic:
    A. *Absidia* sp.
    B. *Mucor* sp.
    C. *Rhizopus* sp.

    ___ 1. Produces rhizoids
    ___ 2. Branching sporangiophores
    ___ 3. Internodal sporangiophores

4. *Epicoccum* sp., *Ulocladium* sp., and *Stemphylium* sp. all demonstrate similar conidia. Describe at least two ways to differentiate them.

5. Circle true or false:

   T F Isolates of *Helminthosporium* are distinguished from *Drechslera* in that *Helminthosporium* possess conidiophores that grow in a bent-knee fashion, while *Drechslera* conidiophores grow straight.

6. Circle true or false:

   T F *Aspergillus fumigatus* produces phialides and phialoconidia only at the end of the vesicle.

7. In these blanks, write the genus identified from each drawing in the right-hand column.

   A. _____

   B. _____

   C. _____

   D. _____

   E. _____

   F. _____

   G. _____

   H. _____

   I. _____

   J. _____

   K. _____

   L. _____

STOP HERE UNTIL YOU HAVE COMPLETED THE ANSWERS.

Look up the answers in the back of the book. If you missed more than three of them, go back and repeat this module. Correctly complete any missed questions before proceeding.

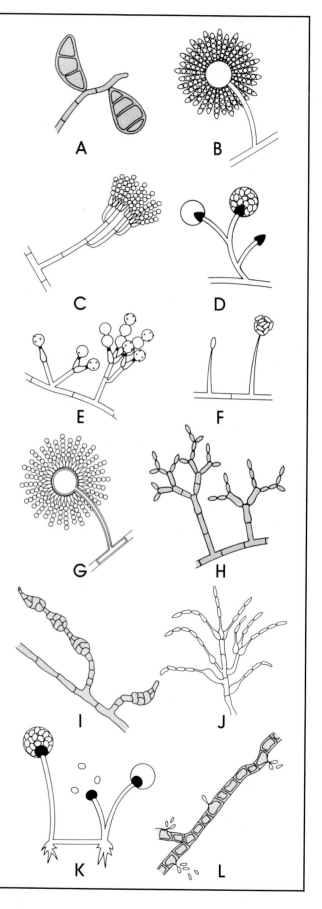

SUPPLEMENTAL RATIONALE

Aspergillosis

Aspergillosis is usually acquired by inhalation of the conidia. It begins as a pulmonary disease, producing **granulomatous** (tumorous) lesions in the lungs or bronchi. These may be spread from the lung tissue into the surrounding blood vessels. Subsequently, the disease disseminates to the rest of the body, including the brain, gastrointestinal tract, and kidneys. This invasive pulmonary form of aspergillosis is being increasingly observed in debilitated patients receiving antibiotic, immunosuppressive, or cancer therapy. The disseminated disease is usually acute and fatal. In two characteristic forms of aspergillosis—otomycosis (external ear infection) and fungus ball (abscess)—there is no tissue invasion. Asthma attacks can be initiated in sensitized individuals by inhalation of *Aspergillus* conidia. Miscellaneous types of aspergillosis include myocarditis, meningitis, osteomyelitis, mycetoma, burn infection, invasion of the nasal sinuses, onychomycosis, mycotic keratitis, and toxin ingestion from eating contaminated foods.

Direct mounts of specimens reveal septate hyphae that branch dichotomously (Y-shaped branching) (Color Plate 33). Specimens from fungus balls may also show the typical *Aspergillus* fruiting heads (Fig. 3-44). Classically, diagnosis is confirmed if repeated cultures of infected material grow large numbers of *Aspergillus* species. However, in cases of invasive pulmonary aspergillosis, only 25 percent of patients may produce positive cultures, and only half of those may possess more than one positive result. Therefore, isolation of *A. fumigatus* or *A. flavus* should not be automatically considered as lab contamination but rather should be judged in light of the patient's medical history. *A. fumigatus* is most commonly isolated from invasive pulmonary aspergillosis, fungus ball, and allergic bronchopulmonary disease. *A. flavus* is seen in invasive pulmonary aspergillosis and allergic bronchopulmonary disease, while *A. niger* produces fungus ball and otomycosis.

Mycotic Keratitis

The cornea of the eye is resistant to infection. However, with predisposing factors, fungi can invade the cornea and cause mycotic keratitis (Fig. 3-45). Such factors include trauma to the eye, use of corticosteroids (anti-inflammatory medication used in conjunction with antibiotics for supposed bacterial infection of the eye), and glaucoma. A white or cream-colored infiltrate develops after the conidia germinate, and hyphal growth forms in the area of trauma. Ulceration occurs in the cornea, eventually scarring and causing blindness. Fungal lesions range from the extremely painful to the unnoticed—unnoticed possibly because of decreased sensation of the eye which follows nerve damage or long-continued wearing of contact lenses. The lesions may elicit an **inflammatory** (pus cell) response as described above, or none at all. Corneal scrapings should be taken for direct mounts and culture. Since the causative organisms are mostly contaminants, a fungus must be repeatedly isolated to be considered etiologically significant. There are over 80 fungi that may cause mycotic keratitis (**see Chart 3-3 on page 109**).

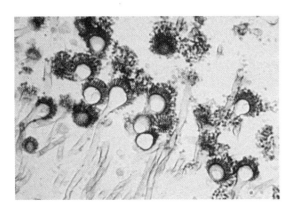

FIGURE 3-44. Aspergillosis, fruiting heads, Gridley's modification of PAS stain. (From: Dolan, D. et al: Atlas of Clinical Mycology. ASCP, Washington, DC, 1976, with permission.)

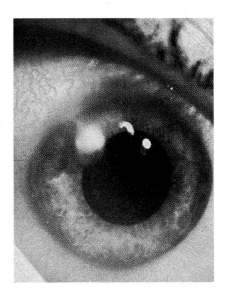

FIGURE 3-45. Mycotic keratitis. (From: Beneke, ES and Rogers, AL: Medical Mycology Manual. Burgess, Minneapolis, 1970, with permission.)

Otomycosis

Otomycosis (Fig. 3-46) is a fungal infection of the external auditory opening or ear canal, with symptoms of inflammation, itching, scaling, and partial deafness due to the ear canal being filled with a hyphal plug. Trauma often starts the disease; the habit of cleaning the ears with matches or similar objects causes abrasions that become readily infected. Fungal infection may be secondary to a bacterial ear infection or to previous use of antibiotics. Too much heat and moisture may predispose the patient to otomycosis. Scrapings and purulent discharge are the specimens of choice for direct mount and culture. Many of the fungal etiologic agents are contaminants and thus must be repeatedly isolated in large numbers before being considered significant. Also, other organisms, such as yeasts or dermatophytes, may cause otomycosis.

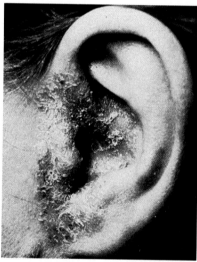

FIGURE 3-46. Otomycosis. (From: Conant, NF, et al.: Manual of Clinical Mycology. WB Saunders, Philadelphia, 1971, with permission.)

Penicilliosis

Penicilliosis is usually acquired by inhaling the conidia of the contaminants *Penicillium, Scopulariopsis,* or *Paecilomyces.* It starts as a pulmonary disease but may spread into the adjacent blood vessels. Subsequently it disseminates to the rest of the body, including the spinal fluid, kidneys *(Penicillium),* and endocardium *(Paecilomyces, Penicillium).* Such total invasion occurs in debilitated patients. Penicilliosis may also include infections of the nails *(Scopulariopsis),* otomycosis *(Penicillium),* mycotic keratitis *(Penicillium, Scopulariopsis),* inguinal ulcers *(Scopulariopsis),* and allergic bronchial asthma in sensitized people *(Penicillium, Scopulariopsis).* Observing hyphae and conidia in direct mounts is in itself not significant unless the organism is also repeatedly isolated in large numbers.

Zygomycosis (Mucormycosis, Phycomycosis)

Zygomycosis (Fig. 3-47) is an acute fungus infection caused by fungi from the subdivision Zygomycotina. These fungi commonly grow on bread and fruits. Spores become airborne and, if the patient is in acidosis, as with uncontrolled diabetes or malnutrition, or is on corticosteroids, antibiotics, or antileukemic drugs, the spores may infect the nasal sinuses and **orbital** (eye) area. The infection rapidly spreads to adjacent blood vessels, causing necrosis and vascular **thrombosis** (blood clots). From here it spreads to the brain and meninges and produces a rapidly fatal meningoencephalitis. The disease may disseminate to the lungs and gastrointestinal tract. Death ensues two to ten days after the initial sinus/eye infection. A chronic, self-limiting form of zygomycosis has been observed in subcutaneous lesions. Direct mounts of specimens from both types of infections show branching, large aseptate hyphae, and round sporangia may be present. Diagnosis is confirmed with repeated isolation of the organism. Since zygomycosis of the sinuses, orbital area, and meninges is so rapidly fatal, the physician should begin treatment as soon as the disease is suspected.

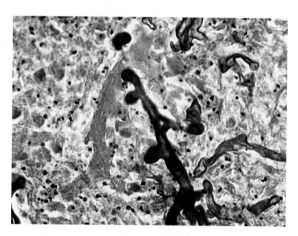

FIGURE 3-47. Zygomycosis, hematoxylin and eosin stain, ×450.

Study Questions—Supplemental Rationale

1. Circle true or false:

   T F In aspergillosis, the etiologic fungus may be isolated only once and still be considered significant.

2. Circle the letter of the correct answer(s).

   Otomycosis involves:

   A. external ear infections.
   B. deep inner ear infections.

3. Circle true or false:

   T F The cornea of the eye is easily susceptible to infection.

For questions 4 through 7, refer to this case study and Figure 3-48.

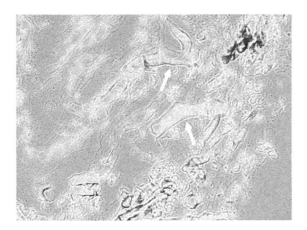

FIGURE 3-48. Case study demonstration, methenamine silver stain, ×450. Arrows indicate hyphae.

A 10-year-old boy was admitted to the hospital in diabetic ketoacidosis. Three days later, he complained of nasal sinus blockage. Stained histologic preparations of material removed from his sinuses showed the wide, ribbonlike hyphae seen in Figure 3-48. On Sabouraud dextrose agar, a white cottony mold rapidly grew.

4. Which disease do you suspect, and why?

5. Circle the letter of the correct answer.

   Three agents of this mycosis are:

   A. *Rhizomucor, Fusarium,* and *Acremonium.*
   B. *Penicillium, Scopulariopsis,* and *Paecilomyces.*
   C. *Absidia, Mucor,* and *Rhizopus.*
   D. *Aspergillus fumigatus, Aspergillus niger,* and *Aspergillus flavus.*
   E. *Cladosporium, Alternaria,* and *Drechslera.*

6. Slide cultures of the mold revealed unbranching sporangiophores at rhizoid nodes.

   Fill in the blank: The causative organism is _____ .

Box continues on next page.

7. Since this is an opportunistic infection, should the physician wait for repeated cultures before initiating treatment? Why or why not?

STOP HERE UNTIL YOU HAVE COMPLETED THE QUESTIONS.

Look up the answers in the back of the book. If you missed more than one, go back and review the Supplemental Rationale section and the section on aseptate contaminants. Correctly complete any missed questions.

CHART 3-1. Flow Diagram for Identification of Septate Fungal Contaminants*

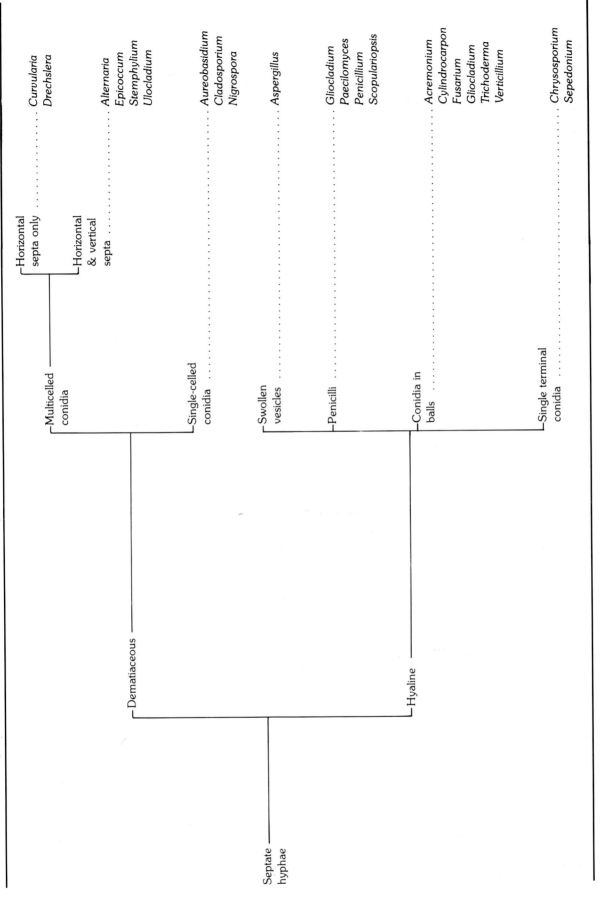

Septate hyphae

Dematiaceous
- Multicelled conidia
  - Horizontal septa only .... *Curvularia* / *Drechslera*
  - Horizontal & vertical septa .... *Alternaria* / *Epicoccum* / *Stemphylium* / *Ulocladium*
- Single-celled conidia .... *Aureobasidium* / *Cladosporium* / *Nigrospora*

Hyaline
- Swollen vesicles .... *Aspergillus*
- Penicilli .... *Gliocladium* / *Paecilomyces* / *Penicillium* / *Scopulariopsis*
- Conidia in balls .... *Acremonium* / *Cylindrocarpon* / *Fusarium* / *Gliocladium* / *Trichoderma* / *Verticillium*
- Single terminal conidia .... *Chrysosporium* / *Sepedonium*

*Modified from Koneman, Roberts, and Wright, 1978

COMMON FUNGAL CONTAMINANTS

CHART 3-2. Identification of the Most Common Species of *Aspergillus**

	A. FUMIGATUS	A. NIGER	A. FLAVUS	A. GLAUCUS	A. TERREUS
PATHOGENICITY	Most common cause of aspergillosis	Usually considered a contaminant but also known to cause disease in the debilitated	Usually a contaminant but also known to cause disease in the debilitated	Commonly known as a contaminant but also known to cause infection under certain conditions	Commonly considered a contaminant but also known to cause infection
MACROSCOPIC MORPHOLOGY[†]	Velvety or powdery, at first white, then turning dark greenish Reverse white to tan	Wooly, at first white to yellow, then turning dark brown to black Reverse white to yellow	Velvety, yellow to green or brown Reverse goldish to red brown	Feltlike; green with yellow areas; occasionally brown Reverse yellowish to maroon (Grown best with 20% sucrose added to the medium)	Usually velvety, cinnamon brown Reverse white to brown
MICROSCOPIC MORPHOLOGY OF CONIDIOPHORES	Short (<300 μm) Smooth	Variable length Smooth	Variable length Rough, pitted, spiny	Variable length Smooth	Short (<250 μm) Smooth
MICROSCOPIC MORPHOLOGY OF PHIALIDES	Single, usually only on upper half of vesicle, parallel to axis of stalk	Double, cover entire vesicle, form "radiate" head	Single and double, cover entire vesicle, point out in all directions	Single, radiate to very loosely columnar, cover entire vesicle (Cleistothecia generally present)	Double, compactly columnar (Round hyaline cells produced on mycelium submerged in agar)

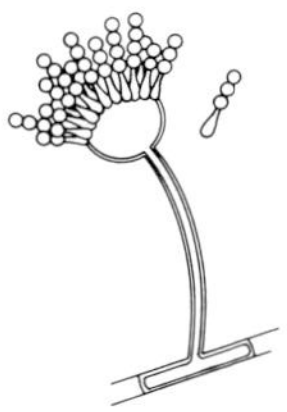

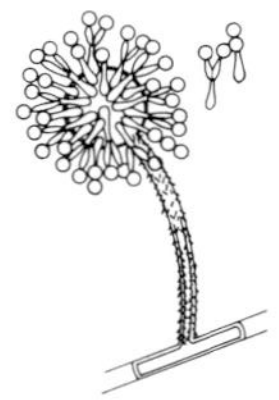

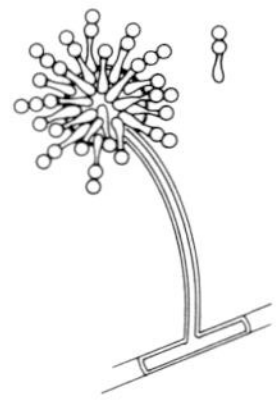

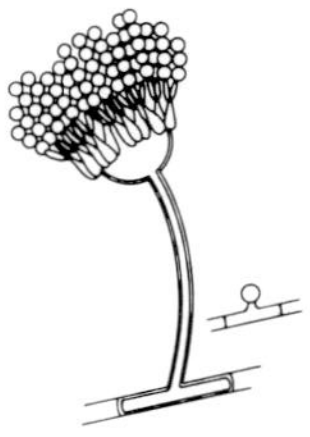

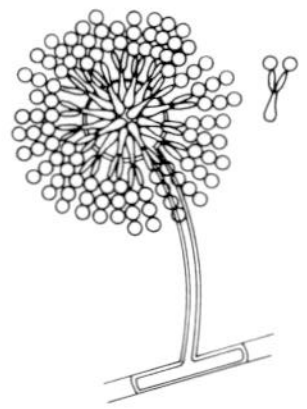

*From Larone, DH: Medically Important Fungi: A Guide to Identification, Harper & Row, Hagerstown, Maryland, 1976.
†Classically studied on Czapek-Dox agar. On Sabouraud dextrose agar most species of aspergillus grow luxuriantly but not always characteristically.

CHART 3-3. Some Organisms that Cause Contaminant-Associated Diseases

ASPERGILLOSIS	MYCOTIC KERATITIS	OTOMYCOSIS	PENICILLIOSIS	ZYGOMYCOSIS
Aspergillus flavus	Absidia sp.	Aspergillus fumigatus	Paecilomyces sp.	Absidia sp.
Aspergillus fumigatus	Acremonium sp.	Aspergillus niger	Penicillium sp.	Cunninghamella sp.
Aspergillus niger	Actinomyces bovis	Aspergillus terreus	Scopulariopsis sp.	Mortierella sp.
Aspergillus terreus	Alternaria sp.	Candida albicans		Mucor sp.
	Aspergillus flavus	Candida tropicalis		Rhizomucor sp.
	Aspergillus fumigatus	Epidermophyton floccosum		Rhizopus sp.
	Aspergillus niger	Fusarium sp.		
	Candida sp.	Mucor sp.		
	Cladosporium sp.	Penicillium sp.		
	Curvularia sp.	Rhizopus sp.		
	Cylindrocarpon sp.	Scopulariopsis sp.		
	Drechslera sp.	Trichophyton violaceum		
	Exophiala jeanselmei			
	Fusarium sp.			
	Graphium sp.			
	Mucor sp.			
	Nigrospora sp.			
	Nocardia sp.			
	Penicillium sp.			
	Phialophora verrucosa			
	Rhizopus sp.			
	Rhodotorula sp.			
	Scedosporium sp.			
	Scopulariopsis sp.			
	Sporothrix schenckii			
	Trichosporon sp.			
	Ustilago sp.			
	Volutella sp.			

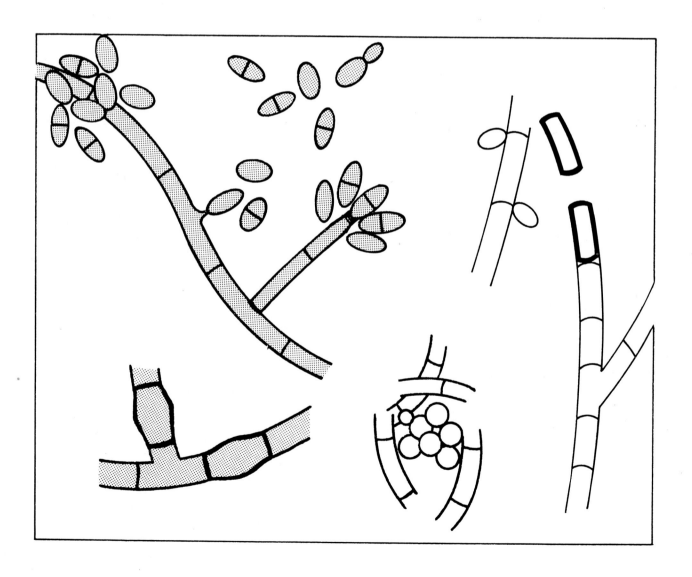

SUPERFICIAL AND DERMATOPHYTIC FUNGI

PREREQUISITES. The learner must possess a good background knowledge in clinical microbiology and must have finished Module 1, Basics of Mycology, and Module 2, Laboratory Procedures for Fungal Culture and Isolation.

BEHAVIORAL OBJECTIVES: Upon completion of this module, the learner should be able to:

1. Compare and contrast:

   Superficial and cutaneous mycoses
   Cutaneous mycoses and dermatomycoses

2. Identify hairs with endothrix invasion, ectothrix invasion, and in vitro perforation.

3. Identify the following fungi from culture, microscopic appearance, biochemical characteristics, and mycosis produced:

   Malassezia furfur
   Exophiala werneckii
   Piedraia hortai
   Trichosporon beigelii
   Microsporum audouinii
   Microsporum canis
   Microsporum gypseum
   Epidermophyton floccosum
   Trichophyton mentagrophytes
   Trichophyton rubrum
   Trichophyton verrucosum
   Trichophyton tonsurans
   Trichophyton schoenleinii
   Trichophyton violaceum

4. Briefly describe the following mycoses and state which organisms listed in number 3 cause each. State common mycosis names where appropriate.

   Pityriasis versicolor
   Tinea nigra
   Black piedra
   White piedra
   Tinea capitis
   Tinea barbae
   Tinea corporis
   Tinea cruris
   Tinea pedis
   Tinea unguium

5. Concerning the three dermatophyte genera:

   A. List them.
   B. State which body sites (skin, nails, ectothrix hair, endothrix hair) are infected by each genus.
   C. Describe the microscopic characteristics, especially macro- and microconidia, that are typical for each genus.

6. Discuss how the type of tinea, hair fluorescence, and growth rate aid in dermatophyte speciation.

7. Describe usefulness of the following in dermatophyte species identification:

   Color on potato dextrose or corn meal agar
   In vitro perforation of autoclaved hair
   Trichophyton agars
   Christenson's urea agar
   Polished rice grains

   Include which organisms are differentiated, how to set up each procedure, and positive and negative results.

CONTENT OUTLINE

I. Introduction
II. Superficial organisms
   A. *Exophiala werneckii*
   B. *Malassezia furfur*
   C. *Piedraia hortai*
   D. *Trichosporon beigelii*
   E. Study questions
III. Dermatophytes
   A. General differential characteristics
      1. Location of the ringworm (tinea)
      2. Hair fluorescence
      3. Growth rate
      4. Microscopic characteristics of each dermatophyte genus
      5. Physiologic tests
      6. Study questions
   B. Dermatophytes pathogenic to man
      1. *Microsporum* species
         a. *Microsporum audouinii*

b. *Microsporum canis*
c. *Microsporum gypseum*
2. *Epidermophyton* species
a. *Epidermophyton floccosum*
3. *Trichophyton* species
a. Ectothrix hair invasion
(1) *Trichophyton mentagrophytes*
(2) *Trichophyton rubrum*
(3) *Trichophyton verrucosum*
b. Study questions
c. Endothrix hair invasion
(1) *Trichophyton schoenleinii*
(2) *Trichophyton tonsurans*
(3) *Trichophyton violaceum*
IV. Final exam

FOLLOW-UP ACTIVITIES

1. **Students may observe colonies and slide culture preparations of fungi that cause superficial and dermatophytic infections.**

2. **Students may be assigned unknown dermatophytes for which they must perform differential identification tests.**

REFERENCES

ARAVIYSKY, AN, ARAVIYSKY, RA, AND ESCHKOV, GA: *Deep generalized trichophytosis.* Mycopathologia 56:47, 1975.

BENEKE, ES AND ROGERS, AL: *Medical Mycology Manual*, ed 4. Burgess Publishing Co., Minneapolis 1980.

CHONG, KC, ADAM, BA, AND SOO-HOO, TS: *Morphology of Piedraia hortai.* Sabouraudia 9:157, 1975.

DELACRETAZ, J, GRIGORIU, D, AND DUCEL, G: *Color Atlas of Medical Mycology.* Hans Huber Publishers, Year Book Medical Publishers (distributor), Chicago, 1976.

EMMONS, CW, BINFORD, CH, UTZ, JP, AND KWON-CHUNG, KJ: *Medical Mycology*, ed 3. Lea & Febiger, Philadelphia, 1977.

FUSARO, M, MILLER, NG, AND KELLY, D: *Tinea pedis caused by Trichophyton violaceum.* Am J Clin Pathol 80:110, 1983.

GRAPPEL, SF, FETHIERE, A, AND BLANK, F: *Macroconidia of Trichophyton schoenleinii.* Sabouraudia 9:144, 1971.

HALEY, LD AND CALLAWAY, CS: *Laboratory Methods in Medical Mycology*, ed 4. U.S. Department of Health, Education, and Welfare, Washington, DC, 1978.

KANE, J AND SMITKA, C: *Early detection and identification of Trichophyton verrucosum.* J Clin Microbiol 8:740, 1978.

KONEMAN, EW, ROBERTS, GD, AND WRIGHT, SF: *Practical Laboratory Mycology*, ed 2. Williams & Wilkins, Baltimore, 1978.

LARONE, DH: *Medically Important Fungi: A Guide to Identification.* Harper & Row, Hagerstown, Md, 1976.

MOK, WY: *Nature and identification of Exophiala werneckii.* J Clin Microbiol 16:976, 1982.

OBERLE, AD, FOWLER, M, AND GRAFTON, WD: *Pityrosporum isolate from the upper respiratory tract.* Am J Clin Pathol 76:112, 1981.

PHILPOT, CM: *The use of nutritional tests for the differentiation of dermatophytes.* Sabouraudia 15:141, 1977.

SHADOMY, HJ AND PHILPOT, CM: *Utilization of standard laboratory methods in the laboratory diagnosis of problem dermatophytes.* Am J Clin Pathol 74:197, 1980.

WEST, BC AND KWON-CHUNG, KJ: *Mycetoma caused by Microsporum audouinii.* Am J Clin Pathol 73:447, 1980.

INTRODUCTION

Superficial and cutaneous fungi are often grouped together, since they infect the same outer areas of the body—skin, hair, and nails. **Superficial mycoses** are noninvasive and basically asymptomatic, involving just the top keratin-containing layers of skin or hair, while **cutaneous mycoses** affect the deeper epidermal layers, producing more tissue destruction and symptoms. Primary cutaneous mycoses are caused by *Candida* sp. or the dermatophytes *Microsporum, Epidermophyton,* and *Trichophyton.* The term **tinea,** or ringworm, is applied to the diseases elicited by these organisms. If the skin is abraded, systemic pathogens, for example, *Coccidioides immitis,* may also rarely produce cutaneous infections without involving the rest of the body. In addition, systemic organisms may exhibit secondary cutaneous manifestations as part of the disseminated disease process. Secondary infections must be carefully differentiated from primary ones, as the prognosis and treatment are quite different. Dermatophyte identification is presented in this module; *Candida* and systemic fungus identification is presented in Modules 5 and 7, respectively.

SUPERFICIAL ORGANISMS

Superficial fungi are primarily observed in tropical climates. However, because they are sometimes seen in the United States, they are included in this text. Skin scrapings and plucked hairs are the specimens of choice. See Module 2 for specimen collection and processing. Key identifying features are in capital letters.

Exophiala (Cladosporium) werneckii (Figs. 4-1 and 4-2)

Culture: On Sabouraud dextrose agar at room temperature, a BLACK, YEASTY colony slowly develops, which later may be covered with short olive-gray mycelium (Color Plate 34).

Microscopic: The yeast portion of the colony contains only DARK, one- or two-celled blastoconidia (Fig. 4-2A). In the older mold portion, hyphae develop with one- or two-celled dark blastoconidia in large clusters along the hyphae (Fig. 4-2B), which resemble *Candida;* small clusters along the hyphae (Fig. 4-2C) resemble the contaminant *Aureobasidium*. Very old colonies produce ANNELLIDES with CLUSTERS or chains of one- or two-celled dark ANNELLOCONIDIA (Fig. 4-2D).

Other comments: *E. werneckii* may easily be mor-

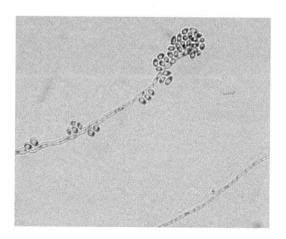

FIGURE 4-1. *Exophiala werneckii,* **lactophenol cotton blue (LPCB) stain, ×450.**

phologically mistaken for *E. jeanselmei* or *W. dermatitidis* (Module 6). However, *E. werneckii* will hydrolyze casein, while the others do not.

Pathogenicity: *Exophiala werneckii* causes **tinea nigra,** in which brown to black, nonscaly patches form primarily on the palms of the hands (Color Plate 35). This organism has rarely been isolated from tinea capitis, tinea pedis, and tinea cruris.

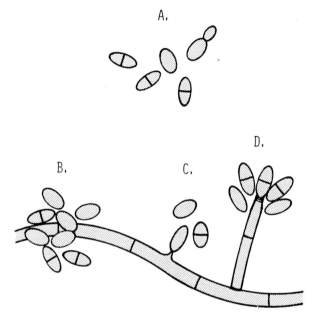

FIGURE 4-2. *Exophiala werneckii.*

Malassezia furfur (Pityrosporum ovale, Pityrosporum orbiculare) (Figs. 4-3 and 4-4)

Culture: *M. furfur* will not grow on routine culture media unless a lipid such as olive oil is layered over it and the culture is incubated at 37°C. Diagnosis is usually made by observing the organism in potassium hydroxide preparations of skin scales.

Microscopic: In potassium hydroxide or stained preparations of skin, *M. furfur* appears as thick, round to oval cells in clusters, accompanied by short, angular hyphae—a SPAGHETTI AND MEATBALLS semblance.

Pathogenicity: This organism causes **pityriasis versicolor,** an asymptomatic skin infection characterized by scaly patches of different colors: reddish brown, brown, and white (Color Plate 36). The patches fluoresce under a Wood's lamp. *Malassezia* has also been reported from a case of nasal sinusitis.

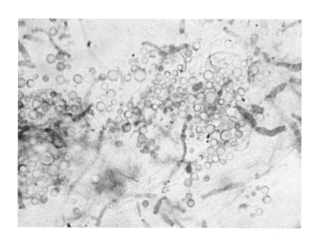

FIGURE 4-3. *Malassezia furfur,* skin scales, PAS stain. (From: Dolan, et al: Atlas of Clinical Mycology. ASCP, Washington, DC, 1976, with permission.)

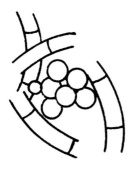

FIGURE 4-4. *Malassezia furfur.*

Piedraia hortai (Figs. 4-5 and 4-6)

Culture: On Sabouraud dextrose agar at room temperature, a compact, greenish-black, heaped, glabrous colony slowly forms.

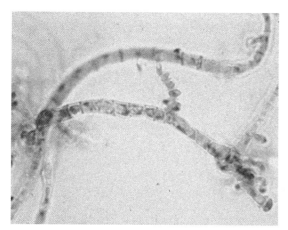

FIGURE 4-5. *Piedraia hortai.* (From: Dolan, et al: Atlas of Clinical Mycology. ASCP, Washington, DC, 1976, with permission.)

Microscopic: P. hortai produces DARK, THICK-WALLED HYPHAE with swellings. ASCI containing ascospores may be present.

Pathogenicity: P. hortai causes **black piedra** (Fig. 4-7), which consists of firmly attached, hard black nodules around the outside of scalp hairs.

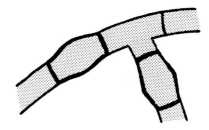

FIGURE 4-6. *Piedraia hortai.*

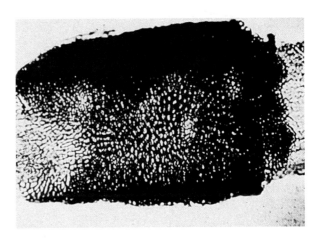

FIGURE 4-7. Black piedra on hair, high power. (Courtesy of Dr. Leanor Haley, Centers for Disease Control, Atlanta.)

Trichosporon beigelii (cutaneum) (Figs. 4-8 and 4-9)

Culture: On Sabouraud dextrose agar at room temperature, a cream-colored, wrinkled, glabrous colony forms within five days (Color Plate 37).

Microscopic: On corn meal-Tween 80 agar, hyaline hyphae with BLASTOCONIDIA and ARTHROCONIDIA are observed. Biochemical tests can be performed to identify this fungus (see Module 5).

Pathogenicity: Trichosporon beigelii produces **white piedra,** which consists of light brown, soft nodules around beard and mustache hairs (Color Plate 38). These nodules are less firmly attached than those of black piedra.

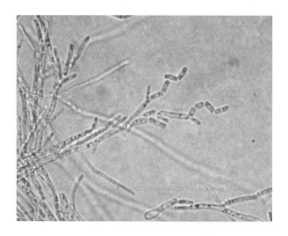

FIGURE 4-8. *Trichosporon beigelii,* corn meal-Tween 80 agar, ×450.

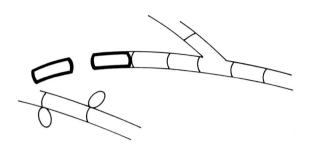

FIGURE 4-9. *Trichosporon beigelii,* corn meal-Tween 80 agar.

Study Questions

Matching: Place the letter(s) of the words in Column B in front of the corresponding words in Column A.

Column A
1. ____ *Trichosporon beigelii*
2. ____ Spaghetti & meatballs
3. ____ Black patches on skin
4. ____ Black piedra

Column B
A. Multicolored patches on skin
B. Tinea nigra
C. Hard, black hair nodules
D. *Malassezia furfur*
E. Light brown hair nodules
F. Black mold mistaken for *Candida* or *Aureobasidium*

STOP HERE UNTIL YOU HAVE COMPLETED THE ANSWERS.

Look up the answers in the back of the book. If you missed more than one, go back and review the superficial organisms. Correctly complete any missed study questions before proceeding further.

DERMATOPHYTES

Dermatophytes are the genera *Microsporum, Epidermophyton,* and *Trichophyton.* They live in the soil, on animals, or on man. Not all dermatophytes are pathogenic to man; one must beware that nonpathogens may be found as contaminants on specimens. Skin scrapings, nail scrapings, and hair stubs (including the roots) are the usual specimens for dermatophyte study. Potassium hydroxide preparations are made and observed for branching septate hyphae in skin and nail scrapings. Arthroconidia are sought in hairs, and it is noted whether they are outside the hair shaft (**ectothrix invasion**) or inside (**endothrix invasion**). Be careful in observing hairs, for ectothrix invasion (Fig. 4-10) begins within the shaft at the base and then moves outside further up the hair. Ectothrix and endothrix (Fig. 4-11) characteristics are seen only in direct mounts, not in hairs that have been cultured.

Dermatophyte test medium* is useful as a screening medium. After incubation at room temperature for 14 days, if the organism is a dermatophyte, it will change the yellow indicator to red. There are a few other fungi, for example, *Cladosporium,* that will also change the color of the medium; slide cultures must thus be performed for definitive identification. Sabouraud dextrose

---

*Oricult, Medical Technology Corp., 71 Veronica Ave., P.O. Box 218, Somerset, NJ 08873.

agar with cycloheximide and chloramphenicol is also satisfactory for isolating dermatophytes. (See Module 2 for further details on specimen collection and processing.)

fects skin and ectothrix hair; *Epidermophyton* invades skin and nails; *Trichophyton mentagrophytes, rubrum,* and *verrucosum* affect skin, nails, and ectothrix hair, while *Trichophyton tonsurans, schoenleinii,* and *violaceum* produce disease in skin, nails, and endothrix hair.

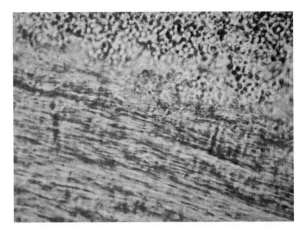

FIGURE 4-10. Ectothrix hair invasion. Hair shaft is in bottom half of photo, while ectothrix arthroconidia are on top. (From: Beneke: Human Mycoses. Upjohn, Minneapolis, 1979, with permission.)

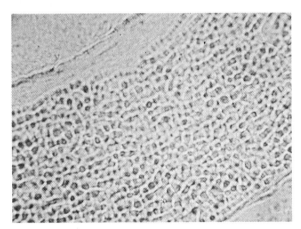

FIGURE 4-11. Endothrix hair invasion. (From: Dolan, et al: Atlas of Clinical Mycology. ASCP, Washington DC, 1976, with permission.)

	Skin	Nail	Ectothrix Hair	Endothrix Hair
Microsporum	+		+	
Epidermophyton	+	+		
Trichophyton mentagrophytes rubrum verrucosum	+	+	+	
tonsurans schoenleinii violaceum	+	+		+

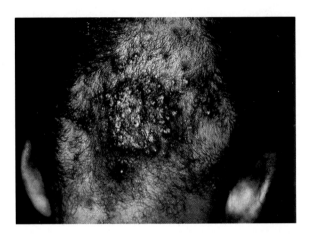

FIGURE 4-12. Tinea capitis. (Courtesy of Dr. Robert Kenney, William Beaumont Medical Center, El Paso, Texas.)

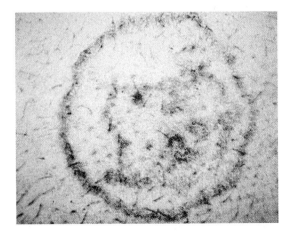

FIGURE 4-13. Tinea corporis. (From: Beneke: Human Mycoses. Upjohn, Minneapolis, 1979, with permission.)

General Differential Characteristics

Microsporum, Epidermophyton, and *Trichophyton* may be identified in many different ways.

LOCATION OF THE RINGWORM (FIGS. 4-12 AND 4-13)

Dermatophytes infect specific body sites, which are the basis for clinical diagnosis. Ringworm location may aid in preliminary fungal identification. **(See Chart 4-1 on page 127 at end of module.)** *Microsporum* sp. in-

117

HAIR FLUORESCENCE

Fungi infecting hairs may make a metabolite, pteridine, which produces a bright greenish-yellow fluorescence under a Wood's lamp (366 nm). (See Color Plate 39.) Organisms that produce this fluorescence are *Microsporum canis, audouinii, distortum,* and *ferrugineum.* Besides helping to tentatively identify the agent responsible for the infection, fluorescence, if present, will help to choose infected hairs (those that fluoresce) from non-infected ones for culture. Note that negative fluorescence of all hairs on the affected body site may still indicate a fungal infection, but by organisms other than those listed above.

GROWTH RATE

Growth rate is helpful in broadly differentiating the dermatophytes. Of the organisms that commonly elicit symptoms in man, *Epidermophyton floccosum, Microsporum canis, Microsporum gypseum,* and *Trichophyton mentagrophytes* form mature colonies in 6 to 10 days (intermediate growers). *Microsporum audouinii, Trichophyton rubrum, Trichophyton schoenleinii, Trichophyton tonsurans, Trichophyton verrucosum,* and *Trichophyton violaceum* form mature colonies in 11 to 21 days (slow growers). Another way to remember this is that all the microsporums listed in this module except *M. audouinii* are intermediate growers, while all the trichophytons except *T. mentagrophytes* are slow growers.

MICROSCOPIC CHARACTERISTICS OF EACH DERMATOPHYTE GENUS

These are the most important criteria for genus identification. **(See Chart 4-2 on page 128 at end of module.)** The microscopic characteristics are rapidly lost with subsequent culture transfers; aerial structures like micro- and macroconidia disappear and only vegetative structures remain. Conidial formation is enhanced by subculturing the organism to media low in nutrients, for example, potato dextrose agar.

With fresh isolates grown on Sabouraud dextrose agar, these are microscopic characteristics for the dermatophyte genera.

Microsporum sp. produce numerous rough, thick- or thin-walled, elliptical or spindle-shaped macroconidia containing three to seven cells. There are few club-shaped microconidia borne singly along the hyphae. The exception is *M. audouinii,* which rarely produces macro- or microconidia.

Epidermophyton contains only one pathogenic species, *E. floccosum,* which develops numerous smooth, thin-walled, club-shaped macroconidia containing two to four cells. Microconidia are absent.

Trichophyton sp. usually form rare thin-walled, pencil-shaped macroconidia containing three to eight cells; some strains produce numerous macroconidia. Numerous round, oval, or club-shaped microconidia are borne in grapelike clusters or singly along the hyphae. The exceptions are *T. schoenleinii* and *T. violaceum,* which do not grow macroconidia under ordinary conditions and rarely form microconidia.

PHYSIOLOGIC TESTS

Recently the use of physiologic, or nutritional, tests to differentiate the *Microsporum, Trichophyton,* and *Epidermophyton* species has been outlined (Philpot, 1977). Urease and assimilation of sugars and nitrogen compounds were used. While this technique holds promise, further work needs to be performed to validate the procedure. Do not confuse these tests with the well-established *Trichophyton* nutritional procedures, which use vitamin requirements for *Trichophyton* sp. differentiation.

STUDY QUESTIONS

1. **Multiple choice. This is a hair shaft with arthroconidia. The dermatophyte genus which is producing this type of hair invasion is:**

   A. *Microsporum*
   B. *Epidermophyton*
   C. *Candida*
   D. *Trichophyton*

Fill in the blanks:

2. **A common name for tinea pedis is**

   _____ .

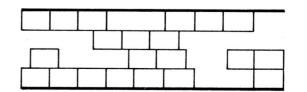

3. **Hair fluorescence is produced from infection with organisms of the** _____ **genus.**

118

Dermatophytes Pathogenic To Man

Below are listed specific characteristics of species that cause most of the tineas in man. Note that there are many other dermatophytes that rarely infect man, and also there are many contaminant dermatophytes that must be differentiated from pathogens. Characteristics especially helpful in identification are in capital letters. **(See Chart 4-3 on pages 129-132 at end of module for an identification scheme.)**

MICROSPORUM SPECIES

Microsporum audouinii (Fig. 4-14)

Culture: On Sabouraud dextrose agar at room temperature, a slow-growing, matted to velvety colony forms, which is light tan with a REVERSE color of SALMON (Color Plates 40 and 41). The salmon color is enhanced if the fungus is cultured on potato dextrose agar. The reverse color tends to turn orange-brown with age; the colony must be observed when it is one to two weeks old for any salmon color to be present.

Microscopic: Rare, irregularly shaped macroconidia exhibit thick, rough walls with two to nine cells. Rare club-shaped microconidia are borne singly along the hyphae. Racquet hyphae, nodular bodies, and TERMI-NAL, usually POINTED, VESICLES (mistaken for chlamydoconidia) are most commonly found.

Other comments: Infected hairs fluoresce. POOR GROWTH on STERILE POLISHED RICE GRAINS (see gray box) helps differentiate *M. audouinii* from other *Microsporum* species, which grow well on rice grains. Adding yeast extract to the slide culture medium may enhance macroconidial production.

Pathogenicity: *M. audouinii* causes tinea corporis and children's epidemics of tinea capitis. There has been one reported case of mycetoma produced by this fungus.

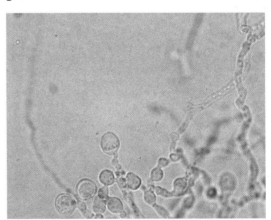

FIGURE 4-14. Terminal vesicles, *Microsporum audouinii*, LPCB stain, ×450.

RICE GRAINS TEST

Medium Preparation
(Commercially available from Remel, 12076 Santa Fe Dr., Lenexa, Kansas 66215)

Polished unfortified white rice*	8.0 gm
Distilled water	25.0 ml

1. Mix together the rice and water in a small screw-capped bottle.
2. Autoclave at 15 psi for 15 minutes and cool.

Box continues on next page.

Microsporum canis (Fig. 4-15)

Culture: On Sabouraud dextrose agar at room temperature, a white, woolly colony with a buff to brown center and bright yellow periphery is formed within one week. The REVERSE is BRIGHT YELLOW to YELLOW ORANGE (Color Plates 42 and 43).

Microscopic: There are numerous rough, thick-walled, SPINDLE-SHAPED (tapered ends) MACROCONIDIA containing 6 to 15 cells. A few one-celled, club-shaped microconidia are borne singly along the hyphae. Racquet hyphae, nodular bodies, and chlamydoconidia may be present.

Other comments: Infected hairs fluoresce. Macroconidial production is enhanced by growth on Emmon's medium or modified corn meal agar.

Pathogenicity: M. canis causes tinea corporis and tinea capitis, which are usually contracted from infected dogs and cats.

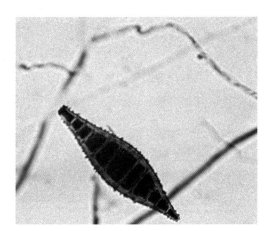

FIGURE 4-15. Macroconidium, *Microsporum canis*, LPCB stain, ×450.

Microsporum gypseum (Fig. 4-16)

Culture: On Sabouraud dextrose agar at room temperature, a powdery, BUFF to CINNAMON colony with a tan reverse forms within one week (see Color Plate 5).

Microscopic: There are numerous rough, THIN-WALLED, ELLIPTICAL MACROCONIDIA containing four to six cells. A few club-shaped microconidia are borne singly along the hyphae.

Pathogenicity: M. gypseum causes an inflammatory tinea corporis and tinea capitis.

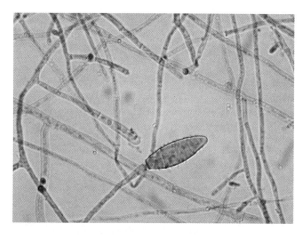

FIGURE 4-16. Macro- and microconidia, *Microsporum gypseum*, LPCB stain, ×450.

EPIDERMOPHYTON SPECIES

Epidermophyton floccosum (Fig. 4-17)

Culture: On Sabouraud dextrose agar at room temperature, a velvety, KHAKI-YELLOW colony with a tan reverse forms within 10 days (see Color Plate 7).

Microscopic: There are numerous CLUB-SHAPED, smooth, thin-walled MACROCONIDIA containing two to four cells. The macroconidia are borne singly or in clusters. No microconidia develop; racquet hyphae, spiral hyphae, nodular bodies, and chlamydoconidia may be present.

Other comments: Macroconidial formation may be enhanced by growing the organism on media with a low sugar content.

Pathogenicity: E. floccosum causes epidemic tinea pedis in summer camps and institutions, tinea cruris, and tinea unguium.

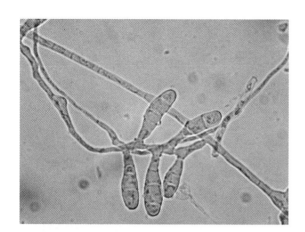

FIGURE 4-17. Macroconidia, *Epidermophyton floccosum*, LPCB stain, ×450.

TRICHOPHYTON SPECIES

The *Trichophyton* species are divided here into groups based on the type of hair invasion. Keep in mind that these fungi also infect skin and nails.

Ectothrix Hair Invasion

TRICHOPHYTON MENTAGROPHYTES (FIGS. 4-18 and 4-19)

Culture: On Sabouraud dextrose agar at room temperature, two colonial textures are seen after 7 to 10 days. Fluffy colonies are white with a colorless to yellow reverse (Color Plate 44). Granular colonies are buff to rose-tan with a brown, red, or yellow reverse (Color Plate 45). Red strains may be mistaken for *Trichophyton rubrum*.

Microscopic: Granular forms usually produce numerous pencil-shaped, smooth, thin-walled macroconidia containing five to eight cells, while fluffy strains demonstrate rare macroconidia. Numerous to few ROUND MICROCONIDIA are found in GRAPELIKE CLUSTERS. Microconidia may also be seen singly along the hyphae but then they are more tear- to club-shaped. Racquet hyphae, spiral hyphae, nodular bodies, and chlamydoconidia may also be present.

Other comments: T. *mentagrophytes* must be differentiated from *T. rubrum;* the former usually forms

NO RED PIGMENT on potato dextrose or corn meal agar. It also produces a POSITIVE UREASE reaction in two to four days on Christenson's urea agar at room temperature (Module 6), while other dermatophytes may be positive after five days. *T. mentagrophytes* PERFORATES AUTOCLAVED HAIR in vitro (see gray box), although other dermatophytes will too. All three tests must be performed in conjunction with each other for a valid interpretation.

Pathogenicity: T. *mentagrophytes* causes inflammatory tinea pedis, tinea corporis, tinea unguium, tinea barbae, and tinea capitis. It is the most common cause of athlete's foot.

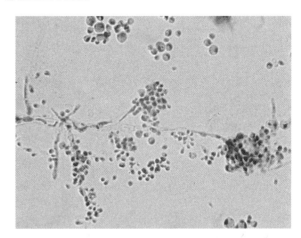

FIGURE 4-18. Grapelike clusters of microconidia, *Trichophyton mentagrophytes*, LPCB stain, ×450.

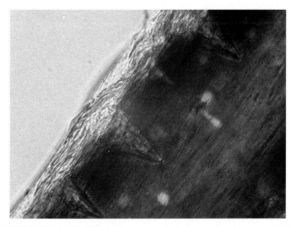

FIGURE 4-19. Wedge-shaped hair perforations, *Trichophyton mentagrophytes*, LPCB stain, ×450.

IN VITRO HAIR PERFORATION TEST

Medium Preparation

10 percent Yeast extract, filter sterilized	0.1 ml
Sterile distilled water	25.0 ml

Box continues on next page.

TRICHOPHYTON RUBRUM (Fig. 4-20)

Culture: On Sabouraud dextrose agar at room temperature, a granular or fluffy white colony with a pink periphery and DEEP RED REVERSE forms in two weeks (Color Plates 46 and 47). The color is best seen on potato dextrose or corn meal agar.

Microscopic: Numerous or few smooth-walled, pencil-shaped macroconidia with three to eight cells are observed. Numerous club-shaped microconidia are borne singly along the hyphae. Chlamydoconidia, racquet hyphae, and nodular bodies may also be present.

Other comments: T. rubrum produces a DEEP RED PIGMENT on potato dextrose or corn meal agar, is UREASE NEGATIVE within seven days, and DOES NOT PERFORATE AUTOCLAVED HAIR. Growth on heart infusion tryptose agar greatly enhances macroconidial formation.

Pathogenicity: T. rubrum causes tinea corporis, tinea pedis, tinea cruris, and tinea unguium.

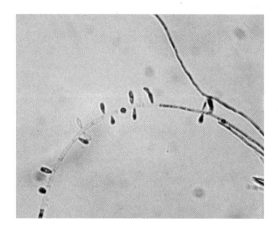

FIGURE 4-20. Microconidia, *Trichophyton rubrum*, LPCB stain, ×450.

TRICHOPHYTON VERRUCOSUM (Fig. 4-21)

Culture: On Sabouraud dextrose agar at room temperature, this organism does not flourish (Color Plate 48). T. verrucosum colonies grow more readily on Sabouraud dextrose agar with yeast extract or on heart infusion tryptose agar with thiamine. On these enriched media at 37°C, a heaped, waxy, white to bright yellow colony with a nonpigmented to yellow reverse forms in two or three weeks.

Microscopic: On plain Sabouraud dextrose agar, only chlamydoconidia in chains are produced. On thiamine enriched media, rare three- to five-celled MACROCONIDIA with an elongated, RAT-TAIL END, and moderate numbers of club-shaped microconidia borne along the hyphae, are observed.

Other comments: In *Trichophyton* nutritional tests (see gray box), T. verrucosum REQUIRES THIAMINE for growth and some strains also require INOSITOL.

Pathogenicity: T. verrucosum causes tinea capitis, tinea barbae, and tinea corporis. The ringworm is usually acquired from cattle.

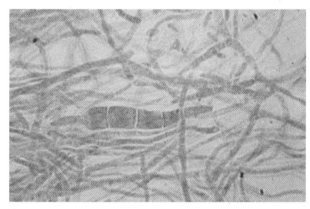

FIGURE 4-21. Rat-tail macroconidium, *Trichophyton verrucosum*. (From: Dolan, et al: Atlas of Clinical Mycology. ASCP, Washington, DC, 1976, with permission.)

TRICHOPHYTON NUTRITIONAL TESTS

Media Preparation

Commercially available (Difco, Remel, 12076 Santa Fe Dr., Lenexa, Kansas 66215)

Basal Medium

Casamino acid, vitamin free	2.5 gm
Glucose	40.0 gm
Magnesium sulfate	0.1 gm
Monobasic potassium phosphate (KH_2PO_4)	1.8 gm
Agar	20.0 gm
Distilled water	1 liter

1. Mix together the above ingredients and adjust the pH to 6.8. Aliquot in tubes.
2. Autoclave at 15 psi for 15 minutes and cool. Refrigerate.

Casein + Thiamine:

Basal medium, above	
Thiamine hydrochloride	0.2 μg/ml of medium

1. Mix together the basal medium and thiamine, heat to dissolve, and put in tubes.
2. Autoclave at 15 psi for 15 minutes. Cool and refrigerate.

Casein + Inositol:

Basal medium, above	
i-Inositol	50.0 μg/ml of medium

1. Mix together the basal medium and inositol, heat to dissolve, and put in tubes.
2. Autoclave at 15 psi for 15 minutes. Cool and refrigerate.

Casein + Inositol + Thiamine:

Basal medium, above	
Thiamine hydrochloride	0.2 μg/ml of medium
i-Inositol	50.0 μg/ml of medium

1. Mix together basal medium, thiamine, and inositol, heat to dissolve, and put in tubes.
2. Autoclave at 15 psi for 15 minutes. Cool and refrigerate.

Procedure

1. Bring media to room temperature. Pick a tiny, uniform amount of the test fungus from Sabouraud dextrose agar. Be careful not to take any SDA along with the fungus, as nutrients may be carried over to the test.
2. Inoculate each *Trichophyton* agar in the center and incubate at 25°C for 2 weeks. If *T. verrucosum* or *T. schoenleinii* is suspected, incubate the agars at 37°C.
3. See Chart 4-4 (on page 133 at end of module) for the amount of growth on each medium, by species.

Study Questions

Fill in the statements below with the letter(s) of the appropriate tests. More than one letter may be used per statement.

A. Urease test
B. Polished rice grains test
C. Red pigment on potato dextrose agar
D. *Trichophyton* nutritional agar tests
E. In vitro hair perforation

1. _____ Test(s) that help differentiate *T. mentagrophytes* from *T. rubrum*

2. _____ Test(s) that help differentiate *M. audouinii* from *M. canis*

3. Circle the letter of the correct answer:

   Features that distinguish *M. gypseum* from *M. canis* and *M. audouinii* are all of the following *except*:

   A. *M. gypseum* macroconidia are thin walled, while *M. canis* and *M. audouinii* are thick.

   B. *M. gypseum* colony reverse is tan, while *M. canis* is yellow, and *M. audouinii* is salmon.

   C. *M. gypseum* macroconidia are smooth walled, while *M. canis* and *M. audouinii* are rough.

   D. *M. gypseum* macroconidia are elliptical, while *M. canis* are spindle shaped and *M. audouinii* are irregularly (aborted) shaped.

4. Circle true or false:

   T   F   *E. floccosum* macroconidia may be confused with those of *T. verrucosum.*

STOP HERE UNTIL YOU HAVE COMPLETED THE ANSWERS.

If you missed more than two, go back and review the *Microsporum, Epidermophyton,* and ectothrix *Trichophyton* sections. Correctly complete any missed questions before proceeding further.

Endothrix Hair Invasion

TRICHOPHYTON SCHOENLEINII (Fig. 4-22)

Culture: On Sabouraud dextrose agar at room temperature, a waxy, heaped, light yellow to buff colony with a colorless to yellow-orange reverse forms in two to three weeks (Color Plate 49).

Microscopic: No macroconidia are exhibited under routine conditions. FAVIC CHANDELIERS are the most prevalent feature; although they may be seen in other species, favic chandeliers are more common in *T. schoenleinii.* Chlamydoconidia and hyphal swellings may be present.

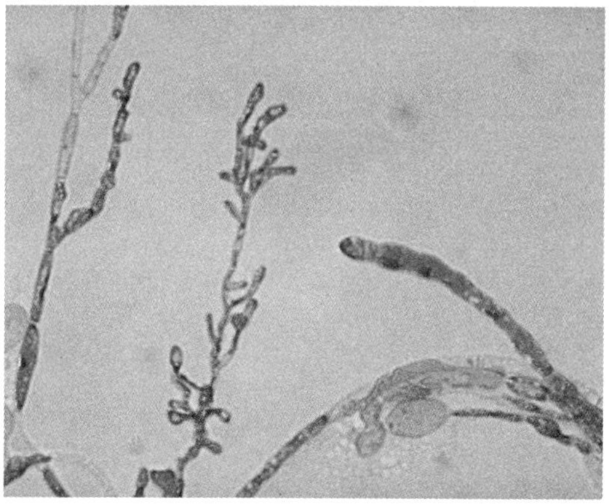

Other comments: Microconidia are formed on rice grains.

Pathogenicity: *T. schoenleinii* causes tinea capitis and rarely tinea corporis and tinea unguium.

FIGURE 4-22. Favic chandeliers, *Trichophyton schoenleinii,* LPCB stain, ×450.

TRICHOPHYTON TONSURANS (Fig. 4-23)

Culture: On Sabouraud dextrose agar at room temperature, three colonial types are formed in one to two weeks: a grey-white, suede front with a mahogany reverse; granular white front with a colorless reverse; and a bright yellow, granular to suede, rugose colony with a yellow reverse (Color Plate 50).

Microscopic: Rare smooth-walled, club-shaped, or aborted macroconidia are observed. Numerous MICROCONIDIA with a GREAT SIZE and SHAPE VARIATION are seen. Chlamydoconidia and racquet hyphae may be present.

Other comments: Isolates may be confused with *T. mentagrophytes; T. tonsurans* is urease positive after four days but does not perforate hair in vitro. In *Trichophyton* nutritional tests, *T. tonsurans* also grows better in the presence of THIAMINE, while *T. mentagrophytes* multiplies well with or without thiamine.

Pathogenicity: *T. tonsurans* causes the black dot type of tinea capitis (appearance due to broken off hair shafts near the scalp). This organism occasionally causes tinea corporis, tinea pedis, and tinea unguium.

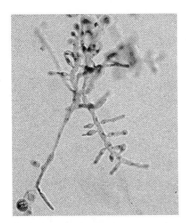

FIGURE 4-23. Micronconidia, *Trichophyton tonsurans*, LPCB stain, ×450.

TRICHOPHYTON VIOLACEUM (Fig. 4-24)

Culture: On Sabouraud dextrose agar at room temperature, a waxy or suede, VIOLET, heaped colony with a lavender reverse forms in two to three weeks (Color Plate 51). The violet color may be lost on subculture. Better growth occurs on Sabouraud dextrose agar with trypticase and thiamine.

Microscopic: Macroconidia are not produced; only chlamydoconidia in chains and hyphal swellings are observed.

Other comments: In *Trichophyton* nutritional tests, *T. violaceum* requires THIAMINE. On thiamine-enriched media, a few microconidia may be formed.

Pathogenicity: *T. violaceum* causes tinea capitis, tinea corporis, rarely tinea unguium, and deep infections.

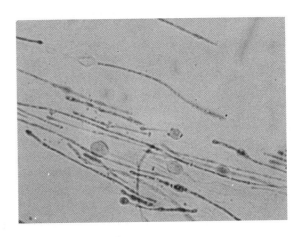

FIGURE 4-24. Chlamydoconidia, *Trichophyton violaceum*, LPCB stain, ×450.

FINAL EXAM

1. **Superficial and cutaneous mycoses are similar in that they involve skin and hair. How do they differ?**

2. Circle true or false:

   T F All dermatophytes infecting man cause cutaneous mycoses, but not all cutaneous mycoses are elicited by dermatophytes.

3. **Circle the letter of the correct answer:**

   This organism is an etiologic agent of epidemic tinea pedis in summer camps and institutions. It does not infect hair.

   A. *Trichophyton mentagrophytes*
   B. *Epidermophyton floccosum*
   C. *Microsporum audouinii*
   D. *Trichophyton violaceum*
   E. *Trichosporon beigelii*

4. **These are the characteristics of a fungus isolated from a patient with tinea capitis:**

Culture: (SDA)	Waxy, buff, reverse colorless
Growth rate:	Slow

   Box continues on next page.

Slide culture: (SDA) Many favic chandeliers, few chlamydoconidia and hyphal swellings

Circle the letter of the correct answer.

This organism most likely is:

A. *Microsporum gypseum*
B. *Trichophyton tonsurans*
C. *Trichophyton mentagrophytes*
D. *Epidermophyton floccosum*
E. *Trichophyton schoenleinii*

5. *Trichophyton verrucosum* and *Trichophyton violaceum* both may cause tinea capitis, are slow growers, may produce only chlamydoconidia in chains on Sabouraud dextrose agar slide cultures, and are enhanced if grown on media containing yeast extract (has thiamine). How may these fungi be differentiated? Give at least two ways.

6. A patient with black nodules on his scalp hairs came to the dermatology clinic. On Sabouraud dextrose agar, a greenish-black, glabrous colony slowly formed. Slide cultures on Sabouraud dextrose agar showed thick, dark-walled, septate hyphae with numerous intercalary swellings. This organism is most likely (circle the letter of the correct answer):

A. *Trichophyton violaceum*
B. *Piedraia hortai*
C. *Trichophyton verrucosum*
D. *Microsporum audouinii*
E. *Exophiala werneckii*

Matching: Place the letter of the answer in *Column B* in front of the words in *Column A*. Answers may be used more than once.

Column A

7. _____ Means ringworm of the nails
8. _____ Variously sized and shaped microconidia
9. _____ Microconidia in grapelike clusters
10. _____ Salmon colony reverse
11. _____ Hairs fluoresce
12. _____ (+) Urease in two to four days

Column B

A. Tinea pedis
B. *Microsporum audouinii*
C. *Trichophyton tonsurans*
D. *Trichophyton mentagrophytes*
E. Tinea unguium
F. *Trichophyton rubrum*

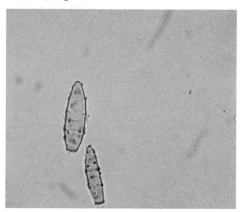

FIGURE 4-25. Final exam demonstration, LPCB stain, ×450.

13. See Figure 4-25. These macroconidia are characteristic of:

A. *Microsporum canis*
B. *Microsporum audouinii*
C. *Epidermophyton floccosum*
D. *Trichophyton rubrum*
E. *Microsporum gypseum*

STOP HERE UNTIL YOU HAVE COMPLETED THE ANSWERS.

If you missed more than three, go back and repeat this module. Make sure that all questions are correctly completed before proceeding further.

CHART 4-1. Human Tineas and Common Causative Organisms

TINEA	OTHER NAMES	CAUSATIVE ORGANISMS
Tinea capitis	Ringworm of the scalp	Any *Microsporum* species Any *Trichophyton* (except *Trichophyton concentricum*) RARELY *Exophiala werneckii*
Tinea corporis	Ringworm of the body	*Microsporum audouinii, Microsporum canis, Microsporum gypseum* *Trichophyton mentagrophytes, Trichophyton rubrum, Trichophyton verrucosum, Trichophyton violaceum* RARELY *Trichophyton tonsurans, Trichophyton schoenleinii*
Tinea barbae	Ringworm of the beard, barber's itch	*Microsporum canis* *Trichophyton mentagrophytes, Trichophyton rubrum, Trichophyton verrucosum, Trichophyton violaceum*
Tinea cruris	Ringworm of the groin, jock itch	*Epidermophyton floccosum* *Trichophyton mentagrophytes, Trichophyton rubrum* *Candida albicans* RARELY *Exophiala werneckii*
Tinea pedis	Ringworm of the foot, athlete's foot	*Epidermophyton floccosum* *Trichophyton mentagrophytes, Trichophyton rubrum* *Candida albicans* RARELY *Trichophyton tonsurans, Trichophyton violaceum, Exophiala werneckii*
Tinea unguium	Ringworm of the nail, onychomycosis	*Epidermophyton floccosum* *Trichophyton mentagrophytes, Trichophyton rubrum* *Candida albicans* RARELY *Trichophyton tonsurans, Trichophyton violaceum, Trichophyton schoenleinii, Microsporum canis, Exophiala werneckii*

CHART 4-2. Microscopic Characteristics of Dermatophyte Genera

	MICROSPORUM	EPIDERMOPHYTON	TRICHOPHYTON
Macroconidia:			
Quantity	Numerous	Numerous	Usually rare
Rough-/smooth-walled	Rough	Smooth	Smooth
Shape	Elliptical/spindle	Club	Pencil
Thick-/thin-walled	Thick or thin	Thin	Thin
Number of cells inside	Usually 3-7	Usually 2-4	Usually 3-8
	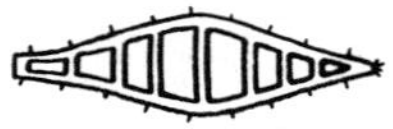	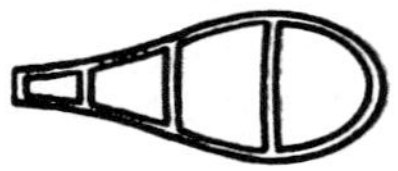	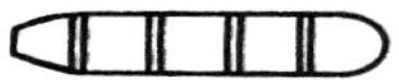
Microconidia:			
Quantity	Few	Absent	Numerous or few
Shape	Club	—	Round, oval, or club
How borne	Singly	—	Singly/grapelike clusters
	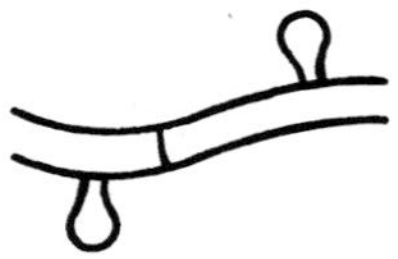		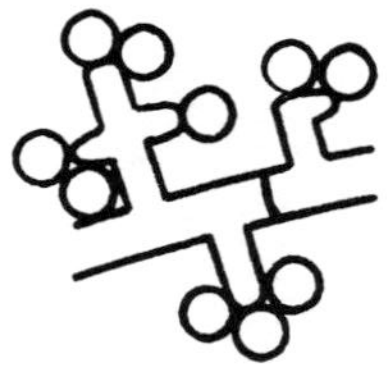

CHART 4-3. Identification of Dermatophytes Commonly Pathogenic to Man

I. Macroconidia observed on Sabouraud dextrose agar slide cultures

  A. Rough-walled

    1. Thin-walled, numerous

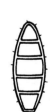

            Microsporum gypseum

            Additional characteristics:
            Elliptical, 4- to 6-celled macroconidia
            Colony powdery, buff to cinnamon, reverse tan
            Few club-shaped microconidia

  A. 2. Thick-walled

    a. Spindle-shaped (tapered ends), numerous

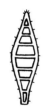

            Microsporum canis

            Additional characteristics:
            Macroconidia contain 6 to 15 cells
            Colony reverse bright yellow to yellow-orange
            Few club-shaped microconidia

    b. Bizarre shaped (aborted), rare

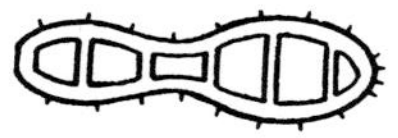

            Microsporum audouinii

            Additional Characteristics:
            Macroconidia contain 2 to 9 cells
            Colony reverse salmon
            Prevalent terminal pointed vesicles
            Poor growth on rice grains

  B. Smooth walled

    1. Club-shaped, numerous

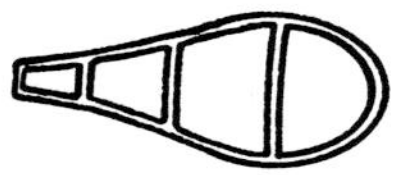

            Epidermophyton floccosum

            Additional characteristics:
            Macroconidia contain 2 to 4 cells
            Colony khaki-yellow
            No microconidia

CHART 4-3. Continued

2. Pencil-shaped, rare or numerous

a.

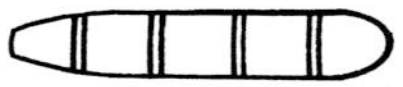

Trichophyton mentagrophytes

Additional characteristics:
Macroconidia contain 5 to 8 cells
Numerous round microconidia, usually in grapelike clusters, although they may appear singly along the hyphae
No red color on potato dextrose agar
Positive urease in 2 to 4 days
Perforates autoclaved hair in vitro

b.

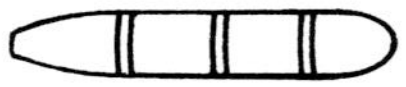

Trichophyton rubrum

Additional characteristics:
Macroconidia contain 3 to 8 cells
Numerous club-shaped microconidia
Red color on potato dextrose agar
Negative urease in 7 days
Does not perforate autoclaved hair in vitro

3. Aborted, rare

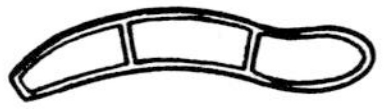

Trichophyton tonsurans

Additional characteristics:
Numerous microconidia with great size and shape variation
Grows better in the presence of thiamine

II. Microconidia observed on Sabouraud dextrose agar slide cultures

A. Numerous

1. Grapelike clusters, round to oval cells

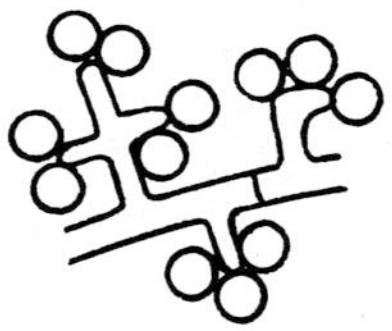

Trichophyton mentagrophytes

Additional characteristics:
Microconidia most commonly in grapelike clusters, although they may appear singly along the hyphae
Rare or numerous, 5- to 8-celled, pencil-shaped, smooth-walled macroconidia
No red color on potato dextrose agar
Positive urease in 2 to 4 days
Perforates autoclaved hair in vitro

CHART 4-3. Continued

2. Borne singly along the hyphae

a. Uniform size and shape

1.

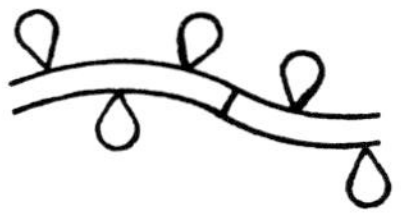

Trichophyton mentagrophytes

Additional characteristics:
Microconidia most commonly round to oval and in grapelike clusters
Rare or numerous, 5- to 8-celled, pencil-shaped, smooth-walled macroconidia
No red color on potato dextrose agar
Positive urease in 2 to 4 days
Perforates autoclaved hair in vitro

2.

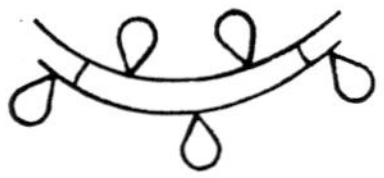

Trichophyton rubrum

Additional characteristics:
Rare or numerous, 3- to 8-celled, pencil-shaped, smooth-walled macroconidia
Red color on potato dextrose agar
Negative urease in 7 days
Does not perforate autoclaved hair in vitro

b. Great size and shape variation

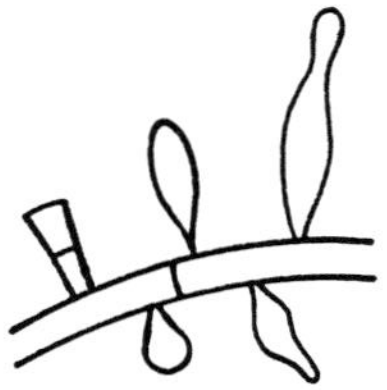

Trichophyton tonsurans

Additional characteristics:
Rare, aborted, smooth-walled macroconidia
Grows better in the presence of thiamine

B. Few microconidia, club shaped

1. Colony cinnamon, reverse tan

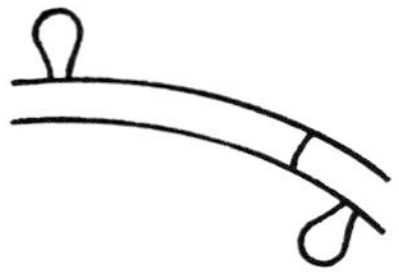

Microsporum gypseum

Additional characteristics:
Numerous rough, thin-walled, elliptical macroconidia containing 4 to 6 cells

CHART 4-3. Continued

2. Colony white with yellow periphery, reverse bright yellow

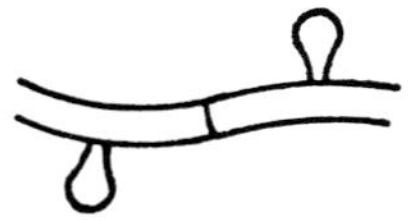

Microsporum canis

Additional characteristics:
Numerous rough, thick-walled, spindle-shaped macroconidia with 6 to 15 cells

C. Rare microconidia, club shaped

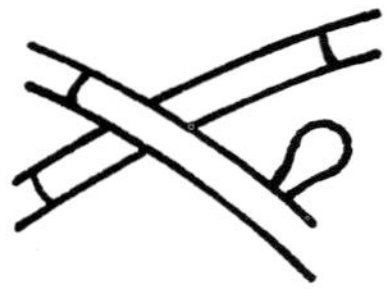

Microsporum audouinii

Additional characteristics:
Colony light tan with salmon reverse
Rare, rough, thick-walled, aborted macroconidia
Prevalent terminal pointed vesicles
Poor growth on polished rice grains

III. No microconidia or macroconidia observed on Sabouraud dextrose agar slide cultures

A. Terminal pointed vesicles

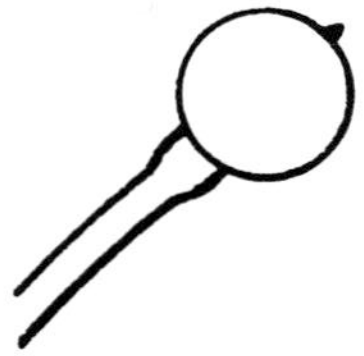

Microsporum audouinii

Additional characteristics:
Colony light tan with salmon reverse
Rare, rough, thick-walled, aborted macroconidia, whose growth is enhanced on media with yeast extract
Rare club-shaped microconidia borne singly along the hyphae
Common racquet hyphae, nodular bodies
Poor growth on polished rice grains

B. Chlamydoconidia in chains

1. Colony violet, reverse lavender

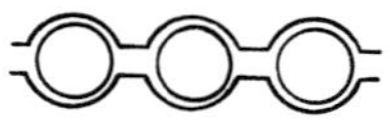

Trichophyton violaceum

Additional characteristics:
No macroconidia produced
Few microconidia form on thiamine enriched media
Grows better in the presence of thiamine

2. Colony white to bright yellow, reverse nonpigmented to yellow

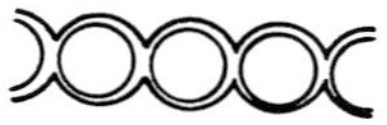

Trichophyton verrucosum

Additional characteristics:
On thiamine-enriched media, rare smooth-walled, rat-tail macroconidia, and moderate club-shaped microconidia are produced
Grows better at 37°C
Requires thiamine for growth
Most strains also require inositol for growth

C. Favic chandeliers prevalent

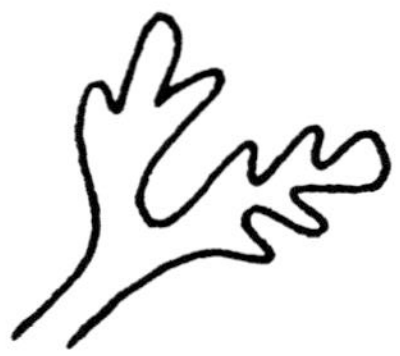

Trichophyton schoenleinii

Additional characteristics:
Colony light yellow to buff, reverse nonpigmented to yellow-orange
No macroconidia produced
Chlamydoconidia and hyphal swellings common
Microconidia form on rice grains
Does not require thiamine for growth

CHART 4-4. *Trichophyton* Nutritional Growth Patterns

	CASEIN BASAL AGAR	CASEIN + INOSITOL	CASEIN + INOSITOL + THIAMINE	CASEIN + THIAMINE
T. verrucosum (37°C) 84%	0	±	4+	0
16%	0	0	4+	4+
T. tonsurans	±−1+	2+	4+	4+
T. violaceum	±−1+	1+	4+	4+
Organisms in which nutritional patterns are not helpful:				
T. mentagrophytes	4+	4+	4+	4+
T. rubrum	4+	4+	4+	4+
T. schoenleinii (37°C)	4+	4+	4+	4+

4+ = rich abundant growth
1+ = submerged growth of approximately 10 mm
± = no growth or growth of approximately 2 mm
Adapted from Koneman, Roberts, and Wright (1978)

133

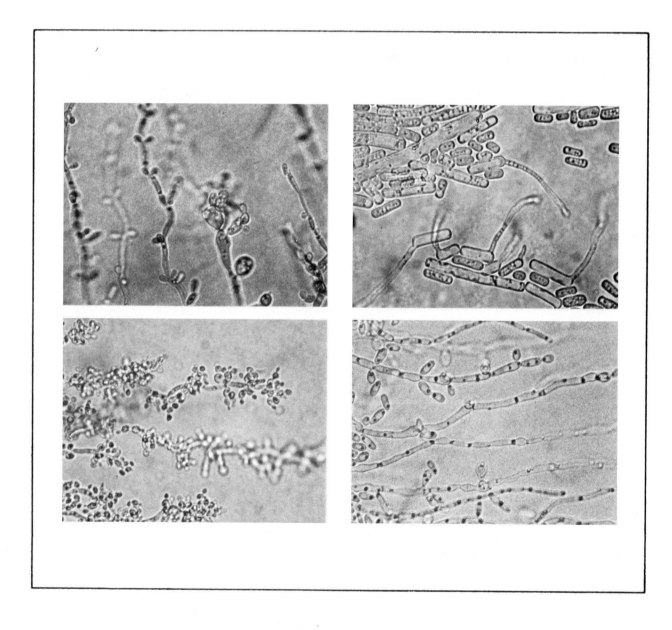

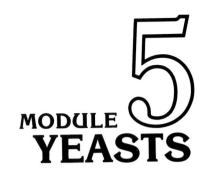

MODULE **5**
YEASTS

PREREQUISITES. The learner must possess a good background knowledge in clinical microbiology and must have finished Module 1, Basics of Mycology, and Module 2, Laboratory Procedures for Fungal Culture and Isolation.

BEHAVIORAL OBJECTIVES. Upon completion of this module, the learner should be able to:

1. Identify, from colonial morphology, corn meal-Tween 80 morphology, and appropriate biochemical tests:

   Candida albicans   Other *Candida* species
   Candida stellatoidea   *Trichosporon* species
   Candida tropicalis   *Geotrichum* species, including *G. candidum*
   Candida parapsilosis   *Rhodotorula* species
   Candida pseudotropicalis   *Cryptococcus* species, including *C. neoformans*
   Candida krusei   *Saccharomyces* species
   Candida guilliermondi

2. Correctly perform and interpret results from the following, including when to use each:

   Corn meal-Tween 80 morphology
   Germ tube test
   Carbohydrate assimilations
   Carbohydrate fermentations
   Urease test
   Rapid nitrate test
   Malt extract for *Trichosporon* and *Geotrichum* blastoconidia
   Malt extract agar for ascospores
   Modified Kinyoun acid-fast stain
   India ink preparation
   Caffeic acid or niger seed agar for *Cryptococcus neoformans*
   TOC medium for germ tubes, chlamydospores, and pigment production

3. Briefly discuss the usefulness of the following procedures for confirming yeast identification: colonial morphology on Sabouraud dextrose or Candida BCG agar, growth at 37°C, and cycloheximide tolerance.
4. Write a schema for identification of each of the organisms in number 1.
5. Briefly discuss candidosis, cryptococcosis, torulopsosis, and geotrichosis including etiologic agents, manifestations, disease incidence (common or rare), and mode of transmission.

CONTENT OUTLINE

I. Introduction
II. Laboratory procedures
  A. Direct examination and cultural isolation
  B. Yeast identification methods
    1. Microscopic morphology on corn meal-Tween 80 agar
    2. Study questions
    3. Germ tube production
    4. Assimilation reactions
    5. Urease production
    6. Capsule production
    7. Ascospore production
    8. Pigment production on niger seed or caffeic acid agar
    9. Nitrate test
    10. Fermentation reactions
    11. Other tests
III. Final exam
IV. Supplemental Rationale
  A. Candidosis
  B. Cryptococcosis
  C. Geotrichosis
  D. Torulopsosis
  E. Study questions

FOLLOW-UP ACTIVITIES

1. Students may compare colonial morphology of yeasts on Sabouraud dextrose agar and Candida BCG agar.

2. Students may look under the microscope at corn meal-Tween 80 preparations of various yeasts.

3. Students may be assigned unknown yeasts for which they must perform differential identification tests.

REFERENCES

ALTERAS, I, ET AL: *Widely disseminated cutaneous candiosis in adults.* Sabouraudia 17:383, 1979.

BARNETT, JA AND PANKHURST, RJ: *A New Key to the Yeasts.* American Elsevier Publishing Co., New York, 1974.

BENEKE, ES AND ROGERS, AL: *Medical Mycology Manual,* ed 4. Burgess Publishing Co., Minneapolis, 1980.

BILLIE, J, STOCKMAN, L, AND ROBERTS, GD: *Detection of yeasts and filamentous fungi in blood cultures during a 10-year period (1972 to 1981).* J Clin Microbiol 16:968, 1982.

CASAL, M AND LINARES, MJ: *The comparison of six media for chlamydospore production by Candida albicans.* Mycopathologia 76:125, 1981.

CASAL, M AND LINARES, MJ: *Preliminary evaluation of a new test for the rapid differentiation of Candida albicans and Candida stellatoidea.* Mycopathologia 81:63, 1983.

CONANT, NF, ET AL: *Manual of Clinical Mycology,* ed 3. WB Saunders, Philadelphia, 1971.

DE CAMARGO, ZP AND FISCHMAN, O: *Prototheca stagnora: An encapsulated organism.* Sabouraudia 17:197, 1979.

DELACRETAZ, J, GRIGORIU, D, AND DUCEL, G: *Color Atlas Of Medical Mycology.* Hans Huber Publishers, Year Book Medical Publishers (distributor), Chicago, 1976.

EMMONS, CW, ET AL: *Medical Mycology,* ed 3. Lea & Febiger, Philadelphia, 1977.

EPSTEIN, JB, PEARSALL, NN, AND TRUELOVE, EL: *Quantitative relationships between Candida albicans in saliva and the clinical status of human subjects.* J Clin Microbiol 12:475, 1980.

FLEMING, WH, HOPKINS, JM, AND LAND, GA: *New culture medium for the presumptive identification of Candida albicans and Cryptococcus neoformans.* J Clin Microbiol 5:236, 1977.

HALEY, LD AND CALLAWAY, CS: *Laboratory Methods in Medical Mycology,* ed 4. U.S. Department of Health, Education, and Welfare, Washington, DC, 1978.

HANSENCLEVER, HF: *The consistent formation of chlamydospores by Candida tropicalis.* Sabouraudia 9:164, 1971.

HINCHEY, WW AND SOMEREN, A: *Cryptococcal prostatitis.* Am J Clin Pathol 75:257, 1981.

HOPFER, RL, ET AL: *Radiometric detection of yeasts in blood cultures of cancer patients.* J Clin Microbiol 12:329, 1980.

HOPKINS, JM AND LAND, GA: *Rapid method for determining nitrate utilization by yeasts.* J Clin Microbiol 5:497, 1977.

KONEMAN, EW, ROBERTS, GD, AND WRIGHT, SF: *Practical Laboratory Mycology,* ed 2. Williams & Wilkins, Baltimore, 1978.

LAND, GA, ET AL: *Rapid identification of medically important yeasts.* Laboratory Medicine 10:533, 1979.

LAND, GA, ET AL: *Improved auxanographic method for yeast assimilations: A comparison with other approaches.* J Clin Microbiol 2:206, 1975.

LARONE, DH: *Medically Important Fungi: A Guide to Identification.* Harper & Row, Hagerstown, Md 1976.

MARTIN, MV: *Germ tube positive Candida tropicalis.* Am J Clin Pathol 71:130, 1979.

MARTIN, MV AND WHITE, FH: *A microbiologic and ultrastructural investigation of germ tube formation by oral strains of Candida tropicalis.* Am J Clin Pathol 75:671, 1981.

McGINNIS, MR: *Laboratory Handbook of Medical Mycology.* Academic Press, New York, 1980.

NGUI YEN, JH AND SMITH, JA: *Use of Autobac 1 for rapid assimilation testing of Candida and Torulopsis species.* J Clin Microbiol 7:118, 1978.

OBLACK, DL, RHODES, JC, AND MARTIN, WJ: *Clinical evaluation of the AutoMicrobic System Yeast Biochemical Card for rapid identification of medically important yeasts.* J Clin Microbiol 13:351, 1981.

QUIRKE, P, HWANG, WS, AND VALIDEN, CC: *Congenital Torulopsis glabrata infection in man.* Am J Clin Pathol 73:137, 1980.

SEGUELA, JP, ET AL: *Carbon assimilation of sugars: Use of Autobac 1 for standardization purpose.* Mycopathologia 76:19, 1981.

SILVA-HUNTER, M AND COOPER, BH: *Medically important yeasts.* In LENNETTE, EH, ET AL (EDS): *Manual of Clinical Microbiology,* ed 3. American Society for Microbiology Washington, DC, 1980.

TIERNO, PM AND MILSTOC, M: *Germ tube positive Candida tropicalis.* Am J Clin Pathol 68:294, 1977.

WEIJMAN, ACM: *Carbohydrate composition and taxonomy of Geotrichum, Trichosporon, and allied genera.* Antonie van Leeuwenhoek 45:119, 1979.

YARROW, D AND MEYER, S: *Proposal for amendment of the diagnosis of the genus Candida Berkhout nom. cons.* International Journal of Systemic Bacteriology 28:611, 1978.

YEN, JHN AND SMITH, JA: *Use of Autobac 1 for rapid assimilation testing of Candida and Torulopsis species.* J Clin Microbiol 7:118, 1978.

INTRODUCTION

In the past, physicians were concerned only about isolation and identification of the yeasts *Candida albicans* and *Cryptococcus neoformans* as disease producers. Now, however, unusual strains are being seen more frequently as infectious agents, especially in patients undergoing surgical procedures, treatment with corticosteroids, catheterization, or immunosuppression, or those in advanced malignancy. Rapid, accurate biochemical tests have been developed which greatly facilitate a quick turn-around time from specimen collecting to reporting culture results. Many commercial yeast identification systems are available.[*]

In addition, automated bacteriologic identification and drug susceptibility systems are being modified to include yeast speciation.[†]

---

[*]Uni-Yeast-Tek System, Flow Laboratories, 25 Lumber Rd., Roslyn, N.Y. 11576.
API System, Analytab Products, 200 Express St., Plainview, N.Y. 11803.
Minitek System, BBL, Cockeysville, Md. 21030.
[†]AutoMicrobic System, Vitek Systems, 595 Anglum Dr., Hazelwood, Mo. 63042.
Autobac 1, General Diagnostics, Division of Warner-Lambert Company, Morris Plains, N.J. 07950.
Quantum II, Abbott Labs, Diagnostics Division, P.O. Box 2020, Irving, Texas 75061.

LABORATORY PROCEDURES

Direct Examination and Cultural Isolation

Yeasts may be isolated from almost any specimen. Saline wet preparations of the specimen will show round to oval budding cells (blastoconidia), and some may be elongated, forming pseudohyphae. Occasionally, arthroconidia, asci, or other structures are observed **(see Chart 1-5 on pages 25-26 at end of Module 1)**. Capsules may be seen around yeast cells on India ink preparations. See Module 2 for specimen collection and direct examination procedures.

Yeasts are best grown at 30°C on Sabouraud dextrose agar, although room temperature is acceptable. Note that cycloheximide or a 37°C incubation inhibits many strains. In two or three days yeasts form cream-colored (rarely, orange), glabrous colonies that are mucoid or waxy, and smooth or wrinkled. When young, yeast colonies may be confused with *Staphylococcus* sp. (For differentiation, see the last paragraph on candidosis in the Supplemental Rationale section of this module.) The suspected yeast should be streaked for isolation on Candida BCG agar* to ensure a pure culture and to observe colonial morphology **(see Chart 5-2 on page 157 at end of module** and Color Plate 55).

*Remel, 12076 Santa Fe Drive, Lenexa, Kansas 66215.

Yeast Identification Methods

Yeast identification is not based on any single criterion; there are a combination of procedures employed to speciate organisms. Each test listed in this section is ordered from most to least generally useful. The first three, corn meal-Tween 80 morphology, germ tube, and assimilations, may be performed concurrently, and the rest performed as required. Be sure to take the purified test yeast from SDA for differential procedures. Antibiotics and dyes in BCG agar, mycobiotic agar, and so forth may inhibit characteristic reactions in differential tests.

MICROSCOPIC MORPHOLOGY ON CORN MEAL-TWEEN 80 AGAR

Corn meal agar without dextrose should be used, with 0.3 percent Tween 80 added. It is highly recommended that rice extract agar with 0.3 percent Tween 80 or TOC (Tween 80, Oxgall, Caffeic Acid) agar (see footnote in gray box), be used in conjunction with corn meal-Tween 80. There is far better chlamydospore development on the rice extract and TOC medium, while blastoconidial development is enhanced on the corn meal. Tubed media are preferred: they can be freshly melted down as needed and poured into biplates. (See gray box.)

MORPHOLOGY ON CORN MEAL-TWEEN 80 AGAR AND RICE EXTRACT-TWEEN 80 AGAR

Media Preparation

Corn meal-Tween 80 agar (Commercially available, Difco, BBL)

Corn meal	50 gm
Agar	15 gm
Distilled water	1 liter
Tween 80	3 ml

Rice extract-Tween 80 agar (Commercially available, Difco, BBL)

Cream of rice	10 gm
Distilled water	1 liter
Agar	10 gm
Tween 80	3 ml

1. **For the commercial media, follow the manufacturer's instructions regarding reconstitution. Go to number 4.**
2. **For homemade corn meal-Tween 80 agar, mix the corn meal in 500 ml distilled water, then autoclave at 15 psi for 10 minutes. Filter through cheesecloth, bring the volume to 1 liter with distilled water, and add the agar. Go to number 4.**
3. **For homemade rice extract-Tween 80 agar, boil 500 ml of distilled water, add the cream of rice, and cook for 30 seconds. Filter through cheesecloth, bring the volume up to 1 liter with distilled water, and add the agar.**

4. **Bring the medium to a boil on a hotplate, using a magnetic stirring rod. Add the Tween 80, mixing well.**
5. **Dispense 10 ml aliquots into screw-capped tubes, autoclave at 15 psi for 15 minutes, cool and refrigerate.**
6. **When needed, boil one tube each of corn meal-Tween 80 agar and rice extract-Tween 80 agar, pour into a sterile labeled biplate, and cool.**

Procedure
1. **Use a very small amount of a young colony. Make two parallel streaks on the agar with an inoculated loop.**
2. **Flame the loop, then move back and forth across the streaks: Do NOT cut into the agar.**
3. **Flame a glass coverslip and place it over the inoculated agar. Tamp down on the coverslip with forceps to remove trapped air.**
4. **After 48 hours at room temperature, remove the Petri dish lid and examine under the coverglass, near the edges, for characteristic features, using the low- and high-power objectives of the microscope. If necessary, reincubate for more growth and examine daily. See Chart 5-1 on pages 154–156 at end of module.**

*TOC-corn meal-Tween 80 biplates are commercially available from Remel, 12076 Santa Fe Dr., Lenexa, Kansas 66215. Germ tube and chlamydospore production of *C.albicans* is observed on TOC, while blastoconidial patterns for other *Candida* spp. are seen on corn meal-Tween 80.

If there are chlamydospores, blastoconidia, and pseudohyphae on corn meal-Tween 80 or rice extract-Tween 80 agar, *Candida albicans* (Fig. 5-1 **and Chart 5-1 on pages 154-156 at end of module**) is probably the organism in question. It is by far the most commonly isolated yeast in clinical specimens. A variant of *Candida albicans* is *Candida stellatoidea*, which forms less numerous chlamydospores. *Candida tropicalis* may also rarely produce chlamydospores.* Perform the germ tube test and carbohydrate assimilations, especially sucrose, for final identification.† Sucrose fermentation may be necessary to rule out *Candida tropicalis*.

	Candida albicans	Candida stellatoidea	Candida tropicalis
Chlamydospores	+	+	Rarely +
Germ tubes in three hours	+	+	Rarely +
Sucrose assim.	+	−	+
Sucrose ferm.	−	−	Gas

If blastoconidia and pseudohyphae are produced on corn meal-Tween 80 or rice extract-Tween 80 agar, various *Candida* species may be suspected (Figs. 5-2 through 5-6). The distinctive morphology of each

*If corn meal-Tween 80 plates are incubated at room temperature and then refrigerated for three days before reading (for example, over a holiday weekend), *Candida tropicalis* will have consistently formed chlamydospores.
†Most, but not all, *Candida albicans* form germ tubes and chlamydospores.

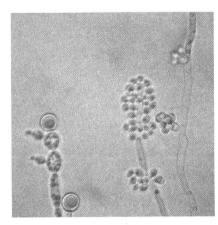

FIGURE 5-1. Clusters of blastoconidia along the pseudohyphae, and terminal chlamydospores, *Candida albicans*, corn meal-Tween 80 (CM-T80) agar, ×450.

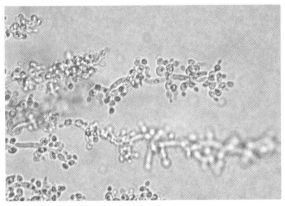

FIGURE 5-2. Clusters of blastoconidia between short pseudohyphae, *Candida guilliermondi*, CM-T80 agar, ×450.

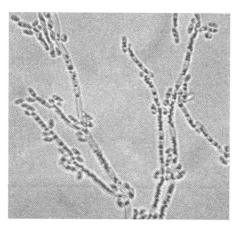

FIGURE 5-3. Cross-matchsticks blastoconidia along pseudohyphae, *Candida krusei,* **CM-T80 agar ×450.**

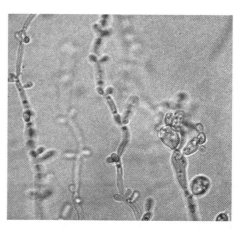

FIGURE 5-4. Giant and thin curved pseudohyphae, *Candida parapsilosis,* **CM-T80 agar, ×450.**

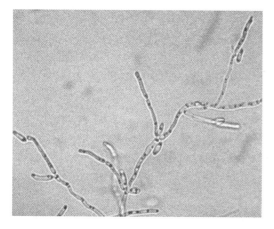

FIGURE 5-5. Logs in a stream blastoconidia along pseudohyphae, *Candida pseudotropicalis,* **CM-T80 agar ×450.**

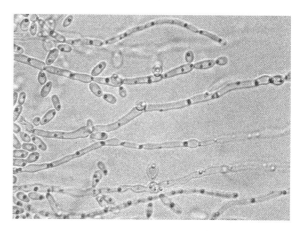

FIGURE 5-6. Sparse blastoconidia along pseudohyphae, *Candida tropicalis,* **CM-T80 agar, ×450.**

greatly aids in speciation, but perform assimilations for confirmatory identification. If there is still difficulty discerning the species, fermentations and colonial morphology on Sabouraud dextrose or Candida BCG agar may be helpful. **(See Chart 5-2 on page 157 and Chart 5-3 on page 158 at end of module.)**

If there are arthroconidia and true hyphae on corn meal-Tween 80 or rice extract-Tween 80 agar, *Trichosporon* species or *Geotrichum* species may be suspected. Perform a urease test: *Trichosporon* is urease positive, while *Geotrichum* is urease negative. On corn meal-Tween 80 agar, *Trichosporon* sp., *Geotrichum (Trichosporon) capitatum,* and *Geotrichum (Trichosporon) penicillatum* produce blastoconidia, although they may be difficult to find. *Geotrichum candidum* (Fig. 5-7) does not produce them. Be careful not to misidentify the corner buds, or germ tubes, extending

from some arthroconidia as blastoconidia. To enhance blastoconidial formation, inoculate malt extract broth with the organism and incubate it at room temperature for three to four days. Examine a wet mount microscopically for the characteristic budding cells. Malt extract broth is a further aid to identification: *Geotrichum* and *Trichosporon* species produce different colony types on this medium. Perform carbohydrate assimilations for confirmation of the species. If there is still difficulty identifying the organism, colonial morphology on Candida BCG agar may be useful.

If there are blastoconidia only (or also rare short pseudohyphae) on corn meal-Tween 80 agar or rice extract-Tween 80 agar, *Cryptococcus* (Fig. 5-8), *Rhodotorula, Saccharomyces* (Fig. 5-9), and *Candida* species may be suspected. Perform a urease test; if it is positive, *Cryptococcus* and *Rhodotorula* are consid-

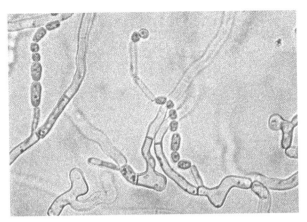

FIGURE 5-7. Arthroconidia, *Geotrichum candidum*, CM-T80 agar, ×450.

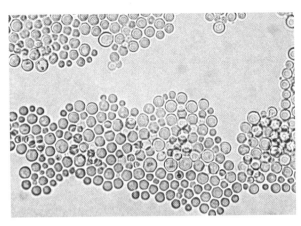

FIGURE 5-8. Round blastoconidia, *Cryptococcus neoformans*, CM-T80 agar, ×450.

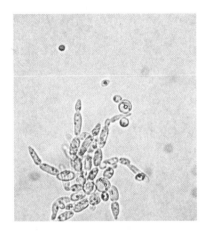

FIGURE 5-9. Blastoconidia and short pseudohyphae, *Saccharomyces cerevisiae*, CM-T80 agar, ×450.

ered. The former produces cream to tan colonies on Sabouraud dextrose agar, while the latter generally produces pink-orange colonies, although *Rhodotorula* may lose its pigment. The uncommon yeast *Sporobolomyces* sp. also possesses a pink-orange color and is urease positive, but on corn meal-Tween 80 agar, blas-

toconidia, **ballistoconidia** (forcibly ejected conidia on denticles), pseudohyphae, and true hyphae are formed. Additionally satellite colonies are produced by the ejected ballistoconidia. Both *Rhodotorula* and *Sporobolomyces* resemble the colonies of the *Serratia* bacteria; a Gram stain must be performed to differentiate them.

Niger seed or caffeic acid agar may be inoculated to help identify *Cryptococcus neoformans*, which is the only yeast to form a dark brown colony on this medium. On an India ink preparation, most *Cryptococcus* and some *Rhodotorula* possess observable capsules. Confirmatory identification of these organisms is based on the assimilation reactions, as fermentations are not useful.

If the urease test is negative on yeasts that produce blastoconidia only on CM-T80 agar, *Saccharomyces* or *Candida* is considered. Inoculate ascospore, assimilation, and fermentation media. The ascosporogenous yeasts, for example, *Saccharomyces*, should be sent to a reference laboratory, since special training is required for identifying these organisms. If no asci are formed on the ascospore medium, read the assimilations and fermentations, which should speciate *Candida (Torulopsis) glabrata*, *Candida famata (Torulopsis candida)*, *Candida guilliermondi*, and other *Candida* species.

Study Questions

1. On a vaginal culture, a cream-colored yeast forms. On corn meal-Tween 80 agar, only small oval blastoconidia are observed. This organism is most likely:

A. *Candida albicans*

B. *Trichosporon beigelii*

C. *Candida glabrata*

D. *Rhodotorula rubra*

E. *Geotrichum candidum*

Box continues on next page.

Matching. Place the letter of the answer in *Column B* in front of the corresponding words in *Column A.*

Column A	Column B
___ 2. Produces asci	A. *Candida parapsilosis*
___ 3. Logs in a stream blastoconidia	B. *Candida krusei*
___ 4. Thick capsule	C. *Candida pseudotropicalis*
___ 5. Cross-matchsticks blastoconidia	D. *Saccharomyces cerevisiae*
___ 6. Giant pseudohyphae	E. *Geotrichum candidum*
	F. *Cryptococcus neoformans*
	G. *Candida guilliermondi*

7. On corn meal-Tween 80 agar, a fungus produces terminal round chlamydospores and clusters of numerous blastoconidia. The organism also forms germ tubes within three hours and assimilates sucrose but does not ferment it. This organism is named _____ .

STOP HERE UNTIL YOU HAVE COMPLETED THE ANSWERS

Look up the answers in the back of the book. If you missed more than one, go back and review this section. Correctly complete any missed study questions before proceeding further.

GERM TUBE PRODUCTION

See gray box. In this procedure, one must be careful not to confuse germ tubes with pseudohyphae:

Germ tubes	*Pseudohyphae*
Parallel sides	Not necessarily parallel
Nonseptate	May be septate
No constriction at point of attachment	Constricted

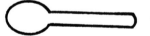 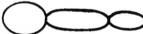

Germ tubes are formed within three hours by *Candida albicans* (Fig. 5-10), *Candida stellatoidea*, and rarely *Candida tropicalis*. Other *Candida* strains may produce them after three hours. Germ tubes may also be produced by arthroconidia, but the arthroconidia should be easily differentiated from blastoconidia. Note that not all *Candida albicans* isolates form germ tubes, especially those from cancer patients on therapy or persons on anti-*Candida* antibiotics. Therefore this test must be combined with other procedures for definitive identification.

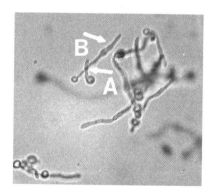

FIGURE 5-10. *Candida albicans* in human serum after 3 hours incubation at 37°C, ×450. Arrow A indicates a germ tube; arrow B points to a pseudohypha.

GERM TUBE PRODUCTION

Media Preparation
1. Place 0.5 ml of rabbit, fetal calf, or human serum into tubes. Rabbit coagulase plasma works well too.

Procedure
1. Inoculate the tube of serum with a small amount of the young test organism. Too large an inoculum will inhibit germ tube formation. Be sure to set up positive and negative controls, particularly if human serum is to be used, to assure that the serum does not possess anti–Candida antibodies and other inhibitory factors.
2. Incubate the tube at 37°C for 3 hours.
3. Place a drop of the suspension on a slide, put on a coverslip, and examine it microscopically for long tubelike projections (germ tubes) extending out from the yeast cells.

ASSIMILATION REACTIONS

These tests formerly were very time consuming and required a lot of technical expertise for interpretation. With the advent of commercial systems (see the introduction to this module), assimilation procedures are now rapid and practical.

Assimilation tests indicate the ability of an organism to use a compound in the presence of oxygen. Each species has its own pattern of compounds assimilated, which is a blueprint for identification. Carbohydrate assimilations (Fig. 5-11) are most commonly performed, and there are two basic techniques for doing these:

a. In separate containers, each carbohydrate is mixed with basal medium. An organism is added to the medium. After incubation, growth in the container indicates assimilation of that particular sugar by the fungus.

b. The organism is mixed in with melted basal agar, and the agar is allowed to solidify. Carbohydrates (liquid or impregnated paper discs) are placed on top of the agar. After incubation, assimilation is

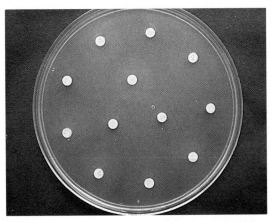

FIGURE 5-11. Plate carbohydrate assimilations. Growth around a sugar-impregnated paper disc indicates assimilation of that compound by the yeast.

indicated by growth around the sugar.

Dye pour plate auxanography uses the second technique, and it is a rapid and sensitive procedure (see gray box).

DYE POUR PLATE AUXANOGRAPHY*

Media Preparation
Basal medium:

Yeast nitrogen base (Difco)	**0.67 gm**
Agar	**20 gm**
Distilled water	**1 liter**
Stock bromcresol purple solution, 1 gm/L (Sigma Chem. Co.)	**20 ml**
0.1 N sodium hydroxide	**4 ml**

1. Mix together the yeast nitrogen base, agar, and distilled water, and bring the medium to a boil on a hot plate, using a magnetic stirrer.
2. Add the bromcresol purple solution and sodium hydroxide, then adjust the pH to 7.0–7.2.
3. Pour 60 ml aliquots into screw-capped bottles, autoclave at 15 psi for 15 minutes, cool, and refrigerate.

Carbohydrate solutions:

Dextrose 30 mg/ml	**Raffinose 100 mg/ml**
Maltose 50 mg/ml	**Inositol 50 mg/ml**
Sucrose 30 mg/ml	**Xylose 100 mg/ml**

Box continues on next page.

Lactose 30 mg/ml

Galactose 30 mg/ml

Cellobiose 100 mg/ml

Trehalose 100 mg/ml

Melibiose 200 mg/ml

Dulcitol 50 mg/ml

1. Prepare the above stock sugar concentrations in distilled water.[†]
2. Adjust the pH to 7.0 and filter sterilize.
3. Dispense 0.1 ml of each carbohydrate onto 0.5-inch wide sterile paper disks, dry, and refrigerate.

Procedure

1. For each organism to be tested, melt two bottles of basal medium and cool them to 45°C.
2. Prepare two suspensions of the organism in 5 ml of sterile distilled water blanks. Adjust the density to a McFarland standard of 4–7.
3. Pour one suspension into each bottle of melted agar, mix, and pour into 150 × 15 mm sterile Petri dishes.
4. After the plates have hardened, place carbohydrate discs on the surface, six to a plate, approximately one inch from the dish edge.
5. Incubate the plates at 30°C for 48 hours. Most yeasts will develop their assimilation patterns in 6–24 hours.
6. Read the results: a positive reaction is a yellow color and growth around the disc, while a negative reaction is a purple color and no growth around the disc. In this procedure, color change is correlated with carbohydrate metabolism.

[*]Land, et al, 1979

[†]Land also suggests using sorbose and melizitose. Sterile carbohydrate impregnated paper discs may be commercially obtained from Difco (Minitek also produces them, but they contain an indicator). However, since the carbohydrate concentrations are not optimal, indicator change cannot be correlated with assimilation, and longer incubation may be required than is stated in this method.

UREASE PRODUCTION

The urease test is especially useful for differentiating the fungi that produce arthroconidia (*Trichosporon*, urease positive; *Geotrichum*, urease negative) and those that produce blastoconidia only on corn meal-Tween 80 agar (*Rhodotorula* and *Cryptococcus*, urease positive; *Saccharomyces* and *Candida*, urease negative).

In the conventional test, a Christenson's urea agar slant is streaked with the organism, incubated at room temperature, and observed for production of a pinkish-purple color within 48 hours, which is a positive test. In a negative test, the medium remains yellow (medium preparation and procedure in gray box, Module 6 page 175). A rapid test for urease production is described in the gray box.

RAPID UREASE TEST*

Medium Preparation

Urea R broth (Difco)

1. Reconstitute a vial of urea R broth according to the manufacturer's instructions.

Procedure

1. Place 0.2 ml of reconstituted urea R broth in a microtiter well and add a heavy inoculum of 3–4 colonies from the test organism. Also inoculate positive and negative controls.
2. Cover the wells with clear tape and incubate at 37°C for 4 hours.
3. Any change to a pink color indicates a positive urease test. If the medium remains yellow, the test is negative.

[*]Land, et al, 1979

CAPSULE PRODUCTION

After mixing the yeast with a drop of saline and a tiny drop of India ink or nigrosin, a positive preparation will show the presence of a clear area, or capsule, around the yeast cell, against a black background. (See Module 2, section on Acid-Fast Stain for more details.)

Most workers associate capsule formation with *Cryptococcus*. However, this genus may possess no discernable capsule, while *Rhodotorula*, some *Candida (Torulopsis)*, *Sporobolomyces*, *Trichosporon beigelii*, and *Prototheca stagnora* (an alga that may be confused with *Cryptococcus*) may be encapsulated. Urease and assimilation reactions are a more reliable guide to identification.

In times of emergency, the physician may reasonably suspect *Cryptococcus neoformans* from positive India ink spinal fluid preparations, and treatment can immediately be instituted. However, any direct mount results need to be confirmed by cultural identification.

ASCOSPORE PRODUCTION

A number of various media for ascospore production have been described in the literature: Gorodkowa ascospore medium, Fowell's acetate ascospore medium, and V-8 medium for ascospores. Wickerham's malt extract agar works well (see gray box). Since most ascosporogenous yeasts require opposite mating types for sexual reproduction, 3 to 4 colonies of the organism must be used to improve the chance of including both types in the inoculum.

ASCOSPORE PRODUCTION

Medium Preparation
  Wickerham's malt extract agar:

Malt extract (Difco, BBL)	20 gm
Agar	12 gm
Distilled water	400 ml

  1. For the commercial medium, follow the manufacturer's directions regarding reconstitution. Go to number 3.
  2. For homemade malt extract agar, mix the agar and water in a flask on a magnetic stirrer, bring to a boil, cool to 50°C, and add the malt extract.
  3. Dispense 10 ml aliquots into screw-capped tubes.
  4. Autoclave at 15 psi for 15 minutes, slant the tubes so that there is a one-inch butt, and allow the medium to harden. Refrigerate.

Procedure
  1. Lightly inoculate a room temperature agar slant with portions of 3–4 young colonies to be tested. Make sure the yeast has been streaked for purity first. Also inoculate positive and negative controls.
  2. Incubate at room temperature for 3–5 days, make a smear of the organism and controls, air dry, heat fix, and stain with the modified Kinyoun acid-fast stain (see gray box on acid-fast stain on page 52 in Module 2). See Color Plate 52.

PIGMENT PRODUCTION ON NIGER SEED OR CAFFEIC ACID AGAR

Caffeic acid is the active component of *Guizotia abyssinica* seed, variously called niger seed, birdseed, and thistle seed. When *Cryptococcus neoformans* is heavily streaked on a medium containing an extract of the seed or caffeic acid, the colonies become dark brown due to phenol oxidase activity of the yeast (Color Plate 53).

Other yeasts, including other *Cryptococcus* species, will retain their original color. TOC (Tween 80, Oxgall, Caffeic acid) is a good medium for *Cryptococcus neoformans* pigment production. There are added advantages in that this medium may be used for *Candida albicans* germ tube and chlamydospore formation, thus making an excellent screening medium. TOC is far superior to rice extract and corn meal agars for chlamydospore production. (See gray box for procedure.)

PIGMENT, GERM TUBE, AND CHLAMYDOSPORE PRODUCTION ON TOC MEDIUM*

Medium Preparation
Tween 80, Oxgall, Caffeic acid (TOC) medium: commercially available (Remel[†])

Oxgall (Difco)	10 gm
Agar	20 gm
10 percent Tween 80 (Fisher)	10 ml
Caffeic acid (Sigma Chemical Co.)	0.3 gm
Distilled water	1 liter

1. Mix together the above ingredients. Autoclave at 15 psi for 15 minutes.
2. Pour into sterile 100 × 15 mm Petri dishes. Allow the agar to harden, then refrigerate.

Procedure
1. Bring the plates to room temperature. Sweep across the surface of the primary isolation plate with a sterile swab, picking up several yeast colonies. If this procedure is not meant to be a screen for *Cryptococcus neoformans* and/or *Candida albicans*, purified isolates may be used. Be sure to run positive and negative controls.
2. Make a heavy streak with the swab on one side of a TOC plate. Adjacent to the heavy streak, lightly inoculate the yeast as for corn meal-Tween 80 morphology.
3. Place a flamed coverglass over the lightly inoculated area, and tamp down with forceps to force out any trapped air bubbles.
4. Incubate the plate at 37°C for 3 hours and observe the coverslipped area microscopically for germ tubes.
5. Reincubate the plate for an additional 18 hours or longer at room temperature and observe the coverslipped area for chlamydospores. Also look for dark brown colonies on the heavy streak.
6. If there are germ tubes and chlamydospores, *Candida albicans* or *Candida stellatoidea* is present. *Candida tropicalis* does not form these structures on TOC medium. If there is dark brown pigment production on the heavy streak, *Cryptococcus neoformans* is present. Note that this medium may NOT be used for microscopic morphology of other filamentous yeasts, for example, other *Candida* species.

*Fleming, et al, 1977
[†]Remel, 12076 Santa Fe Drive, Lenexa, Kansas 66215

NITRATE TEST

The nitrate assimilation test, although time consuming, is a classic procedure. The nitrate reduction test of Hopkins and Land, 1977, is rapid and gives comparable results (see gray box).

RAPID NITRATE TEST*

Reagent Preparation
Nitrate medium: (nitrate swabs commercially available from Remel, 12076 Santa Fe Dr., Lenexa, Kansas 66215)

Potassium nitrate (KNO_3)	2.0 gm
Monosodium phosphate, hydrated ($NaH_2PO_4 \cdot H_2O$)	11.7 gm
Disodium phosphate (Na_2HPO_4)	1.14 gm
17 percent Zephiran chloride	1.2 ml
Distilled water	200 ml

1. Mix together the above ingredients, adjusting the pH to 5.8–6.0.
2. Saturate cotton-tipped swabs with the mixture, dry at 37°C overnight, then autoclave at 15 psi for 15 minutes.

0.5 percent α-Naphthylamine:
Dimethyl-α-Naphthylamine	0.5 gm
5 N acetic acid (1 part glacial acetic acid to 2.5 parts distilled water)	100 ml

0.8 percent sulfanilic acid:
sulfanilic acid	0.8 gm
5 N acetic acid (1 part glacial acetic acid to 2.5 parts distilled water)	100 ml

Procedure
1. Sweep one of the treated swabs across several young yeast colonies from a pure culture, then swirl the swab against the bottom of an empty test tube to assure contact between organisms and medium. Do the same for positive and negative controls.
2. Incubate the tubes and swabs for 10 minutes at 45°C.
3. Transfer each swab to another tube containing two drops each of 0.5 percent α-naphthylamine and 0.8 percent sulfanilic acid.
4. If nitrate reductase is produced by the yeast, the tip of the swab will turn a bright cherry red, a positive test. No color may be a negative test; confirm the negativity by adding zinc dust. Zinc artificially reduces any remaining nitrate to nitrite, thus a red color forms with its addition. If no color appears with the zinc, the organism produced so much nitrate reductase that it completely reduced the nitrate to non–color-forming ammonia; therefore, this is also a positive test.

$$\text{Nitrate source} \xrightarrow[\text{or Zinc}]{\text{Yeast nitrate reductase}} \text{Nitrite (red)} \xrightarrow{\text{Yeast nitrate reductase}} \text{Ammonia (colorless)}$$

*Hopkins and Land, 1977

CARBOHYDRATE FERMENTATION REACTIONS (Fig. 5-12)

These are applied as a backup if there is difficulty identifying an organism by assimilation reactions. Fermentations, which measure the ability to use a compound anaerobically, are rather time consuming to perform. They involve inoculating a set of tubes containing basal media and a different carbohydrate in each. The top is overlaid with vaspar (equal amounts of Vaseline and paraffin) or, prior to sterilization, a Durham tube is inverted in the medium. After five or more days of incubation, the tubes are observed for gas production. Either the vaspar plug is raised above the medium or there is a bubble in the top of the inverted Durham tube. Color change to yellow indicates acid production; however, this only signifies that the sugar was assimilated, while gas formation indicates fermentation. Note that bacterial fermentation media may not be used for yeast fermentations. (See gray box.)

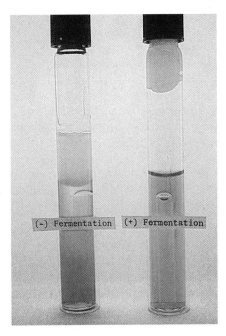

FIGURE 5-12. Carbohydrate fermentation. In a positive test, the vaspar plug is raised and a bubble is present in the Durham tube.

WICKERHAM FERMENTATION METHOD

Media Preparation

  Basal medium:

Yeast extract	4.5 gm
Peptone	7.5 gm
Distilled water	1 liter
Bromthymol blue	

1. Mix together the yeast extract, peptone, and distilled water.
2. Add enough bromthymol blue to produce a dense green color, then pour the medium in 2 ml aliquots into screw-capped tubes.
3. Invert a Durham tube in each aliquot, and autoclave at 15 psi for 15 minutes. Cool.

Carbohydrate solutions:

Dextrose	Lactose
Maltose	Galactose
Sucrose	Trehalose

1. Prepare 6.0 percent aqueous solutions of each sugar.
2. Filter sterilize.
3. After the basal medium has cooled, aseptically add to each tube 1.0 ml of one of the sugar solutions, and swirl to mix. Refrigerate.

Procedure

1. Suspend a young colony of the test organism in sterile distilled water so that the density is less than or equal to a No. 1 McFarland standard.
2. Place 0.1 ml of the suspension into each of the room temperature sugar fermentation broths mentioned above.
3. Incubate at 30°C and gently agitate the tubes daily, taking care not to let any air bubbles into the Durham tube. Read for gas production (liquid displaced out of the Durham tube by a gas bubble) every 2–3 days up to 14 days.

OTHER TESTS

The following tests may be performed as backup to those already mentioned.

Colonial morphology: Sabouraud dextrose or Candida BCG agar are inoculated and examined for typical colonial appearance (Color Plates 6, 54, and 55.) **See Chart 5-2 on page 157 at end of module for descriptions of organisms on both media.** This along with corn meal-Tween 80 microscopic morphology may enable you to make a preliminary identification. However, interpreting colonial appearances takes a lot of practice, and confirmatory identification should come from more reliable results, for example, assimilation patterns.

Growth at 37°C: This may help speciate an organism **(Chart 5-3 on page 158 at end of module).** In the past it was used to differentiate *Cryptococcus neoformans*, which grows at 37°C, from nonpathogenic *Cryptococcus* sp., which usually do not grow at 37°C. Now that there is a need to identify *Cryptococcus* down to species, growth temperature should mainly be used to decide the optimal incubation temperature of organisms for other tests.

Cycloheximide tolerance: Growth in the presence of cycloheximide may be used to help speciate fungi. This test has fallen somewhat into disfavor, as there is a great strain variation within species.

FINAL EXAM

Circle T if the statement is true and F if the statement is false.

1. **T F** All *Candida albicans* produce germ tubes and chlamydospores.

2. **T F** A germ tube is constricted at its point of attachment to the mother cell.

3. **T F** In the dye pour plate auxanography test for sugar assimilations, growth around the disc indicates utilization of the sugar.

4. **T F** In the rapid nitrate test, if the swab turns red when zinc dust is added, nitrate reductase was produced by the organism.

5. **T F** In the Wickerham fermentation test, a positive reaction is indicated by a color change of the medium to yellow.

For numbers 6 through 9, write the letter of the tests that are most helpful in identifying each of the fungi below.

A. Corn meal-Tween 80

B. Germ tube

C. Malt extract broth

D. Assimilations

E. Urease

F. Fermentations

G. Ascospore production

H. Pigment production on caffeic acid agar

I. Capsules on India ink mount

6. ___ *Cryptococcus neoformans*

7. ___ *Trichosporon* sp.

8. ___ *Saccharomyces* sp.

9. ___ *Candida tropicalis*

10. TOC medium is indicated for what three parameters? What are the limitations of this medium? What are the advantages?

11. See Color Plate 56. This yeast is grown on Sabouraud dextrose agar. On corn meal-Tween 80 agar, only blastoconidia are observed. What is the genus of the organism?

12. See Figure 5-13. This corn meal-Tween 80 microscopic morphology is characteristic of the fungus _____ _____ (genus and species). Note: There are no blastoconidia.

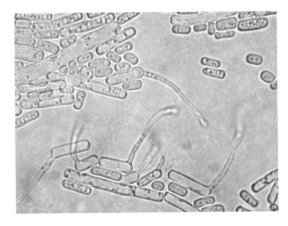

FIGURE 5-13. Final exam demonstration, CM-T80 agar, ×450.

STOP HERE UNTIL YOU HAVE COMPLETED THE ANSWERS.

Look up the answers in the back of the book. If you missed more than three of them, go back and repeat this module. Correctly complete any missed questions before proceeding.

SUPPLEMENTAL RATIONALE

Candidosis (Fig. 5-14)

Candidosis (candidiasis, moniliasis) is primarily caused by *Candida albicans,* although other *Candida* species are becoming increasingly important as disease agents. *Candida albicans* is seen as normal flora in the throat, vulvovaginal area, skin, and stool. When something happens to upset the normal balance of body flora, for example, prolonged antibiotic therapy, debilitating illness with lowered resistance, malignancy, lupus erythematosus, diabetes mellitus, tuberculosis, treatment with corticosteroids or cytotoxic drugs, and so forth, the yeast may proliferate and cause an infection.

Oral candidosis **(thrush)** is commonly observed in infants whose mothers have vaginal candidosis and in elderly patients who are taking antibiotic or steroid therapy for chronic, debilitating diseases such as tuberculosis or cancer. Diabetes, oral contraceptives, and a deficiency of riboflavin, a vitamin, also predispose to prolific growth of *Candida albicans.* White, creamy patches are seen on the mucous membranes and corners of the mouth. Under 400 *Candida* colonies per milliliter of saliva are considered normal, while numbers over 400 signify oral candidosis.

Vaginal candidosis (vulvovaginitis) is often seen in pregnant or diabetic patients. It is thought that the increased sugar in vaginal tissue, blood, and urine of these people makes them more susceptible to infection. Many *Candida* must be repeatedly isolated to be significant.

Cutaneous candidosis (Fig. 5-15) may be localized to one area or it may involve the entire body. Local manifestations are red, inflamed patches with distinct margins, a burned skin appearance. They usually appear at body sites exposed to constant irritation, for example, under the arms, in the groin or perianal area, and between the toes. Diabetics or individuals whose jobs require frequent immersion in water are particularly susceptible. Other predisposing factors are debilitating disease, obesity, alcoholism, vascular problems, and profuse sweating. The generalized disease is usually found in premature babies with immunologic deficiency whose mothers exhibit vaginal candidosis. Because *Candida* may be normal skin flora, especially in the perianal area, these organisms must be often isolated in large numbers before being considered the causative agents.

Candidosis of the nail (onychomycosis; Fig. 5-16) produces a thickening and hardening of the nail material. Often the skin around the nail is also involved.

Bronchopulmonary candidosis is mainly observed as a secondary infection resulting from antibiotic treatment for bacterial pulmonary disease. The patient has an irri-

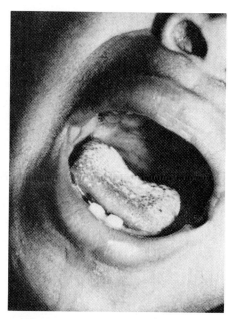

FIGURE 5-14. Candidosis of the tongue. (From: Rippon: Medical Mycology. WB Saunders, Philadelphia, 1982, with permission.)

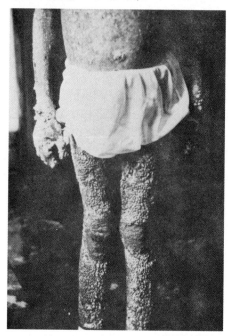

FIGURE 5-15. Generalized cutaneous candidosis. (From: Rippon: Medical Mycology. WB Saunders, Philadelphia, 1982, with permission.)

tating cough and produces mucoid sputum. Chest x-rays are typical of a pneumonia.

Urinary tract infections are often caused by vulvovaginal candidosis. *Candida* may be transmitted sexually, so treatment should begin as soon as possible. One hundred thousand colonies or more per milliliter of urine indicate a yeast infection, although less than this may be significant, depending on the patient's clinical status.

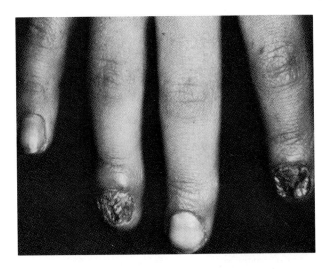

FIGURE 5-16. Candidal onychomycosis. (From: Rippon: Medical Mycology. WB Saunders, Philadelphia, 1982, with permission.)

Intestinal candidosis is usually caused by antibiotic treatment, which destroys the normal bacterial flora and allows *Candida,* normally present in small numbers, to take over and establish an infection. Stool cultures will reveal many yeast colonies.

Systemic candidosis follows hematologic spread of a localized infection, particularly observed in debilitated patients. Some manifestations are endocarditis (usually caused by *C. parapsilosis),* meningitis, and brain abscesses. *Candida tropicalis* is emerging as a significant systemic pathogen, although *C. albicans* is still the most prevalent. Budding yeasts with pseudohyphae and true hyphae are observed on blood smears in patients with candidemia. Unfortunately, yeasts are detected in less than 50 percent of blood cultures from these patients. Researchers are developing assays for measuring blood levels of candidal polysaccharides as a more rapid, reliable means of diagnosing invasive candidosis. Systemic candidosis is life-threatening and must be rapidly treated. Direct mount results, when positive, are very helpful to the physician; however, the organism must be culturally confirmed.

In the laboratory, specimens should be cultured quickly or refrigerated. *Candida* multiplies rapidly, giving a falsely elevated colony count on the culture. On a blood agar plate for routine bacteriology, after 24 hours incubation, *Candida* colonies are small and white, resembling *Staphylococcus epidermidis.* They are also catalase positive and coagulase negative. Be sure to perform a Gram stain to differentiate the two organisms. By 48 hours incubation, the yeasts will be larger and waxier than *Staphylococcus,* providing a better discrimination. With blood cultures for *Candida,* periodically vent all media and use biphasic brain heart infusion media to improve yeast detection.

Cryptococcosis

Cryptococcosis is caused by *Cryptococcus neoformans var. neoformans* (Serotypes A and D), and *Cryptococcus neoformans var. gattii* (Serotypes B and C). These yeasts are easily isolated from pigeon and other bird droppings but are seen elsewhere in nature: fruits, milk, plants, and feces of normal humans. They are usually breathed in and produce a mild, often subclinical respiratory infection. Primary pulmonary cryptococcosis can occur. If the patient is debilitated, especially if he has cancer or tuberculosis or is immunosuppressed, *Cryptococcus* may spread to the brain and meninges, for which it has a predilection. Here it will produce a chronic meninigitis that is fatal if not treated. The yeast may also disseminate to other parts of the body: back to the lungs where lesions may mimic tuberculosis, or to the bone, skin, or subcutaneous tissues. It has also been reported in a case of granulomatous prostatitis.

In the laboratory, India ink mounts of specimens show budding yeasts with large capsules. The capsules are also evident in tissue sections stained in histology (Color Plate 57), particularly with Mayer's mucicarmine stain. This yeast grows well at 37°C, is inhibited by cycloheximide, and produces dark brown colonies on caffeic acid agar. Serology tests, especially the latex agglutination test for cryptococcal antigen in cerebrospinal fluid and serum, are extremely useful for rapid identification of *C. neoformans.*

Geotrichosis

Geotrichosis is caused by *Geotrichum candidum.* The organism is seen as a contaminant in soil, cottage cheese, milk, decaying food, tomatoes, and as normal human flora in the mouth, skin, and stool. It rarely produces infection except in debilitated people. Oral geotrichosis is characterized by white patches that resemble oral candidosis, while intestinal disease results in colitis and bloody stools. Bronchial manifestations are the most common form of *Geotrichum candidum* infection; the chronic cough and the mucoid, bloody sputum simulate tuberculosis. Vaginal infections, which must be differentiated from candidosis, have been reported. Rarely, systemic disease, with organisms isolated from blood, has been observed. Other miscellaneous sites include tumefaction in the hand and skin lesions.

In the laboratory, direct mounts reveal fragmenting hyphae with unalternating rectangular arthroconidia possessing rounded ends. *Geotrichum candidum* must be distinguished from *Coccidioides immitis,* which usually exhibits alternating arthroconidia. In cultures of throat, stool, sputum, and vaginal specimens, many colonies must be repeatedly isolated before *G. candidum* is considered the etiologic agent of infection. Any organisms from blood are important.

Torulopsosis

Since the name of the etiologic yeast, *Torulopsis glabrata*, has been changed to *Candida glabrata*, torulopsosis could be included under candidosis. To date, however, most literature treats the disease as a separate entity. The organism is isolated from soil and is normal human flora in the oral cavity, urogenital area, and gastrointestinal tract. *Candida glabrata* is an opportunistic pathogen, usually eliciting disease in debilitated patients. The lungs and kidneys are primarily affected, although the fungus can disseminate through the blood to the rest of the body, causing fungemia and septic shock. A case of congenital transfer has been reported.

In the laboratory, lung tissue may show budding yeast cells inside macrophages, similar to *Histoplasma capsulatum*. However, *Candida glabrata* has no mold phase, and the isthmus between the budding yeast cells is wider than in *Histoplasma*. Many organisms may be observed in sputum during a lung infection. On urine cultures, 100,000 *C. glabrata* colonies per milliliter of urine are significant but less than this may also be significant, depending on the patient's clinical condition. Any organisms from blood or spinal fluid are important.

Study Questions—Supplemental Rationale

For questions 1 to 4, refer to the following case study:

A 45-year-old pigeon breeder, who recently received a renal transplant (thus was on immunosuppressive steroids), complained to his physician of headache, dizziness, blurred vision, and a stiff neck. Cultures of purulent cerebrospinal fluid were sent to your microbiology lab. A carefully examined Gram stain of the CSF sediment was negative; however, on Sabouraud dextrose agar at 30°C, a white, mucoid yeast rapidly grew. The organism was inhibited on Sabouraud dextrose agar with cycloheximide and chloramphenicol.

1. **Which disease do you suspect? Circle the letter of the correct answer.**

   A. **Candidosis**

   B. **No disease—organism was a laboratory contaminant**

   C. **Histoplasmosis**

   D. **Cryptococcosis**

   E. **Coccidioidomycosis**

2. **Give three reasons for choosing your answer to number 1.**

3. **If the yeast was significant, why was it not observed on the CSF Gram stain?**

4. **If your answer to number 1 was not B, what three tests would you perform to speciate the yeast?**

5. On a urine bacteriology culture blood agar plate at 24 hours, over 100,000 small, white colonies are observed. They are catalase positive and a slide coagulase test is negative. Your next step is to (circle the letter of the correct answer):

A. Report out over 100,000 *Staphylococcus epidermidis*/ml of urine

B. Perform a Gram stain

C. Inoculate a Gram-positive urine antibiotic susceptibility battery

D. Set up a tube coagulase test

E. Ask for a repeat culture

6. Circle the letter of the correct answer. *Candida (Torulopsis) glabrata* may be normal flora of:

A. Stool

B. Vagina

C. Throat

D. All of the above

E. A and C

STOP HERE UNTIL YOU HAVE COMPLETED THE QUESTIONS.

Look up the answers in the back of the book. If you missed more than one, go back and repeat this module.

CHART 5-1. Yeast Microscopic Morphology on Corn Meal-Tween 80 Agar

I. Chlamydospores, blastoconidia, and pseudohyphae

A. Terminal, circular, thick-walled chlamydospores; clusters of numerous or few blastoconidia at septa of pseudohyphae; true hyphae may be present

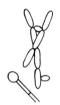

Candida albicans or *Candida stellatoidea*
Perform germ tube, assimilations, and fermentations (especially sucrose)
Backup: serology (see Module 2)

B. Rare terminal, round or variously shaped, thin-walled chlamydospores; sparse single or short-chained blastoconidia anywhere along the pseudohyphae

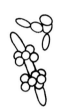

Candida tropicalis
Perform germ tube, assimilations, and fermentations (especially sucrose)

II. Blastoconidia and pseudohyphae

A. Oval blastoconidia in chains from the septa of thin pseudohyphae; or clusters of numerous blastoconidia at the septa of short pseudohyphae; often few pseudohyphae produced; great morphologic variation

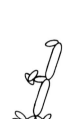

Candida guilliermondi
Perform assimilations
Backup: fermentations, colonial morphology on Sabouraud dextrose or Candida BCG agar

B. Treelike branching of abundant blastoconidia from the septa of elongated pseudohyphae; alternatively said to have a cross-matchsticks appearance

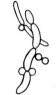

Candida krusei
Perform assimilations
Backup: fermentations, colonial morphology on Sabouraud dextrose or Candida BCG agar

C. Few single or small clustered blastoconidia at or between septa of thin curved pseudohyphae. Sometimes giant pseudohyphae may be observed.

Candida parapsilosis
Perform assimilations
Backup: fermentations, colonial morphology on Sabouraud dextrose or Candida BCG agar

154

CHART 5-1. Continued

D. Branched pseudohyphae with chains of elongated blastoconidia at the septa; logs in a stream arrangement of broken up blastoconidia positioned parallel to each other

Candida pseudotropicalis
Perform assimilations
Backup: fermentations, colonial morphology on Sabouraud dextrose or Candida BCG agar

E. Sparse single or short-chained blastoconidia, at or between septa of pseudohyphae

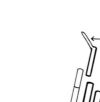

Candida tropicalis
Perform assimilations
Backup: fermentations, colonial morphology on Sabouraud dextrose or Candida BCG agar

III. Arthroconidia and true hyphae

A. Urease positive
Blastoconidia also produced, but they may be difficult to find on corn meal-Tween 80 agar

Trichosporon species
Inoculate malt extract broth (observe colonial and microscopic morphology), and perform assimilations
Backup: colonial morphology on Candida BCG agar

B. Urease negative
Blastoconidia may (*Geotrichum capitatum* and *Geotrichum penicillatum*) or may not (*Geotrichum candidum*) be produced

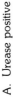

Geotrichum species
Inoculate malt extract broth (observe colonial and microscopic morphology), and perform assimilations
Backup: colonial morphology on Candida BCG agar

IV. Blastoconidia only, or with rare short pseudohyphae

A. Urease positive

1. Pink-orange colony on Sabouraud dextrose agar; corn meal-Tween 80 morphology exhibits oval budding cells with occasional rudimentary pseudohyphae; sometimes a faint capsule is observed

Rhodotorula species
Perform assimilations
Backup: colonial morphology on Sabouraud dextrose or Candida BCG agar

155

CHART 5-1. Continued

2. Cream-tan colony on Sabouraud dextrose agar; corn meal-Tween 80 morphology exhibits round (*Cryptococcus neoformans*) or oval budding cells with a thick capsule (sometimes none is observed); usually there are no pseudohyphae

Cryptococcus species
Perform assimilations and inoculate niger seed or caffeic acid agar
Backup: colonial morphology on Sabouraud dextrose or Candida BCG agar, serology (see Module 2)

B. Urease negative

1. Asci on ascospore medium
Corn meal-Tween 80 morphology exhibits oval cells which may have multiple budding; few short pseudohyphae may form

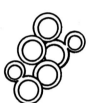

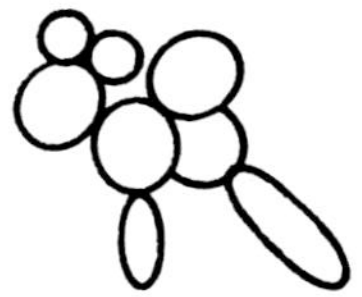

Saccharomyces species, etc.
Send to reference laboratory for identification

2. No asci on ascospore medium
Corn meal-Tween 80 morphology exhibits small oval budding cells; pseudohyphae may or may not be observed, depending on the species

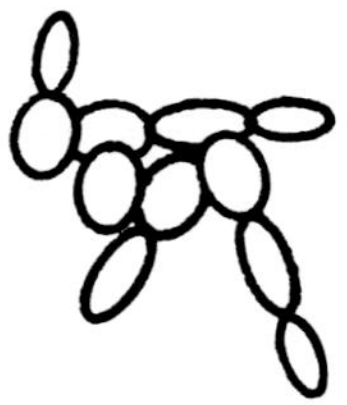

Candida species, esp. C. glabrata
Perform assimilations
Backup: fermentations, colonial morphology on Sabouraud dextrose or Candida BCG agar

CHART 5-2. Colonial Morphology of Yeasts on Sabouraud Dextrose and Candida BCG Agar After 48–72 Hours at 30°C

ORGANISM	SABOURAUD DEXTROSE AGAR	CANDIDA BCG AGAR
Candida albicans	White, creamy, shiny, and moist; variants may be dry and wrinkled	Raised, smooth, soft; white or light yellow color on the front and back; entire periphery
Candida glabrata	Small, white, shiny, and smooth	Small, raised, smooth with an entire periphery; colonies are bile-green with dark green backs
Candida guilliermondi	White, dull, center moist, wrinkles radiating out from center to edge, lacey looking, indented periphery	Flat, soft with an entire periphery; colonies are off shade white with pin-point sized bluish-green domes and greenish backs
Candida krusei	Flat, dry, spreading, ground-glass appearance; variants dull and nonspreading	Large, flat, dry with a delicate feathery periphery; colonies have a yellowish or yellowish-green tinge and bluish-green backs
Candida parapsilosis	Shiny, creamy, moist, wrinkled, turning rust colored at the periphery with age	Slightly flat and somewhat dry with a raised corrugated ring on the surface; colonies possess bluish or greenish-blue domes with greenish-blue backs
Candida pseudotropicalis	White, shiny, becoming dull and wrinkled with age	Large, raised, soft with an entire periphery; colonies are yellow with a tinge of green on the front and back
Candida tropicalis	Dull, dry, semiwhite color, filamentous periphery, wrinkled or smooth	Large, raised, soft; marked feathery periphery; white with an occasional bluish-green center on the front and/or back of the colony
Cryptococcus neoformans	Cream colored, shiny, may or may not be mucoid, entire margin, smooth, raised	Small, raised, and shiny like pearls; capsule may not be obvious; entire periphery, colonies are yellow or bluish-green with bluish-green backs
Geotrichum species	Flat, finely wrinkled, glabrous or covered with short white mycelium	*Geotrichum penicillatum*: Very large (5–7 mm) with large amount of aerial mycelium around periphery; color is bluish on front and back
Rhodotorula species	Pink-orange (may be white), shiny, smooth, entire margin, becoming waxy with age	Small and bluish; capsule may not be obvious; pink color develops in approximately 72 hours
Saccharomyces species	Heaped, wrinkled, shiny, white to gray, numerous other variations	*Saccharomyces cerevisiae*: Small, raised, soft; colonies have a greenish-yellow color on the front and back
Trichosporon species	Dry, wrinkled, brown-white, variants may develop a cottony mycelium	*Trichosporon beigelii*: Large, dry, and slightly raised; delicate feathery edge; colonies are bluish-green with blue backs
		Trichosporon pullulans: Thin, flat, and very feathery; colonies are bluish

Some characteristics compiled from Koneman, Roberts, and Wright (1978), Haley and Callaway (1978), and the Centers for Disease Control Developmental Manual for Yeast Identification.

CHART 5-3. Yeast Reaction Patterns

	ASSIMILATIONS														FERMENTATIONS							
	Dextrose	Maltose	Sucrose	Lactose	Galactose	Cellobiose	Raffinose	Inositol	Xylose	Trehalose	Melibiose	Dulcitol	KNO₃	Urease	Dextrose	Maltose	Sucrose	Lactose	Galactose	Trehalose	Growth at 37°C	Pellicle in malt extract broth
Candida albicans	+	+	+	–	+	–	–	–	+	+	–	–	–	–	G	G	–	–	G	G	+	–
Candida famata (Torulopsis candida)	+	+	+	+	+	+	+	–	+	+	+	+	–	–	G	G	G	–	G	G	+	–
Candida (Torulopsis) glabrata	+	–	–	–	–	–	–	–	–	+	–	–	–	–	G	–	–	–	–	G	+	–
Candida guilliermondi	+	+	+	–	+	+	+	–	+	+	+	+	–	–	G	–	G	–	G*	G	+	–
Candida krusei	+	–	–	–	–	–	–	–	–	+	–	–	–	+*	G*	–	–	–	–	G*	+	+
Candida parapsilosis	+	+	+	–	+	+	–	–	+	+	*	–	–	–	G	–	–	–	G*	G	+	–
Candida pseudotropicalis	+	–	–	+	+	–	+	–	+	–	+	–	–	–	G	–	G	G	G	–	+	–
Candida stellatoidea	+	+	–	–	+	–	–	–	+	+	–	–	–	–	G	–	G	G	G	–	+	–
Candida tropicalis	+	+	+	–	+	+	–	–	+	+	–	–	–	–	G	–	G	–	G	G	+	+
Cryptococcus albidus var. albidus	+	+	+	+*	+*	+	+	+	+	+	*	+	+	–							*	–
Cryptococcus albidus var. diffluens	+	+	+	–	+	+	+	+	+	+	*	+	+	–							+	–
Cryptococcus gastricus	+	+	*	*	*	+	*	–	+	+	+	+	+	–							–	–
Cryptococcus laurentii	+	+	+	+	+	+	+	+	+	+	+	+	+	+							+*	*
Cryptococcus luteolus	+	+	+	+	+	+	+	–	+	+	*	+	+	+							–	–
Cryptococcus neoformans	+	+	+	–	+	+	*	+	+	*	*	+	+	+							+*	*
Cryptococcus terreus	+	*	–	*	+*	*	*	–	+	*	*	*	–	+							+*	–
Cryptococcus uniguttulatus	+	+	–	–	+	+	–	+	+	–	–	–	+	+							–	–
Geotrichum candidum	+	–	–	–	+	–	–	–	+	–	–	–	–	–							+	–
Geotrichum (Trichosporon) capitatum	+	–	–	–	+	–	–	–	+	–	–	+	–	–							+	Pellicle or white islets
Geotrichum (Trichosporon) penicillatum	+	–	+	–	+	+	–	–	+	+	–	+	–	–							+	Wrinkled pellicle; may be submerged
Rhodotorula glutinis	+	+	+	–	+	*	+	–	+	+	–	–	+	+							+	–
Rhodotorula rubra	+	+	+	–	+	*	+	–	+	+	–	–	+	+							*	white wrinkled pellicle
Saccharomyces cerevisiae	+	+	+	–	+	–	+	–	–	*	+	–	–	–	G	G	G	–	G	G*	+	–
Trichosporon beigelii (cutaneum)	+	+*	+*	+*	+	+*	+*	+*	+*	+*	+*	+*	*	*							+*	Pellicle or ring; blastoconidia seen
Trichosporon pullulans	+	+	+	+*	+	+	+*	–	+*	+	+	+	+	+							+*	Pellicle or ring with islets

+ = Positive   – = Negative   * = Strain variation   G = Gas produced, i.e., fermentation

Adapted from Silva-Hunter and Cooper: Medically important yeasts. In Lennette, Balows, Hausler, and Truant (1980).

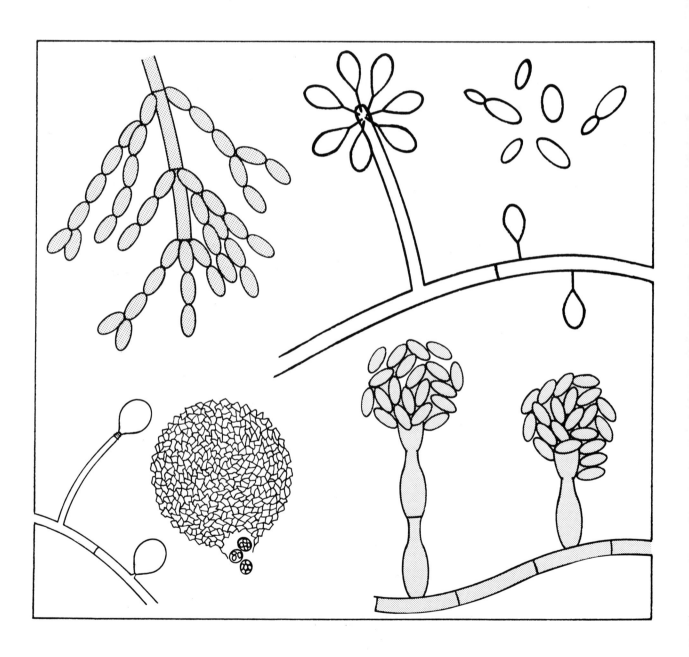

6
ORGANISMS CAUSING
SUBCUTANEOUS MYCOSES

PREREQUISITES. The learner must possess a good background knowledge in clinical microbiology and must have finished Module 1, Basics of Mycology, and Module 2, Laboratory Procedures for Fungal Culture and Isolation.

BEHAVIORAL OBJECTIVES. Upon completion of this module, the learner should be able to:

1. Describe the granules from chromoblastomycosis, eumycotic mycetoma, actinomycotic mycetoma, and actinomycosis. Include granule colors, microscopic appearance, causative organisms, and ways to distinguish them from bacterial granules.

2. From culture, microscopic characteristics, and mycosis elicited, recognize the following:

   Cladosporium trichoides   *Fonsecaea pedrosoi*
   Cladosporium carrionii   *Phialophora verrucosa*
   Exophiala jeanselmei   *Wangiella dermatitidis*
   Fonsecaea compacta   *Scedosporium apiospermum*
                                       Sporothrix schenckii

3. Differentiate the black yeasts *Exophiala* and *Wangiella* by cultural, microscopic, physiologic, and clinical means.

4. Distinguish between the similar-appearing molds *Cladosporium carrionii* and *Cladosporium trichoides*.

5. Compare and contrast microscopic attributes of *Fonsecaea pedrosoi* and *Fonsecaea compacta*.

6. Discriminate between *Sporothrix schenckii* and the similar-appearing contaminant *Acremonium* sp.

7. Define, identify, or discuss the significance of:

   Sclerotic bodies
   Cigar bodies
   Daisy head

Two stages of *Scedosporium apiospermum*
Two phases of *Sporothrix schenckii*
Actinomycete

8. Compare and contrast oxygen requirements, acid-fastness, macro- and microscopic appearance, and odor of the following:

   Nocardia sp.
   Streptomyces sp.
   Group IV Mycobacteria
   Actinomyces sp.

9. Briefly describe four physiologic procedures for aerobic actinomycete identification. Include a description of positive and negative results.

10. Concerning anaerobic actinomycetes, list preliminary identification procedures and results recommended prior to sending the organism to a reference laboratory.

11. Briefly describe chromoblastomycosis, phaeohyphomycosis mycetoma, nocardiosis, actinomycosis, and sporotrichosis, including causative organisms, "dot" or granule characteristics, and mode of transmission.

CONTENT OUTLINE

I. Introduction
II. Molds
   A. Dematiaceous molds
      1. *Cladosporium carrionii*
      2. *Cladosporium trichoides*
      3. *Fonsecaea compacta*
      4. *Fonsecaea pedrosoi*
      5. *Phialophora verrucosa*
      6. *Exophiala jeanselmei*
      7. *Wangiella dermatitidis*
   B. Hyaline molds
      1. *Scedosporium apiospermum*
      2. *Sporothrix schenckii*
   C. Study questions
III. Funguslike bacteria
   A. Aerobic actinomycetes
      1. *Nocardia* sp.
      2. *Streptomyces* sp.
      3. Tests for aerobic actinomycetes
   B. Mycobacteria
   C. Anaerobic actinomycetes
IV. Final exam
V. Supplemental Rationale
   A. Actinomycosis
   B. Chromoblastomycosis
   C. Mycetoma
   D. Nocardiosis
   E. Phaeohyphomycosis
   F. Sporotrichosis
   G. Study questions

FOLLOW-UP ACTIVITIES

1. Students may perform the modified Kinyoun acid-fast stain on *Nocardia* sp. and *Mycobacterium fortuitum,* and compare microscopic features.

2. Students may observe colonies and slide culture preparations of fungi that produce subcutaneous mycoses.

3. Students may convert *Sporothrix schenckii* from the mold to yeast phase.

REFERENCES

BENEKE, ES AND ROGERS, AL: *Medical Mycology Manual,* ed 4. Burgess Publishing Co., Minneapolis, 1980.

BRYAN, CS: *Petriellidium boydii infection of the sphenoid sinus.* Am J Clin Pathol 74:846, 1980.

CONANT, NF, ET AL: *Manual of Clinical Mycology,* ed 3. WB Saunders, Philadelphia, 1971.

EMMONS, CW, ET AL: *Medical Mycology,* ed 3. Lea & Febiger, Philadelphia, 1977.

GEORG, LK, ROBERSTAD, GW, AND BRINKMAN, SA: *Identification of species of Actinomyces.* J Bacteriol 88:477, 1964.

GORDON, MA: *Anaerobic pathogenic actinomycetaceae.* In LENNETTE, EH, SPAULDING, EH, AND TRUANT, JR (EDS): *Manual of Clinical Microbiology,* ed 2. American Society for Microbiology Washington, DC, 1974.

HALEY, LD AND CALLAWAY, CS: *Laboratory Methods in Medical Mycology,* ed 4. U.S. Department of Health, Education, and Welfare, Washington, DC, 1978.

HIRONAGA, M, ET AL: *Annellated conidiogenous cells in Exophiala dermatitidis: Agent of phaeohyphomycosis.* Mycologia 73:1181, 1981.

HOLLICK, GE: *Nocardiosis.* Am J Med Tech 1:267, 1984.

KONEMAN, EW, ROBERTS, GD, AND WRIGHT, SF: *Practical Laboratory Mycology,* ed 2. Williams & Wilkins, Baltimore, 1978.

KWON CHUNG, KJ AND deVRIES, GA: *A comparative study of an isolate resembling Banti's fungus with Cladosporium trichoides.* Sabouraudia (in press).

LARONE, DH: *Medically Important Fungi: A Guide to Identification.* Harper & Row, Hagerstown, Md, 1976.

LOWE, RM, ET AL: *Acid fast actinomyces in a child with pulmonary actinomycosis.* J Clin Microbiol 12:124, 1980.

LUFF, RD, ET AL: *Pelvic actinomycosis and the intrauterine contraceptive device: A cyto-histomorphologic study.* Am J Clin Pathol 69:581, 1978.

McGINNIS, MR, D'AMATO, RF, AND LAND, GA: *Pictorial Handbook of Medically Important Fungi and Aerobic Actinomycetes.* Praeger Publishers, New York, 1982.

McGINNIS, MR: *Chromoblastomycosis. Check-Sample.* Advanced Microbiology AMB 82-3,4 (AMB-39,40). American Society for Clinical Pathology, Chicago, 1982.

McGINNIS, MR: *Chromoblastomycosis and phaeohyphomycosis: New concepts, diagnosis, and mycology.* J Am Acad Derm 8:1, 1983.

MISHRA, SK, GORDON, RE, AND BARNETT, DA: *Identification of nocardiae and streptomycetes of medical importance.* J Clin Microbiol 11:728, 1980.

MOK, WY: *Nature and identification of Exophiala werneckii.* J. Clin Microbiol 16:976, 1982.

NISHIMURA, K AND MIYAJI, M: *Studies on a saprophyte of Exophiala dermatitidis isolated from a humidifier.* Mycopathologia 77:173, 1982.

RIPPON, JW AND KATHURIA, SK: *Actinomyces meyeri presenting as an asymptomatic lung mass.* Mycopathologia 84:187, 1984.

SONNENWIRTH, AC AND DOWELL, VR: *Gram-positive, nonsporeforming anaerobic bacilli.* In LENNETTE, EH, ET AL (EDS): *Manual of Clinical Microbiology,* ed 3. American Society for Microbiology Washington, DC, 1980.

STANECK, JL, ET AL: *Infection of bone by Mycobacterium fortuitum masquerading as Nocardia asteroides.* Am J Clin Pathol 76:216, 1981.

STANECK, JL AND ROBERTS, GD: *Simplified approach to identification of aerobic actinomycetes by thin layer chromatography.* Applied Microbiol 28:226, 1974.

INTRODUCTION

Subcutaneous mycoses may develop when the skin is punctured or abraded with thorns or other vegetation contaminated with fungi that live in the soil. The organisms establish themselves in the skin and produce a localized infection in the surrounding underlying tissue and lymph nodes. Rarely does the infection disseminate. Subcutaneous lesions are characterized by chronic, nonhealing, hard, lumpy, crusted, ulcerated areas which periodically exude fluid. The extremities, especially the feet, are often involved, since they come into more frequent contact with thorns and so forth. Although subcutaneous mycoses are common in the tropics, they are found worldwide.

In addition to higher fungi, the funguslike bacteria are covered in this module. The latter may produce disease manifestations other than subcutaneous mycoses as primary infections. For lack of a better place to put them, the nonsubcutaneous diseases caused by funguslike bacteria are included here.

Because the causative organisms of subcutaneous infections are ubiquitous in nature, cultural isolation alone is not significant. Tissue invasion must be demonstrated via potassium hydroxide and histopathology preparations.

Specimens are taken from active lesions. If small (0.5 to 2.0 mm), variously colored granules (Fig. 6-1) or black dots are observed on the lesion surface or in oozing fluid, these are also collected. Note the color of the dots and granules, as the color may indicate which organism is producing the infection. **(See Chart 6-1 on page 184 at end of module.)**

In histologic stains or potassium hydroxide-dimethyl sulfoxide (KOH-DMSO) preparations, crushed black dots from chromoblastomycosis appear as thick walled, dark brown, round sclerotic bodies, with a single cell or multiple cells formed by cross-walls (Fig. 6-2). Granules from mycetoma exhibit two morphologies: those from higher fungi **(eumycotic mycetoma)** contain pigmented hyphae 2 to 5 μm wide, sometimes accompanied by chlamydoconidia (Fig. 6-3); those from funguslike bacteria **(actinomycotic mycetoma)** contain a center of necrotic debris and peripheral fine, one-micrometer wide, branching, interwoven filaments often surrounded by a gelatinous sheath (Fig. 6-4). The sheath makes the filaments appear club shaped at the granule edge. Dots and granules are not observed in phaeohyphomycosis or sporotrichosis, and only rarely in nocardiosis.

Specimens are processed as in Module 2. Wash the granules several times in sterile saline to remove contamination before plating. Inoculate specimens to Sabouraud dextrose agar with and without antibiotics. Since *Nocardia asteroides* is sometimes inhibited by Sabouraud agar, a plain brain heart infusion agar is additionally inoculated. If the physican suspects *Actinomyces*, inoculate a brain heart infusion plate anaerobically or a thioglycollate broth. Incubate the Sabouraud agars at room temperature or 30°C, and the brain heart infusion agars or thioglycollate at 37°C.

Organisms causing subcutaneous mycoses are dematiaceous molds, hyaline molds, and funguslike bacteria. Dematiaceous molds may require three or four weeks to develop, while the light-colored ones grow more rap-

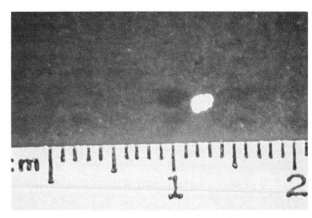

FIGURE 6-1. White granule. (From Dolan, et al: Atlas of Clinical Mycology. ASCP, Washington, DC, 1976, with permission.)

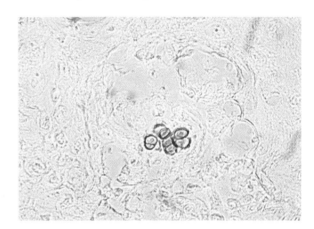

FIGURE 6-2. Sclerotic bodies in tissue, Gridley stain, ×450.

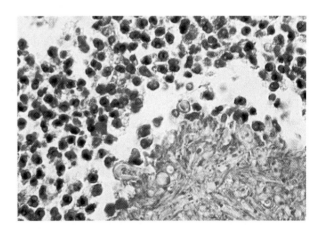

FIGURE 6-3. Eumycotic granule (bottom half of photo), hematoxylin and eosin stain, ×450.

idly. Funguslike bacteria, which possess dry, glabrous, chalky colonies resembling mycobacteria, vary from rapid to intermediate growing, depending on the species. Mold identification is largely dependent on microscopic morphology. Speciation of funguslike bacteria incorporates a battery of physiologic tests.

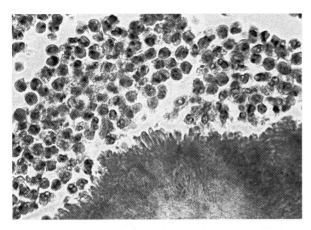

FIGURE 6-4. Actinomycotic granule with clubbed filaments (bottom half of photo), hematoxylin and eosin stain, ×450.

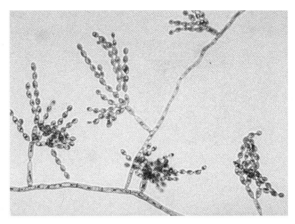

FIGURE 6-5. *Cladosporium carrionii*, lactophenol cotton blue (LPCB) stain, ×450.

MOLDS

Dematiaceous Molds

These organisms may appear as black yeasts at first on Sabouraud dextrose agar, then later form short, velvety aerial hyphae and conidia. On slide cultures, potato dextrose or corn meal agar is excellent for promoting conidial formation.

The dematiaceous molds are grouped by similar microscopic morphology:

a. Branching chains of conidia
  1. *Cladosporium carrionii*
  2. *Cladosporium trichoides*
b. More than one type of conidial formation
  1. *Fonsecaea compacta*
  2. *Fonsecaea pedrosoi*
c. Balls of conidia
  1. *Phialophora verrucosa*
  2. *Exophiala jeanselmei*
  3. *Wangiella dermatitidis*

Important characteristics for each mold are in capital letters. Disease entity, presence of sclerotic bodies or granules, and granule morphology are also important distinguishing features for speciating similar fungi.

Branching Chains of Conidia

CLADOSPORIUM CARRIONII
(Figs. 6-5 and 6-6)

Culture: On Sabouraud dextrose agar at room temperature, SLOW-GROWING black colonies develop dark velvety mycelium.

Microscopic: The hyphae are dark. Long or short conidiophores support REPEATEDLY BRANCHING SHORT CHAINS OF BLASTOCONIDIA (4.8 to 5.2 μm in diameter). On certain media, phialides with

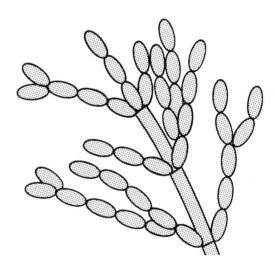

FIGURE 6-6. *Cladosporium carrionii.*

balls of phialoconidia, similar to *Phialophora*, may be observed.

Other comments: C. carrionii DOES NOT GROW AT 42°C and has NO NEUROTROPIC PROPENSITY. *Cladosporium carrionii* and *trichoides* are very similar morphologically. Growth rate, blastoconidial size, growth temperature, and site of infection should differentiate them. C. carrionii does not hydrolyze gelatin.

Pathogenicity: *Cladosporium carrionii* causes chromoblastomycosis.

CLADOSPORIUM TRICHOIDES
(Figs. 6-7 and 6-8)

Culture: On Sabouraud dextrose agar at room temperature, a black, compact colony forms MODERATELY RAPIDLY. The reverse is black.

165

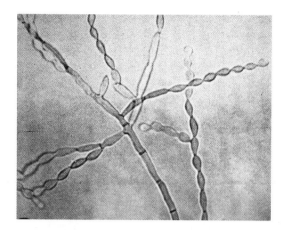

FIGURE 6-7. *Cladosporium trichoides,* ×690. (From Emmons, et al: Medical Mycology. Lea & Febiger, 1977, Philadelphia, with permission.)

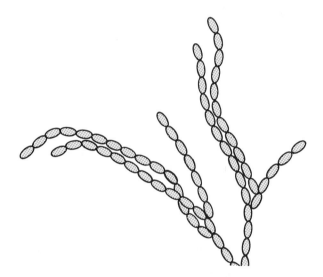

FIGURE 6-8. *Cladosporium trichoides.*

Microscopic: The hyphae are dark. Long or short conidiophores support SPARSELY BRANCHING LONG CHAINS OF BLASTOCONIDIA (7.3 to 7.6 μm in diameter).

Other comments: *C. trichoides* GROWS AT 42°C and has a tendency to INVADE NEURAL TISSUE in animal studies. It does not hydrolyze (liquefy) gelatin: in the past, contaminant *Cladosporium* species were differentiated from the pathogenic strains mentioned in this module by the contaminants' ability to hydrolyze gelatin. This test is unreliable and diagnosis should be made on clinical grounds instead.

Pathogenicity: *Cladosporium trichoides* causes subcutaneous and systemic phaeohyphomycosis.

More Than One Type of Conidial Formation

FONSECAEA COMPACTA (Figs. 6-9 and 6-10)

Culture: On Sabouraud dextrose agar at room temperature, a VERY SLOW-GROWING, small black colony develops low, dark velvety mycelium.

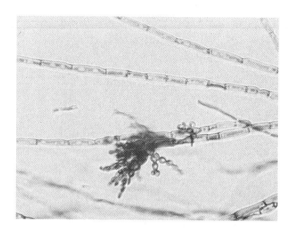

FIGURE 6-9. *Fonsecaea compacta,* LPCB stain, ×450.

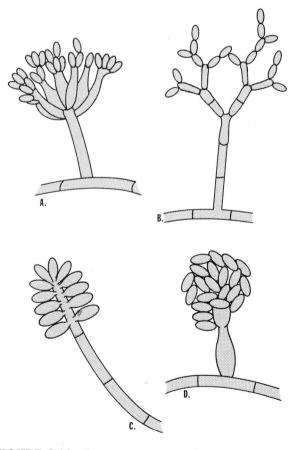

FIGURE 6-10. *Fonsecaea compacta.*

Microscopic: The hyphae are dark. PRIMARY BLASTOCONIDIA at the tip of conidiophores each support one to four SECONDARY CONIDIA, which in turn may produce one to four TERTIARY CONIDIA (Fig. 6-10A). This arrangement culminates in COMPACT CONIDIAL HEADS, while those in similar-appearing *F. pedrosoi* are more loosely organized. Three other types of conidial formation may be less commonly seen: branching chains of blastoconidia as in *Cladosporium* sp. (Fig. 6-10B); one-celled conidia arising opposite each other at the conidiophore tip, the old-named acrotheca sporulation as in *Rhinocladiella* sp. (Fig. 6-10C); and flask-shaped phialides with balls of phialoconidia, as in *Phialophora* sp. (Fig. 6-10D). In the past, identification was based upon observation of at least two of the three less common types of conidial arrangements. Now the key morphologic form, the first description above, is employed instead.

Pathogenicity: Fonsecaea compacta causes chromoblastomycosis.

FONSECAEA PEDROSOI
(Figs. 6-11 and 6-12)

Culture: On Sabouraud dextrose agar at room temperature, a SLOW-GROWING, black colony with low, dark olive to black aerial mycelium is formed (see Color Plate 4).

Microscopic: The hyphae are dark. PRIMARY BLASTOCONIDIA at the tip of the conidiophores each support one to four SECONDARY CONIDIA, which in turn may produce one to four TERTIARY CONIDIA (Fig. 6-12A). This arrangement culminates in LOOSELY ORGANIZED CONIDIAL HEADS, while those of *F. compacta* are more compact. Three other types of conidial formations may be less commonly

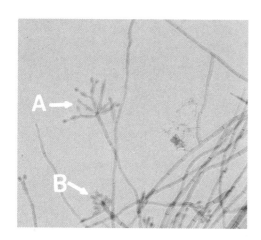

FIGURE 6-11. *Fonsecaea pedrosoi,* **LPCB stain, ×450. Arrow A indicates the key morphologic form; arrow B points to a *Rhinocladiella*like conidial arrangement.**

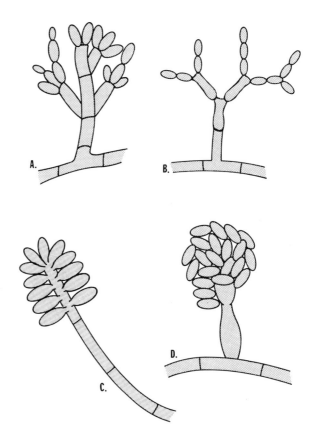

FIGURE 6-12. *Fonsecaea pedrosoi.*

seen: branching chains of blastoconidia as in *Cladosporium* sp. (Fig. 6-12B); one-celled conidia arising opposite each other at the conidiophore tip, the old-named acrotheca sporulation as in *Rhinocladiella* sp. (Fig. 6-12C); and flask-shaped phialides with balls of phialoconidia, as in *Phialophora* sp. (Fig. 6-12D). In the past, identification was based upon observation of at least two of the three less common types of conidial arrangements. Now the key morphologic form, the first description above, is employed instead.

Pathogenicity: F. pedrosoi causes chromoblastomycosis and occasionally systemic phaeohyphomycosis.

Balls of Conidia

PHIALOPHORA VERRUCOSA
(Figs. 6-13 and 6-14)

Culture: On Sabouraud dextrose agar at room temperature, a slow-growing black colony with matted dark mycelium is produced (Color Plate 58).

Microscopic: The hyphae are dark. Flask-shaped PHIALIDES with a distinct CUP-SHAPED COLLARETTE elicit terminal BALLS of oval PHIALOCONIDIA. Phialides may form on the tips of conidiophores or directly off the sides of the hyphae.

Pathogenicity: *Phialophora verrucosa* causes chromoblastomycosis, subcutaneous phaeohyphomycosis, and rarely mycotic keratitis.

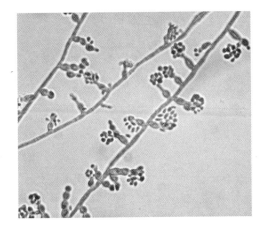

FIGURE 6-13. *Phialophora verrucosa,* **LPCB stain,** ×450.

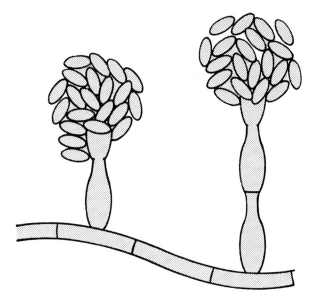

FIGURE 6-14. *Phialophora verrucosa.*

EXOPHIALA (PHIALOPHORA) JEANSELMEI (Figs. 6-15 and 6-16)

Culture: On Sabouraud dextrose agar at room temperature, a BLACK YEAST forms, which slowly develops dark velvety mycelium (Color Plate 59).

Microscopic: At first, only dark budding yeasts are observed (Fig. 6-16A.). With age, ANNELLIDES on annellophores produce CLUSTERS of oval ANNELLOCONIDIA at the tips (Fig. 6-16B); then the annelloconidia tend to fall down the sides of the stalk. This second morphology resembles that of *Wangiella* and *Phialophora.* The conidiogenous cell of *Wangiella* is

tubed like *Exophiala,* but annellations are usually not present. In *Phialophora,* the conidiogenous cell is a vase-shaped phialide. The annellide rings of *Exophiala* may be difficult to discern,* but phase contrast and scanning electron microscopy aid greatly in diagnosis. Clusters of conidia may also form off short denticles on the sides of the hyphae (Fig. 6-16C).

Pathogenicity: *Exophiala jeanselmei* causes mycetoma, subcutaneous and systemic phaeohyphomycosis, and mycotic keratitis.

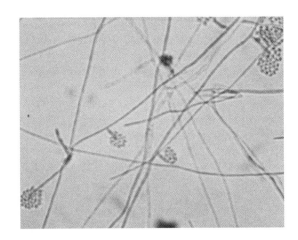

FIGURE 6-15. *Exophiala jeanselmei,* **LPCB stain,** ×450.

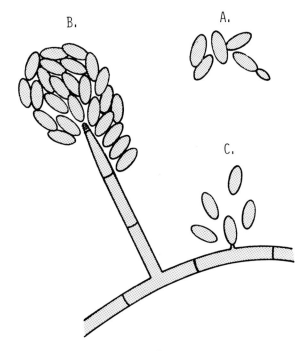

FIGURE 6-16. *Exophiala jeanselmei.*

E. jeanselmei is morphologically easily mistaken for *E. werneckii* (Module 4) and *W. dermatitidis.* The reactions listed on the chart at the top of the next page may differentiate them. (See Mok (1982) for further information.)

168

	Decomposition of		NaNO$_3$ utilization	Max. growth temp. (°C)
	Casein	Tyrosine		
E. werneckii	+	−	+	42
E. jeanselmei	−	+	+	38
W. dermatitidis	−	+	−	42

WANGIELLA (PHIALOPHORA) DERMATITIDIS (Figs. 6-17 and 6-18)

Culture: On Sabouraud dextrose agar at room temperature, colonies are initially shiny BLACK and YEASTY. With time, the periphery develops a dark velvety mycelium.

Microscopic: At first, dark budding yeasts are observed (Fig. 6-18A). With age, a few tubelike PHIALIDES WITHOUT A COLLARETTE and usually without annellations* elicit terminal BALLS of CONIDIA (Fig. 6-18B). The conidia tend to fall down the sides of the phialides. Clusters of conidia may also form off short denticles on the sides of the hyphae (Fig. 6-18C). The yeast form remains predominant.

Other comments: W. dermatitidis morphologically resembles E. jeanselmei, but the former remains more yeastlike, GROWS AT 42°C (E. jeanselmei does not) and is NITRATE NEGATIVE (E. jeanselmei is nitrate positive). See Mok (1982) for further details.

Pathogenicity: Wangiella dermatitidis causes phaeohyphomycosis.

Hyaline Molds

Although the hyaline molds listed below may produce dark-colored colonies and conidia, the hyphae and conidia are usually blue in lactophenol cotton blue

---

*Hironaga et al (1981) and Nishimura and Miyaji (1982) argue that the genus Wangiella should be included with Exophiala, since annellations are present under electron microscopy. McGinnis (1980) feels that Wangiella should stay separate because of its conspicuous yeastlike form and thermotolerance, the inability to observe the annellations with a light microscope, and that phialides rather than annellides are the most distinct, stable, and unique form.

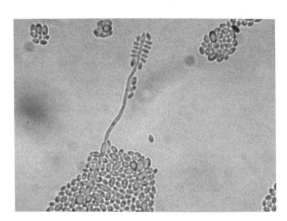

FIGURE 6-17. *Wangiella dermatitidis,* LPCB stain, ×450.

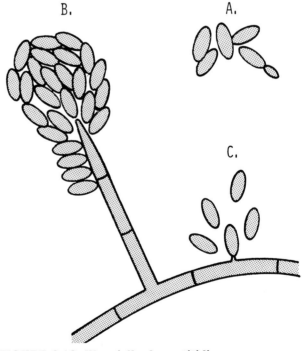

FIGURE 6-18. *Wangiella dermatitidis.*

mounts. Some common light-colored organisms causing subcutaneous disease follow, with key identifying features capitalized.

SCEDOSPORIUM (MONOSPORIUM) APIOSPERMUM (Fig. 6-19)

Culture: On Sabouraud dextrose agar at room temperature, a white fluffy colony develops moderately rapidly, later turning gray with a gray reverse (Color Plate 60).

Microscopic: In the asexual stage, large, SINGLE or small clustered, oval ANNELLOCONIDIA are TERMINALLY produced on long or short annellophores. The annellophores are at the end or on the sides of the hyphae. This asexual morphology is similar to that of the contaminant *Chrysosporium* sp. (Module 3) and the mold phase of the dimorphic fungus *Blastomyces dermatitidis* (Module 7). *Scedosporium* may be differentiated by the diseases it causes and its inability to convert to a yeast phase at 37°C.

Pseudallescheria (Petriellidium, Allescheria) boydii (Figs. 6-20 and 6-21), the sexual stage, may sometimes be observed on potato dextrose or corn meal agar. Large brown CLEISTOTHECIA, 50 to 200 μm in diameter, are seen, which when ruptured disperse ASCI containing 8 light brown, oval ASCOSPORES.

Other comments: With age, the conidia may become slightly dark.

Pathogenicity: *Scedosporium apiospermum* is the most likely agent of mycetoma in the United States. This organism also may cause pulmonary disease, sinusitis, fungus ball, mycotic keratitis, prostatitis, chronic otomycosis, meningomycosis, and systemic disease.

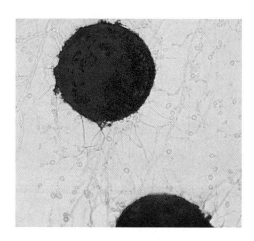

FIGURE 6-20. Sexual stage cleistothecia, *Pseudallescheria boydii.* In the background is the asexual stage, *Scedosporium apiospermum.* (From Dolan, et al: Atlas of Clinical Mycology. ASCP, Washington, DC, 1976, with permission.)

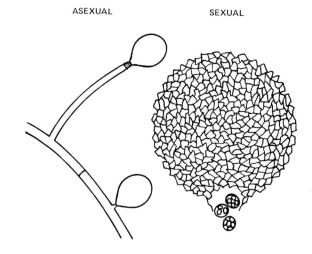

ASEXUAL   SEXUAL

FIGURE 6-21. (Left) Asexual stage, *Scedosporium apiospermum;* (Right) sexual stage, *Pseudallescheria boydii.*

SPOROTHRIX SCHENCKII (Fig. 6-22 and 6-23)

Culture: On Sabouraud dextrose agar at room temperature, this DIMORPHIC fungus forms a cream-colored, wrinkled, leathery colony which may later turn black. The black color is enhanced on potato dextrose or corn meal agar. The mold phase may resemble the glabrous forms of *Acremonium* sp. (Module 3), but the latter does not turn black with age. The 37°C yeast phase colonies are soft and white to cream colored. (See Color Plates 61 to 63.)

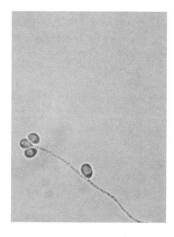

FIGURE 6-19. Asexual stage, *Scedosporium apiospermum,* LPCB stain, ×450.

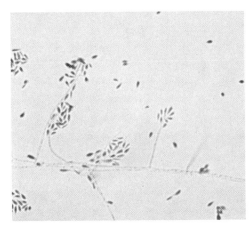

FIGURE 6-22. Mold phase, *Sporothrix schenckii*, LPCB stain, ×450.

Microscopic: At room temperature, the MOLD appears as small oval hyaline or dematiaceous conidia arranged singly along the hyphae, and as a DAISY HEAD, or flowerette, at the ends of short, unbranched conidiophores. The conidia are attached to the conidiophore by minute hairlike structures, not visible except under oil immersion. The flowerette is not as closely packed as the conidia of the similar-appearing *Acremonium*. Also the latter cannot be converted to a yeast phase.

Sporothrix schenckii YEASTS are small, elliptical, budding cells resembling cigars; hence the name CIGAR BODIES has been used to describe them (Color Plate 64). Note that some hyphae may be observed along with the cigar bodies when the fungus is converted in vitro to the yeast phase.

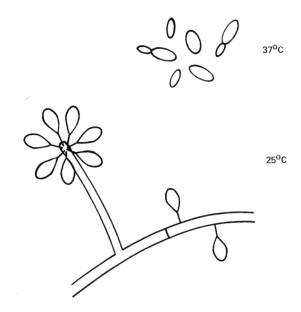

37°C

25°C

FIGURE 6-23. Mold and yeast phases, *Sporothrix schenckii*.

Other comments: The mold is converted to a yeast by subculturing from Sabouraud dextrose agar to brain heart infusion agar, with or without 10 percent blood, at 37°C in 5 percent CO_2 for three to five days. The medium must be kept moist, and one or two rapid serial subcultures may be necessary for yeast formation. Conversion does not need to be complete—in fact, it is very difficult in vitro. Any typical yeast cells indicate dimorphism.

Pathogenicity: *Sporothrix schenckii* causes sporotrichosis and rarely mycotic keratitis.

Study questions

1. **Circle the letter of the correct answer.**

   Cladosporium trichoides and *Cladosporium carrionii* appear very similar culturally and microscopically. They may be speciated by all of the following *except:*

   A. *C. trichoides* grows at 42°C; *C. carrionii* does not.

   B. *C. trichoides* produces sclerotic bodies; *C. carrionii* does not.

   C. *C. trichoides* has a predilection for neural tissues; *C. carrionii* does not.

   D. *C. trichoides* grows more rapidly than *C. carrionii.*

   E. *C. trichoides* exhibits larger blastoconidia than *C. carrionii.*

2. **Fill in the chart below, using colonial, microscopic, physiologic, and clinical attributes.**

Wangiella dermatitidis Similarities	*Exophiala jeanselmei* Similarities
1. _____	1. _____
2. _____	2. _____
3. _____	3. _____

Box continues on next page.

Differences

1. _____

2. _____

3. _____
_____

Differences

1. _____

2. _____

3. _____
_____

3. Which of the following may demonstrate phialoconidia and cup-shaped collarettes as seen in Figure 6-24? Circle the letter(s) of the correct answer.

   A. *Exophiala jeanselmei*
   B. *Fonsecaea pedrosoi*
   C. *Scedosporium apiospermum*
   D. *Fonsecaea compacta*
   E. *Wangiella dermatitidis*
   F. *Phialophora verrucosa*

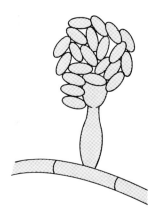

FIGURE 6-24. Study question demonstration.

4. Circle the correct answer. *Fonsecaea compacta* and *Fonsecaea pedrosoi* may be differentiated from each other in that:

   A. *F. pedrosoi* conidial heads are more loosely arranged.
   B. Both may exhibit four separate conidial designs.
   C. Only *F. compacta* produces chromoblastomycosis.
   D. *F. compacta* is a rapid grower.
   E. *F. pedrosoi* colonies are initially cream-colored and leathery, and later turn black with age.

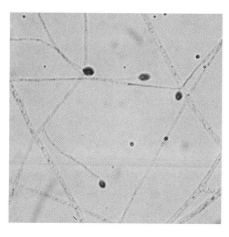

FIGURE 6-25. Study question demonstration, LPCB stain, ×450.

5. See Figure 6-25. This fungus is the leading cause of eumycotic mycetoma in the U.S. (circle the correct letter):

   A. *Cladosporium carrionii*
   B. *Sporothrix schenckii*
   C. *Scedosporium apiospermum*
   D. *Fonsecaea pedrosoi*
   E. *Fonsecaea compacta*

6. Regarding question 5, what other reproductive structure could you expect to observe?

STOP HERE UNTIL YOU HAVE COMPLETED THE ANSWERS.

Look up the answers in the back of the book. If you missed more than two, go back and repeat the Introduction, Dematiaceous, and Hyaline Fungi sections of this module. Correctly complete any missed questions before proceeding.

FUNGUSLIKE BACTERIA

Funguslike bacteria are microorganisms not classified with the true fungi, but rather with the bacterial subdivision Schizomycotina, order Actinomycetales (see Chart 1-2 and Supplemental Rationale section of Module 1). The term **actinomycete** is used to denote all the Actinomycetales except the family Mycobacteriaceae. Colonies and the microscopic, thin (one micrometer in diameter) mycelia or filaments are typical of bacteria, but the organisms branch, produce conidia, and cause mycoticlike diseases, thus also resembling fungi. The actinomycetes include the genera *Nocardia*, *Streptomyces*, and *Actinomyces*.

Aerobic Actinomycetes

NOCARDIA SPECIES

Nocardia sp. are PARTIALLY ACID-FAST (see gray box in Module 2, page 52, for the modified Kinyoun acid-fast stain). 7H10 and 7H11 agars enhance the acid-fast properties of *Nocardia*, while Sabouraud dextrose, brain heart infusion, and blood agars do not; therefore, take suspected isolates from the former media for the stain.

Nocardia sp. survive mycobacterial concentration procedures and grow rapidly on mycobacterial media. Colonies may be mistaken for mycobacteria: they are chalky, brittle, verrucose, and white to orange, or pink to red* (see Color Plates 9 and 65). However, with *Nocardia*, short aerial hyphae are usually observed under a dissecting microscope and an EARTHY ODOR, similar to the smell of mud after a rainfall, is exuded. Microscopically, branching filaments may fragment into bacillary forms. Tiny CONIDIA may be produced in older cultures, although not in *N. brasiliensis*. *Nocardia asteroides*, *Nocardia brasiliensis*, and *Nocardia caviae* cause nocardiosis and occasionally actinomycotic mycetoma. Tissue granules are not usually observed in the first disease, but they are common in the second. *Nocardia (Actinomadura) madurae* and *Nocardia (Actinomadura) pelletierii* produce actinomycotic mycetoma with white or red granules, respectively. *Nocardia (Actinomadura) dassonvillei* has been cultured from ulcerative, granulomatous lesions and especially pulmonary sites; no granules have been reported.

STREPTOMYCES SPECIES

Streptomyces sp. are NON–ACID-FAST (though conidia of contaminant strains may be) and grow rapidly on most primary isolation media, including mycobacterial inhibitory egg medium. Do not use media with cy-

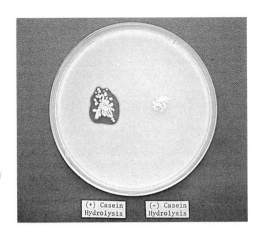

FIGURE 6-26. Casein hydrolysis. In a positive test, the medium around the colony is clear, or hydrolyzed.

cloheximide and chloramphenicol. Colonies resemble *Nocardia* and exude an EARTHY ODOR. Short aerial hyphae are usually observed. Microscopically, branching filaments do not fragment easily, and CONIDIA may be produced with age. *Streptomyces somaliensis* causes actinomycotic mycetoma, with white to yellow granules. *Streptomyces griseus* has occasionally been isolated from subcutaneous abscesses and mycetomas. Most *Streptomyces* sp. are nonpathogenic contaminants.

---

*Note that isolation media must not contain cycloheximide or chloramphenicol, as these antibiotics suppress funguslike bacteria. Also some strains of *N. asteroides* may be inhibited on Sabouraud dextrose agar. Once purified, aerobic actinomycetes can be cultured on Czapek-Dox agar to enhance colony color and microscopic conidial formation.

Mycobacterium fortuitum can be misdiagnosed as *Nocardia asteroides*:

	N. asteroides	M. fortuitum
Acid-fast	+	+
Colonial morphology	variable	variable
Growth at 45°C	±	−
Catalase	+	+
Casein hydrolysis	−	−
Tyrosine	−	−
Xanthine	−	−
Cell wall sugars	Arabinose-galactose	Arabinose-galactose
Gelatin	−	−
DAP in cell wall	meso	meso
INH resistance	+	+

Therapy for these two infections is quite different, with *N. asteroides* requiring sulfa, minocycline, or doxycycline, and *M. fortuitum* requiring antimycobacterial agents. Thus it is imperative for the two organisms to be correctly identified. Perform lipid chromatography: *N. asteroides* contains LCN-A, while *M. fortuitum* does not. See Staneck et al (1981) for further details.

Since *Nocardia* and *Streptomyces* are so similar culturally and microscopically, speciation is primarily dependent on physiologic tests.

Tests for Aerobic Actinomycetes

The casein (Fig. 6-26), tyrosine, xanthine, and urease tests, plus microscopic appearance on tap water agar, will usually speciate the organism (gray boxes and **Chart 6-2 on page 185).** Also *N. asteroides* grows at 45°C, while *N. brasiliensis* does not. If there is still difficulty identifying the funguslike bacterium, starch hydrolysis, gelatin hydrolysis, sugar assimilations, DAP chromatography, and lipid chromatography may be performed. (See Haley and Callaway (1978), Staneck and Roberts (1974), and Mishra et al (1980) for further information.)

CASEIN, TYROSINE, AND XANTHINE HYDROLYSIS FOR AEROBIC ACTINOMYCETES

Media Preparation
Commercially available (Remel, 12076 Santa Fe Drive, Lenexa, Kansas 66215)

Casein agar:
  Solution A
Dehydrated or instant nonfat skim milk	10.0 gm
Distilled water	100.0 ml

  1. Dissolve the milk in water, tube in 10 ml aliquots, autoclave at 15 psi for 15 minutes, and cool.

  Solution B
Agar	2.0 gm
Distilled water	100.0 ml

  1. Heat the agar and water to dissolve, tube in 10 ml aliquots, autoclave at 15 psi for 15 minutes, and cool.
  2. Mix one tube each of Solution A and Solution B together in a Petri dish and allow to harden.

Xanthine and Tyrosine agar:
Nutrient agar	23.0 gm
Demineralized water	1 liter
Xanthine OR	4 gm OR
Tyrosine	5 gm

1. Combine the agar, half the water, and either xanthine or tyrosine crystals. Add the rest of the water.
2. Adjust the pH to 7.0 and autoclave at 15 psi for 15 minutes.
3. Cool until the medium is almost solidified and pour into Petri dishes that have been refrigerated for 30 minutes prior to pouring. This last step prevents the crystals from settling out. Make sure the crystals are evenly distributed in the plates. Allow the agar to harden.

Procedure
1. Inoculate a 5-mm area on each of the above plates with the test organism. Be sure to include positive and negative controls on the same plate.
2. Incubate at room temperature for up to four weeks and observe for clearing (or hydrolysis) of the medium around the colony—a positive test. No clearing is a negative test.

UREASE TEST*

Medium Preparation

Commercially available as Christenson's urea agar slants (Difco, BBL)

Urea agar base (Difco, BBL)	**29 gm**
Distilled water	**100 ml**
Agar	**15 gm**
Distilled water	**900 ml**

1. Dissolve the urea in water and filter sterilize.
2. Dissolve the agar in water and autoclave at 15 psi for 15 minutes.
3. After the agar has cooled to 50°C, add the urea agar base solution, mix well, and aseptically put in tubes. Slant the tubes so that there is a one-inch butt and allow them to harden. Refrigerate.

Procedure

1. Inoculate a 5-mm area on the slant of a tube that has been warmed to room temperature. Be sure to inoculate a positive and negative control.
2. Incubate the tubes at room temperature for up to four weeks.
3. A pink-purple color is a positive test; no color change is a negative test.

*This procedure may be used for differentiation of yeasts, aerobic actinomycetes, and some *Trichophyton* species.

MORPHOLOGY ON TAP WATER AGAR

Medium Preparation

Agar	**15 gm**
Tap water	**1000 ml**

1. Add the agar to water and autoclave at 15 psi for 15 minutes.
2. Pour into Petri dishes, and allow to harden.

Procedure

1. Streak a purified isolate onto the plate.
2. Incubate 24–72 hours at 35°C, or up to 1 week at room temperature.
3. Invert the plate and observe it under low power on the microscope. Submerged filaments will appear fine and delicate; aerial hyphae will be coarse and black.

Mycobacteria

Group IV rapid-growing mycobacteria are not funguslike bacteria, but they are easily confused with the aerobic actinomycetes. It is desirable to learn some distinguishing characteristics of the former in order to rule them out. Mycobacteria are aerobic, growing well on TB media and sometimes on fungal media. Colonies are brittle or smooth, beige to yellow-orange, and no aerial hyphae are produced on tap water agar. An earthy odor is not present. Mycobacteria are acid-fast, even after decolorizing for three minutes. Microscopically, short bacillary filaments rarely branch and no conidia are produced. Physiologic tests give reactions characteristic for each mycobacterial species. These organisms do not cause mycetoma.

Anaerobic Actinomycetes

Anaerobic actinomycetes are ANAEROBIC, facultatively anaerobic, or microaerophilic; they are not acid-fast in culture and grow in 7 to 10 days. On brain heart infusion agar at 37°C under an atmosphere of 95 percent N_2 and 5 percent CO_2, colonies are small, white, and flat or centrally indented, resembling a MOLAR TOOTH (Color Plate 66). In thioglycollate broth (Fig.

175

6-27), pure cultures present a BREAD CRUMB or diffuse appearance. Microscopically, long or short BRANCHING FILAMENTS and DIPHTHEROID FORMS are observed. On Gram stains of clinical material (Fig. 6-28), *Actinomyces* may appear as Gram-positive rods or coccobacilli due to fragmentation, and the organism can be mistaken for diphtheroids. No conidia are produced.

Actinomyces israelii and *naeslundii* are isolated as normal flora from saliva and tonsillar crypts. Sputum may contain anaerobic actinomycetes, reflecting colonization rather than infection; thus, for suspected pulmonary actinomycosis, specimens of choice are lung biopsy, pulmonary needle aspiration, or pleural fluid. *Actinomyces israelii*, *Actinomyces bovis*, *Actinomyces naeslundii*, *Actinomyces meyeri*, *Actinomyces viscosus*, *Arachnia propionica*, and *Bifidobacterium adolescentis* (*Actinomyces eriksonii*) may cause actinomycosis. The characteristic sulfur-colored granules associated with this disease are produced by some but not all *Actinomyces* sp. and *Arachnia propionica*, while *Bifidobacterium adolescentis* does not exhibit them. Note that bacteria may form granules resembling those of funguslike bacteria, and the causative organisms must be differentiated physiologically. *Actinomyces israelli* and *bovis* may cause actinomycotic mycetoma, with oozing sinuses containing sulfur granules.

Examine streaked anaerobic plates under a dissecting microscope at 48 hours and again at 7 to 10 days to observe the colonial morphology. Perform a Gram stain and inoculate three brain heart infusion slants with an isolated colony of the test organism. Incubate one slant aerobically. After 24 to 48 hours at 37°C, or when aerobically. After 29 to 48 hours at 37°C, or when there is good colony formation, compare the growth in each tube. **See Chart 6-3 on page 186 at end of module for results.**

Perform a catalase test by adding 3 percent H_2O_2 to the brain heart infusion slant with the best growth. Be sure to wait at least 30 minutes after removing the slant from anaerobic incubation before adding H_2O_2. Bubbles indicate a positive test, while absence of bubbles indicates a negative result. Anaerobic diphtheroids, *Pro-*

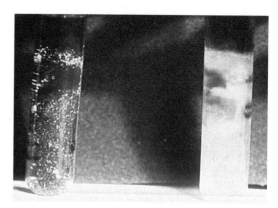

FIGURE 6-27. Bread crumb and diffuse colonies of *Actinomyces* in thioglycollate broth. (From Jones, et al: Atlas of Medical Mycology. ASCP, Washington, DC, 1976, with permission.)

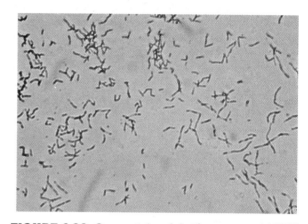

FIGURE 6-28. Gram stain of *Actinomyces*, ×1000.

pionibacterium sp., are catalase-positive, and anaerobic actinomycetes are catalase-negative.

At this point, send the organism to a reference laboratory for further identification, or perform nitrate reduction, starch hydrolysis, and mannitol and mannose fermentation tests (gray boxes). Other tests that may be performed as needed are gelatin liquefaction, litmus milk reaction, more sugar fermentations, indole production, and gas-liquid chromatography. (See Gordon (1974) and the paper by Georg et al (1964) for further details.)

NITRATE REDUCTION TEST FOR ANAEROBIC ACTINOMYCETES

Medium and Reagent Preparation
  Nitrate medium:

Heart infusion broth (Difco)	**25 gm**
Yeast extract	**5 gm**
Casitone (Difco)	**4 gm**
Potassium nitrate	**1 gm**
Distilled water	**1 liter**

    1. Mix the above ingredients together, adjust the pH to 7.0, tube, cotton plug, and autoclave at 15 psi for 15 minutes. Cool and refrigerate.

Sulfanilic acid solution: same as for yeast rapid nitrate test

Glacial acetic acid	100 ml
Sulfanilic acid	2.8 gm
Distilled water	250 ml

    1. Add the acetic acid to water, then dissolve the sulfanilic acid.

α-Naphthylamine solution: same as for yeast rapid nitrate test

Dimethyl-α-naphthylamine	1.75 gm
Glacial acetic acid	100 ml
Distilled water	250 ml

    1. Add the acetic acid to water, then dissolve the naphthylamine.

Procedure

1. Bring the nitrate medium to room temperature. Inoculate a tube with a pure culture of the test isolate, and incubate at 37°C anaerobically, or aerobically with pyrogallol-carbonate seals.*

2. Every 5 days, remove a small amount of broth to a clean tube, add 2 drops each of sulfanilic acid solution and α-naphthylamine solution, and mix.

3. Observe for a red color—a positive test. If there is no red color, add zinc dust. If the medium now turns red, the remaining nitrates were reduced by the zinc and the test is negative. If the medium remains colorless after the zinc addition, the nitrate was reduced by the organism to ammonia, also a positive test.

4. If the nitrate test is negative, reincubate the rest of the broth, testing it every 5 days for a total of 2 weeks.

*Pyrogallol-carbonate seals may be used instead of anaerobic incubation. To a small piece of cotton, add 5 drops each of pyrogallol solution (150 ml water and 100 gm pyrogallic acid) and 10 percent sodium carbonate. Plug the inoculated tube with the cotton, then insert a rubber stopper into the cotton. The tube may now be incubated aerobically.

STARCH HYDROLYSIS TEST FOR ANAEROBIC ACTINOMYCETES

Medium Preparation

Heart infusion broth (Difco)	25 gm
Yeast extract	5 gm
Casitone (Difco)	4 gm
Soluble starch	5 gm
Agar	15 gm
Distilled water	1 liter

    1. Mix together the above ingredients; adjust the pH to 7.0.

    2. Tube in 8 ml aliquots, then autoclave at 15 psi for 15 minutes.

    3. Slant and allow to harden.

Procedure

1. Streak the surface of the slant and incubate it aerobically with a pyrogallol-carbonate seal (see gray box, Nitrate Reduction Test for Anaerobic Actinomycetes), or anaerobically.

2. After 5–10 days at 37°C, add Gram's iodine. If the area around the colonies remains clear, starch was hydrolyzed (a positive test). If the area turns blue, the test is negative.

FERMENTATION TESTS FOR ANAEROBIC ACTINOMYCETES

Medium Preparation
  Fermentation medium:

Heart infusion broth (Difco)	25 gm
Yeast extract	5 gm
Casitone (Difco)	4 gm
Bromcresol purple, 0.04 percent	15 ml
Distilled water	1 liter
Mannitol OR mannose (filter sterilized, 0.05 gms/ml)	1 ml per tube of medium

  1. Mix together the above ingredients, then adjust the pH to 7.0.
  2. Tube in 9 ml aliquots; autoclave at 15 psi for 15 minutes.
  3. Cool and aseptically add 1 ml of mannitol OR mannose to each tube. Refrigerate.

Procedure
  1. Bring a tube of mannitol and mannose to room temperature. Inoculate them with a pure culture of the test organism, and pyrogallol-carbonate seal them (see gray box on Nitrate Reduction Test for Anaerobic Actinomycetes).
  2. Incubate for 1 month at 37°C, checking periodically for acid production, a yellow color, which indicates a positive test. If the tubes remain purple, the test is negative.

FINAL EXAM

Place the letter(s) of the genera below in front of the corresponding characteristics.

  A. *Actinomyces* sp.

  B. *Streptomyces* sp.

  C. *Nocardia* sp.

  D. *Mycobacterium* sp.

1. _____ Acid-fast

2. _____ Anaerobic

3. _____ Earthy odor

4. _____ Conidia

5. _____ Molar tooth appearance on agar

6. Circle true or false.
   T F Only fungi and funguslike bacteria may produce granules in tissue.

7. Red granules are observed in a foot lesion. Microscopically, the crushed granules contain fine, one-micrometer wide, branching filaments radiating out from a center of necrotic material. The patient most likely has: (circle the letter of the correct answer)

  A. Chromoblastomycosis

  B. Eumycotic mycetoma

  C. Actinomycotic mycetoma

  D. Actinomycosis

  E. Sporotrichosis

8. *Sporothrix schenckii* resembles *Acremonium*, a contaminant which may cause mycetoma. How may they be differentiated? Describe two ways.

9. **Circle the correct letter. Which of the following exhibits polymorphism, in which more than one type of conidial arrangement may be observed?**

    A. *Cladosporium carrionii*

    B. *Phialophora verrucosa*

    C. *Fonsecaea pedrosoi*

    D. *Fonsecaea compacta*

    E. A,C, and D

    F. All of the above

10. **Draw an arrow from the organisms on the left to the appropriate test(s) on the right:**

    Anaerobic actinomycetes
    Aerobic actinomycetes

    Casein, tyrosine, xanthine
    Gelatin liquefaction
    KOH-DMSO prep for sclerotic
       bodies
    Catalase, fermentations

STOP HERE UNTIL YOU HAVE COMPLETED THE ANSWERS.

Look up the answers in the back of the book. If you missed more than two of them, repeat this module. Correctly complete any missed questions before proceeding further.

SUPPLEMENTAL RATIONALE

Actinomycosis

Unlike the other subcutaneous mycoses, actinomycosis has an endogenous origin: the main causative agents are normal anaerobic flora of the mouth. When the oral mucous membranes become injured (for example, after a tooth extraction), the organisms infect the adjacent face and neck areas, producing swollen, hard, lumpy, draining abscesses (**lumpy jaw** Fig. 6-29). If the funguslike bacteria are aspirated into the lungs, they produce pulmonary or thoracic actinomycosis characterized by cough, fever, mucopurulent bloody sputum, and multiple draining lung sinuses, which may contain sulfur-colored granules. Pulmonary disease may simulate tuberculosis. If *Actinomyces* are swallowed, they produce abdominal disease with symptoms of appendicitis or carcinoma. Primary pelvic actinomycosis associated with the intrauterine device has recently been noted. Systemic spread from the jaw, lungs, or gastrointestinal tract may include the skin, kidneys, genital tract, liver, ovaries, bones, joints, and central nervous system. Draining pus contains sulfur-colored granules or masses of Gram-positive branching filaments. The

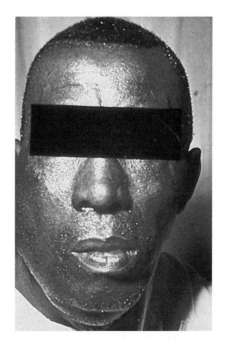

FIGURE 6-29. Actinomycosis of jaw. (From Dolan, et al: Atlas of Clinical Mycology. ASCP, Washington, DC, 1976, with permission.)

179

prognosis is very good if the disease is diagnosed early. Unfortunately, physicians often do not suspect actinomycosis, and many laboratories do not routinely inoculate anaerobic fungal media. Organisms causing the disease are *Actinomyces israelii, Actinomyces bovis, Actinomyces naeslundii, Actinomyces meyeri, Actinomyces viscosus, Bifidobacterium adolescentis (eriksonii),* and *Arachnia propionica.*

Chromoblastomycosis (Fig. 6-30)

This infection is almost always limited to the lower extremities, though it has occurred on the hands, face, ear, neck, chest, shoulders, and buttocks. Puncture with contaminated vegetation produces an initial ringwormlike lesion which very slowly becomes hard, dry, and raised. Many lumps form on top, providing a cauliflower semblance. Usually the eruption is dry but it may ulcerate. Black dots are found in the deep part of the lesion. New eruptions spread down the lymphatic drainage, sometimes blocking the lymphatics and producing elephantiasis; bone is not involved. Lesions itch but are basically painless unless secondary bacterial infection ensues. Up to 15 years may elapse before an entire extremity is involved. Fungi causing chromoblastomycosis are all dematiaceous: *Fonsecaea pedrosoi, Fonsecaea compacta, Phialophora verrucosa, Cladosporium carrionii, Rhinocladiella aquaspersa,* and *Cladophialophora ajelloi.*

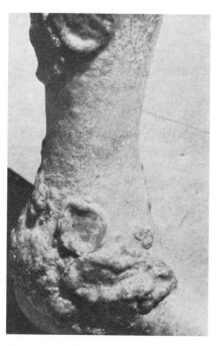

FIGURE 6-30. Cauliflower lesions of chromoblastomycosis. (From Rippon: Medical Mycology. WB Saunders, Philadelphia, 1982, with permission.)

Mycetoma (Fig. 6-31) (Maduromycosis, Madura foot)

Mycetoma resulting from puncture or abrasion with contaminated material is usually limited to the feet but may be seen on the hands and buttocks. Nodules that periodically exude oily fluid containing white, yellow, red, or black granules slowly progress to involve the entire leg. Infection caused by the higher fungi (eumycotic mycetoma) elicits bored out, punched in lesions, with little pain or bone destruction, while that caused by funguslike bacteria (actinomycotic mycetoma) shows blown out, conelike lesions, like pimples erupting, with a lot of exudate and painful bone involvement. The extremity becomes greatly enlarged and deformed. As long as 10 to 15 years may ensue before the entire leg is infected. Agents of human eumycotic mycetoma are *Scedosporium apiospermum, Acremonium falciforme, Acremonium recifei, Exophiala jeanselmei, Madurella mycetomii,* and *Madurella grisea.* Organisms producing actinomycotic mycetoma are *Nocardia asteroides, Nocardia brasiliensis, Nocardia caviae, Nocardia madurae, Nocardia pelletierii, Streptomyces somaliensis, Actinomyces israelii,* and *Actinomyces bovis.*

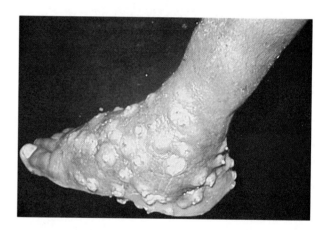

FIGURE 6-31. Mycetoma of foot. (From Dolan, et al: Atlas of Clinical Mycology. ASCP, Washington, DC, 1976, with permission.)

Nocardiosis (Fig. 6-32)

This infection is being seen with increased frequency, especially in patients with cancer or those on corticosteroids. After breathing in the organism, manifestations are initially pulmonary, resembling tuberculosis or bacterial pneumonia. Purulent sputum contains acid-fast branching filaments. Early spread of the disease results in scattered subcutaneous draining abscesses involving the brain and skin, and less frequently, the pleura and heart. Granules are usually not observed. Nocardiosis should be considered whenever the physician suspects tuberculosis, since the clinical manifestations may be very similar, the funguslike bacteria are acid-fast, and generalized nocardiosis has a high mortality. Organisms implicated in this disease are *Nocardia asteroides, Nocardia caviae,* and rarely, *Nocardia brasiliensis.*

Note that *Nocardia* does not take up the hematoxylin and eosin tissue stain; the periodic acid-Schiff and Gridley stains are also not dependable. Thus, diagnosis may be missed in histologic sections. *Nocardia* is effectively demonstrated in the Gomori methenamine silver and Brown and Brenn stains. On sputum smears in the microbiology laboratory, the Gram and modified Kinyoun stains are useful.

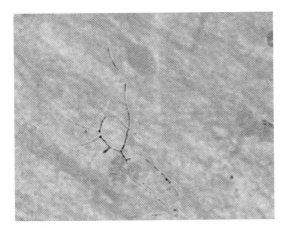

FIGURE 6-32. *Nocardia* **in Gram stain of sputum, ×1000.**

Phaeohyphomycosis (Chromoblastomycosis in part, Cladosporiosis)

Phaeohyphomycosis represents a broad spectrum of dematiaceous fungal infections, ranging from superficial involvement to deep organ disease. In the past, there has been considerable confusion surrounding the terms phaeohyphomycosis and chromoblastomycosis, as the former was designated a special entity of chromoblastomycosis. Now phaeohyphomycosis is described as a separate disease because sclerotic bodies (and also granules) are not evident in tissue; instead, dark yeast-like cells, pseudohyphaelike fungal elements, hyphae, or a combination of these structures appear in the tissue.

McGinnis (1983) has proposed the following four categories for classifying phaeohyphomycosis, which should clarify the confusion if universally accepted.

A. Superficial—includes black piedra and tinea nigra

B. Cutaneous and corneal—includes dermatomycoses, mycotic keratitis, and onychomycosis produced by dematiaceous fungi

C. Subcutaneous—usually localized abscesses caused by traumatic implantation. *E. jeanselmei* and *W. dermatitidis* are the most common etiologic agents.

D. Systemic—initial inhalation of the fungus leads to lung infection, which then disseminates to other organs. The brain is often involved, with *C. trichoides* as the most common agent.

Sporotrichosis (Fig. 6-33)

This infection usually is a result of puncture with contaminated materials such as rose thorns, hay, and wood. Subcutaneous, hard, black, ulcerating lesions are most often seen on the extremities, and they may progress along the lymphatics. Pulmonary sporotrichosis is being observed more frequently, and it must be differentiated from tuberculosis, coccidioidomycosis, histoplasmosis, and sarcoidosis. Rarely, disseminated sporotrichosis may occur. No granules are present in any of the manifestations. Budding yeasts, called cigar bodies, are observed in specimen direct mounts, although the yeasts are not plentiful. Hyphae and conidia are seen on media at room temperature. Conversion of the mold to the yeast phase in vitro is required for identification of the etiologic agent, *Sporothrix schenckii.*

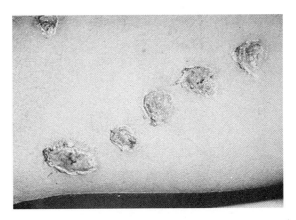

FIGURE 6-33. Sporotrichosis of arm. (From Dolan, et al: Atlas of Clinical Mycology. ASCP, Washington, DC, 1976, with permission.)

Study Questions—Supplemental Rationale

Circle true or false:

1. T F Granules are seen in mycetoma caused by *Nocardia,* yet, in nocardiosis, granules are usually not observed.

2. T F Characteristic sulfur-colored granules are usually present in both actinomycosis and mycetoma produced by the same organisms.

3. T F In the past, phaeohyphomycosis was considered a part of chromoblastomycosis. Now the two are separated by the lack of sclerotic bodies in phaeohyphomycosis.

4. Chromoblastomycosis and mycetoma are both slowly progressing infections which affect the extremities. Describe two ways they may be differentiated.

5. Circle the correct letter.

   The subcutaneous disease with an endogenous (within self) origin is:

   A. Sporotrichosis
   B. Actinomycosis
   C. Phaeohyphomycosis
   D. Eumycotic mycetoma
   E. Chromoblastomycosis

For the next three questions, refer to this case study.

A 35-year-old rose gardener noticed a hard, unmovable lump under the skin of his index finger but decided to ignore it. A month later, the lump ulcerated to present a black, necrotic appearance, and two more lesions developed further up the wrist and forearm. At this point, he visited his physician. A histologic stain of material from deep in the lesions showed rare elongated yeast cells resembling cigars. On Sabouraud dextrose agar at room temperature, a cream-colored leathery colony grew relatively rapidly, and after 9 days it started to turn black.

6. What disease is suspected and why? Give two reasons.

7. What would you expect to see in microscopic mounts from the SDA? Circle the letter of the correct answer.

   A. Hyaline cigar bodies
   B. Dematiaceous annellides with terminal conidia
   C. Hyaline daisy head flowerettes of conidia
   D. Single terminal, hyaline conidia
   E. Hyaline, tapering conidiophores with terminal balls of conidia

8. The etiologic agent is ubiquitous in nature. How did the patient probably contract the fungus?

For the next two questions, refer to this case study.

Black sclerotic bodies were observed on crusty, cauliflowerlike foot lesions of a 30-year-old male Indian patient from South America. Culture of the crushed black dots on Sabouraud dextrose agar revealed a slow-growing black, velvety colony. Microscopically, there was only the conidial arrangement seen in Figure 6-34.

9. What disease is suspected and why? Give two reasons.

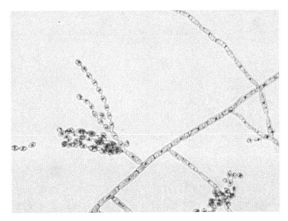

FIGURE 6-34. Study question demonstration, LPCB stain, ×450.

10. The etiologic agent is most likely: (circle the letter of the correct answer)

A. *Cladosporium trichoides*

B. *Fonsecaea pedrosoi*

C. *Fonsecaea compacta*

D. *Exophiala jeanselmei*

E. *Cladosporium carrionii*

STOP HERE UNTIL YOU HAVE COMPLETED THE QUESTIONS.

Look up the answers in the back of the book. If you missed more than three, go back and repeat this module. Correctly complete any missed questions.

CHART 6-1. Black Dot and Granule Colors and Associated Diseases

DOT/GRANULE COLOR AND ORGANISMS	CHROMOBLASTOMYCOSIS (BLACK DOTS)	EUMYCOTIC MYCETOMA (GRANULES)	ACTINOMYCOTIC MYCETOMA (GRANULES)	ACTINOMYCOSIS (GRANULES)
Brown to black				
Sclerotic bodies:				
Fonsecaea pedrosoi	X			
Fonsecaea compacta	X			
Phialophora verrucosa	X			
Cladosporium carrionii	X			
Other:				
Exophiala jeanselmei		X		
White to yellow:				
Scedosporium apiospermum		X		
Acremonium falciforme		X		
Nocardia asteroides			X	
Nocardia brasiliensis			X	
Nocardia caviae			X	
Nocardia madurae			X	
Streptomyces somaliensis			X	
Actinomyces israelii			X	X
Actinomyces bovis			X	X
Arachnia propionica			X	X
Red to pink:				
Nocardia pelletieri			X	

CHART 6-2. Some Properties of Aerobic Funguslike Bacteria*

	CONIDIA	AERIAL HYPHAE	ACID-FASTNESS	CASEIN HYDROLYSIS	TYROSINE HYDROLYSIS	XANTHINE HYDROLYSIS	UREASE	MORPHOLOGY ON TAP WATER AGAR
Nocardia:								
asteroides	32% +	100% +	61% +	0% +	1% +	0% +	96% +	Extensive treelike branching; thick aerial hyphae
brasiliensis	0	100	78	93	99	0	99	Extensive treelike branching; thick aerial hyphae
caviae	26	100	65	2	14	100	95	Extensive treelike branching; thick aerial hyphae
madurae	15	45	0	98	91	0	0	Branching to a variable extent; sparse aerial hyphae
pelletierii	0	24	0	100	100	0	0	Branching to a variable extent; sparse aerial hyphae
dassonvillei	67	91	0	98	100	100	39	Usually extensive branching; abundant aerial hyphae
Streptomyces:								
somaliensis	14	54	0	100	100	0	0	Extensive branching; abundant aerial hyphae
griseus	91	96	0	100	100	97	92	Extensive branching; abundant aerial hyphae
spp. (contaminants)			0	+	+	±	±	
Mycobacterium:								
fortuitum (for comparison only)	−	−	+	−	−	−	+	Moderate short branches at oblique angles with no aerial hyphae
Rhodococcus (for comparison only)	+	−	+	−	±	−	±	Minimal branching, diphtheroid-like; no aerial hyphae

*Compiled from Mishra et al (1980). Morphology on tap water agar and *Rhodococcus* characterization courtesy of Joseph L. Staneck, Ph.D. and Geoffrey A. Land, Ph.D. (personal communications).

CHART 6-3. Identification of Anaerobic Actinomycetes*

	ACTINOMYCES ISRAELII	ACTINOMYCES BOVIS	ACTINOMYCES NAESLUNDII	BIFIDOBACTERIUM ADOLESCENTIS	ARACHNIA PROPIONICA
Aerobic growth	1+	2+	2+ (best grown in 5% CO_2)	0	1-2+
Anaerobic growth	4+	4+	4+	4+	4+
48-hour colony on BHI agar, anaerobically incubated (examine under microscope)	Spidery, dense mycelial center with lacey border	Circular, granular to smooth; slightly raised center with an entire edge	Resembles A. israelii (spidery form with dense center)	Flat, granular with dense hyphal core	Resembles A. israelii
7-10-day colony on BHI agar (anaerobic)	Raised, rough; lobular; like a molar tooth	Flat to convex; opaque with smooth to pebbly edges	May resemble A. israelii or A. bovis; most often similar to A. bovis	Resembles A. bovis; usually has scalloped edge	Resembles A. bovis; smooth and flat
Growth in thioglycollate broth, 37°C	Discrete, bread crumb colonies without turbidity	Turbidity with dense sediment	Rough colonies or soft diffuse growth; somewhat cloudy	Soft colonies, diffuse growth	Diffuse or turbid growth
Microscopic morphology (all are Gram +)	Branching, diphtheroid forms	Diphtheroid forms most usual; branching rarely seen	Branching, diphtheroid forms	Branching, diphtheroid forms	Branching, diphtheroid forms; long branching forms with age
Catalase	0	0	0	0	0
Nitrate reduction	80% +	0	90% +	0	+
Starch hydrolysis	0 or ±	4+	0 or ±	4+	0
Mannitol fermentation	V	0	0	A	±
Mannose fermentation	A	0 or ±	A	A	A
Other test results:					
Gelatin hydrolysis	0 (occasionally late +)	0	0	0	0
Glucose fermentation	A	A	A	A	A
Xylose fermentation	80% A	0^v	0	A	0
Raffinose fermentation	V	0	80% A	A	A

*Compiled from Larone (1976) and Beneke and Rogers (1980).

A = Acid
V = Variable
0 = Negative
+ = Positive
± = Weak reaction

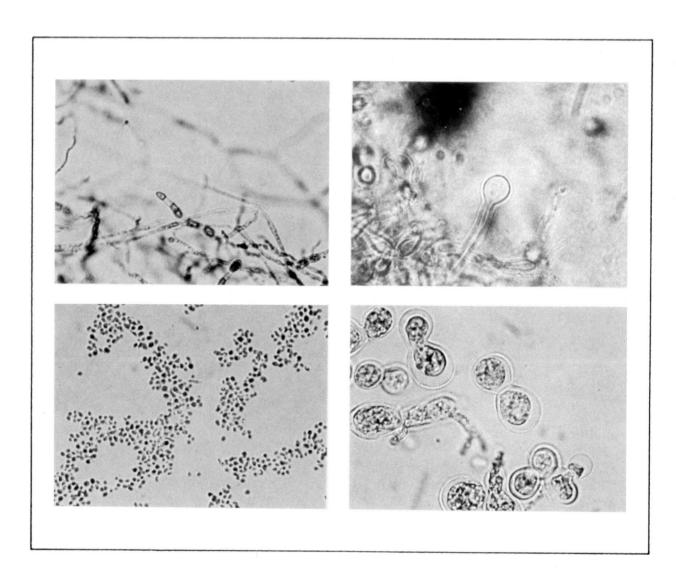

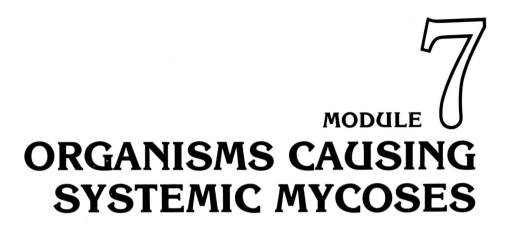

MODULE 7
ORGANISMS CAUSING SYSTEMIC MYCOSES

PREREQUISITES. The learner must possess a good background knowledge in clinical microbiology and must have finished Module 1, Basics of Mycology, and Module 2, Laboratory Procedures for Fungal Culture and Isolation.

BEHAVIORAL OBJECTIVES. Upon completion of this module, the learner should be able to:

1. List two properties that *Blastomyces dermatitidis*, *Paracoccidioides brasiliensis*, *Histoplasma capsulatum*, and *Coccidioides immitis* all share.

2. Discuss safety precautions when working with systemic pathogens.

3. List two reasons why direct mounts are especially useful when working with suspected systemic fungi.

4. From specimen direct mounts, identify characteristic fungal structures associated with the systemic agents in number 1.

5. Convert *Blastomyces*, *Paracoccidioides*, or *Histoplasma* from the mold to yeast phase and discuss special conditions necessary for conversion.

6. Identify from culture, microscopic preparations, and disease descriptions the organisms listed in number 1.

7. Differentiate the systemic pathogens from other similar-appearing organisms.

Box continues on next page.

> 8. Briefly describe blastomycosis, paracoccidioidomycosis, histoplasmosis, and coccidioidomycosis, including any special epidemiologic (geographic) associations, mode of transmission, causative agents, and main clinical types of infection.

CONTENT OUTLINE

I. Introduction
II. Organisms
  A. *Blastomyces dermatitidis*
  B. *Coccidioides immitis*
  C. *Histoplasma capsulatum*
  D. *Paracoccidioides brasiliensis*
III. Final exam
IV. Supplemental Rationale
  A. Blastomycosis
  B. Coccidioidomycosis
  C. Histoplasmosis
  D. Paracoccidioidomycosis
  E. Study questions

FOLLOW-UP ACTIVITIES

1. Students may observe room temperature colonies, 37°C colonies, and tease preparations of fungi causing systemic mycoses.

2. Students may convert *Blastomyces dermatitidis* from the mold to yeast phase.

REFERENCES

AL-DOORY, Y, AND PAIRON, R: *A bibliography of blastomycosis and paracoccidioidomycosis.* Mycopathologia 56:159, 1975.

BENEKE, ES: *Human Mycoses: A Scope Publication.* Upjohn Company, Kalamazoo, Mich., 1979.

BENEKE, ES, AND ROGERS, AL: *Medical Mycology Manual,* ed 4. Burgess Publishing Co., Minneapolis, 1980.

CONANT, NF, ET AL.: *Manual of Clinical Mycology,* ed 3. WB Saunders, Philadelphia, 1971.

DELACRETAZ, J, GRIGORIU, D, AND DUCEL, G: *Color Atlas of Medical Mycology.* Hans Huber Publishers, Year Book Medical Publishers (distributor), Chicago, 1976.

DOLAN, CT, ET AL.: *Atlas of Clinical Mycology.* American Society of Clinical Pathologists, Commission on Continuing Education, Chicago, 1975.

EL-ANI, AS, PICKREN, JW, AND FITZPATRICK, JE: *Coccidioidomycosis in a patient with lymphoma: Spherulation in human pleural fluid medium.* Am J Clin Pathol 70:423, 1978.

EMMONS, CW, ET AL.: *Medical Mycology,* ed 3. Lea & Febiger, Philadelphia, 1977.

HALEY, LD, AND CALLAWAY, CS: *Laboratory Methods in Medical Mycology,* ed 4. U.S. Department of Health, Education, and Welfare, Washington, DC, 1978.

KAUFMAN, L: *Serodiagnosis of fungal diseases.* In ROSE, NR, AND FRIEDMAN, H (EDS): *Manual of Clinical Immunology,* ed 2. American Society for Microbiology, Washington, DC, 1980.

KONEMAN, EW, ROBERTS, GD, AND WRIGHT, SF: *Practical Laboratory Mycology,* ed 2. Williams & Wilkins, Baltimore, 1978.

MCGINNIS, MR: *Laboratory Handbook of Medical Mycology.* Academic Press, New York, 1980.

ROBERTS, JA, COUNTS, JM, AND CRESELIUS, HG: *Production in vitro of Coccidioides immitis spherules and endospores as a diagnostic aid.* Ann Rev Resp Dis 102:811, 1970.

SMITH, CD, AND GOODMAN, NL: *Improved culture method for the isolation of Histoplasma capsulatum and Blastomyces dermatitidis from contaminated specimens.* Am J Clin Pathol 63:276, 1975.

SUN, SH, HUPPERT, M, AND VUKOVICH, KR: *Rapid in vitro conversion and identification of Coccidioides immitis.* J Clin Microbiol 3:186, 1976.

INTRODUCTION

In this module, those organisms that classically cause systemic mycoses, that is, *Blastomyces dermatitidis, Paracoccidioides brasiliensis, Histoplasma capsulatum,* and *Coccidioides immitis,* are described. Note that these fungi may also produce cutaneous manifestations without systemic involvement. Also, many opportunistic fungi may elicit systemic disease under the proper conditions, for example, in debilitated or immunosuppressed patients. Opportunists are covered in other modules.

Specimens are collected as described in Module 2. Direct mounts are a must; because the four fungi listed above are dimorphic and the mold phase of all but *Coccidioides* are slow growing, a rapid preliminary identification is facilitated by observing the tissue phases in these mounts. The tissue phases can be seen in unstained wet preparations of specimens, for example, in sputum, although histology stains such as PAS, GMS, and H&E are more definitive. *Blastomyces* exhibits thick-walled budding yeasts, with a broad base of attachment between the mother and daughter cell. *Coccidioides* spherules are difficult to grow in vitro and thus may be seen only in direct mounts (Color Plate 67) unless animal studies are performed, which are beyond the scope of most clinical laboratories. Animal studies also require a longer turn around time than is useful for the physician and patient. In histoplasmosis a Wright stain of infected blood or bone marrow will reveal pseudoencapsulated yeast forms of *Histoplasma capsulatum,* with a narrow isthmus between mother and daughter cells. The yeasts will be observed inside reticuloendothelial cells (monocytes and neutrophils). Regular histology stains of various tissues will show the same morphology as the Wright stain (Color Plate 68). Although rare in the United States, *Paracoccidioides* should not be overlooked; multiple thick-walled daughter yeasts bud off a large mother cell (Color Plate 13).

Serologic procedures are important in systemic diseases. Paired acute and convalescent sera may be tested by several methods to determine if there is a fourfold rise in titer against one of the test antigens, which are derived from the four organisms discussed above **(see Chart 2-7 on page 83).** Also, once the fungus has grown in culture, it may be serologically identified by using antisera from animals inoculated with the systemic fungi. Each serologic procedure has its advantages and disadvantages, which is beyond the scope of this text. (*See* Kaufman (1980) for more details.)

Sabouraud dextrose agar plus brain heart infusion agar, sabhi agar, or yeast extract phosphate agar* is inoculated. Antibiotics may be added to the medium to inhibit contaminants. If specimens are respiratory in origin, they must be decontaminated and concentrated (Module 2) before inoculating to media. Slants are preferred over plates for all systemic fungi, especially *Coccidioides,* because there is less chance for the mold phase to become airborne and infect laboratory personnel.[†] Media are incubated at room temperature for up to 12 weeks.

With the exception of *Coccidioides,* which is an intermediate grower, the other systemic pathogens grow slowly at 25°C, requiring 3 to 6 weeks to form a mature culture. Colonies are initially membranous but later develop white to tan aerial mycelia. Lactophenol tease mounts reveal septate hyphae and conidia or arthroconidia. Do not inoculate slide cultures with suspected systemic molds for safety reasons. Conversion to the tissue phase is the confirmatory identification for dimorphic fungi (gray box).

---

*Smith, CD and Goodman, NL: Improved culture method for the isolation of *Histoplasma capsulatum* and *Blastomyces dermatitidis* from contaminated specimens. Am J Clin Pathol 63:276, 1975.

†Mold forms of systemic organisms are highly infective. Wear mask and gloves while working under a microbiologic hood. It is preferable to pour 10 percent formalin over the culture and let it sit overnight before preparing tease mounts, but first transfer some of the colony to media at 25°C and 37°C to maintain viable colonies for further studies.

CONVERSION OF DIMORPHIC FUNGI FROM THE MOLD TO YEAST PHASE

Medium Preparation
Brain heart infusion agar with 10 percent blood: see Module 2

Procedure
1. Place a small amount of the test mold on a slant of brain heart infusion agar with 10

ORGANISMS

Key identifying features are in capital letters.

Blastomyces dermatitidis (Figs. 7-1 and 7-2)

Culture: On Sabouraud dextrose agar at room temperature, a yeastlike colony initially develops. With time, the center becomes prickly and later the entire colony is fluffy white or tan (Color Plate 69).

On brain heart infusion agar with blood at 37°C, colonies are waxy, wrinkled, and cream to tan colored (Color Plate 70). Conversion from the mold to yeast phase takes four to five days.

Microscopic: Tease mounts of the room temperature colony (MOLD phase) show SINGLE smooth-walled, round to oval CONIDIA at the ENDS of short conidiophores or directly on the hyphae. The mold phase may microscopically resemble the contaminant *Chrysosporium* sp. (Module 3) or the subcutaneous pathogen *Scedosporium apiospermum* (Module 6). *Blastomyces dermatitidis* may be differentiated by its slow growth rate (*Chrysosporium*=rapid, *Scedospo-*

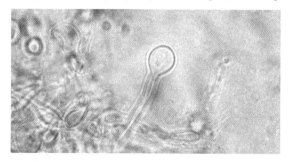

FIGURE 7-1. Mold phase, *Blastomyces dermatitidis*, lactophenol cotton blue (LPCB) stain, ×1000.

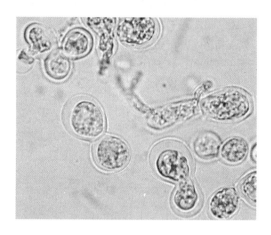

FIGURE 7-2. Yeast phase, *Blastomyces dermatitidis*, LPCB stain, ×1000.

rium=intermediate) and by its ability to convert to a yeast phase (neither of the others can do this).

The 37°C YEAST phase microscopically appears as large, round, THICK-WALLED, SINGLE-BUDDING yeast cells with a BROAD ISTHMUS where the daughter cell attaches to the mother. **(See Chart 7-1 on page 199 at end of module.)**

Pathogenicity: *Blastomyces dermatitidis* causes blastomycosis.

Coccidioides immitis (Fig. 7-3)

Culture: On Sabouraud dextrose agar at room temperature or 37°C, a moist white colony initially forms which is later covered with white fluffy mycelium (Color Plate 71). Colonies form in 5 to 7 days, although diagnostic arthroconidia require about 2 weeks.

Microscopic: Tease mounts of the colony reveal hyphal branching at 90-degree angles and many

THICK-WALLED, BARREL-SHAPED or rectangular ARTHROCONIDIA ALTERNATING WITH EMPTY DISJUNCTOR CELLS. The contaminants *Gymnoascus uncinatus*, *Auxarthron* sp. and *Malbranchea* sp. **(see Chart 1-11 on page 36)** also produce alternating arthroconidia, and *Geotrichum candidum* and *Trichosporon* sp. (Module 5) produce adjacent arthroconidia. Demonstration of spherules with endospores being released is therefore required for final identification, or a positive immunodiffusion test using known antibodies to *Coccidioides immitis* and an extract of the unknown mold as antigen.

The tissue phase of this organism may only be grown under special in vitro conditions (El-ani, Pickren, and Fitzpatrick, 1978; Roberts, Counts and Creselius, 1970; or Sun, Huppert, and Vukovich, 1976) or animal inoculations. Round, THICK-WALLED SPHERULES (sporangia) filled with small ENDOSPORES are observed on conversion and also on specimen direct mounts. Young spherules with undeveloped endospores may resemble yeast cells of *Blastomyces dermatitidis*. With a Vaseline-sealed coverslip over the specimen, spherules will form multiple germ tubes after a 24-hour incubation at 37°C, while *Blastomyces* will exhibit only broad-based budding cells.

Pathogenicity: *Coccidioides immitis* produces coccidioidomycosis.

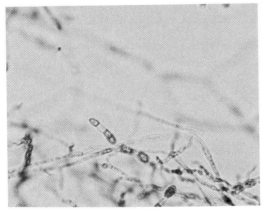

FIGURE 7-3. Mold phase, *Coccidioides immitis*, LPCB stain, ×450.

Histoplasma capsulatum (Figs. 7-4 and 7-5)

Culture: On brain heart infusion agar with blood at room temperature, the slow-growing colony is initially moist and later develops a low, white to brown aerial mycelium. The texture of mature colonies may be glabrous, velvety, or woolly (Color Plate 72). Once the colony has initially formed on brain heart infusion agar with blood, transfer it to a less nutritious medium, for example, Sabouraud dextrose agar, so that characteristic microscopic structures will develop.

On brain heart infusion agar with blood at 37°C, a rough, mucoid, cream to tan colony forms (Color Plate 73). Several transfers may be necessary to convert the mold to yeast phase.

Microscopic: Tease mounts of the room temperature MOLD phase from Sabouraud dextrose agar reveal condiophores at 90-degree angles to the hyphae, which support large round MACROCONIDIA (chlamydoconidia) with smooth, spiny, or FINLIKE (tuberculate) EDGES. Small, round to teardrop, smooth or rough MICROCONIDIA are along the sides of the hyphae. Variants may be observed where macroconidia alone, microconidia alone, or sterile hyphae are present. *Histoplasma capsulatum* macroconidia closely resemble those of the contaminants *Sepedonium* sp. and rough-walled *Chrysosporium* sp. (Module 3). However, *Histoplasma* is slow growing and can be converted to a yeast phase, while the contaminants are rapid growing and do not possess a yeast phase.

The 37°C yeast phase microscopically appears as SMALL, single-budding YEAST cells.

Pathogenicity: *Histoplasma capsulatum* causes histoplasmosis.

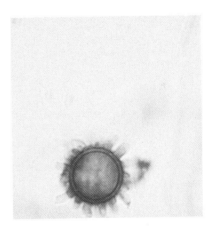

FIGURE 7-4. Macroconidium, mold phase, *Histoplasma capsulatum*, LPCB stain, ×1000.

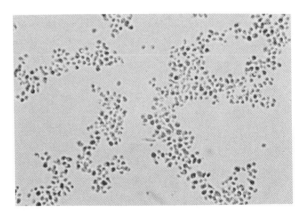

FIGURE 7-5. Yeast phase, *Histoplasma capsulatum*, LPCB stain, ×450.

Paracoccidioides brasiliensis (Figs. 7-6 and 7-7)

Culture: On Sabouraud dextrose agar at room temperature, colonies grow very slowly—2 cm in three weeks. They are smooth at first and later become covered with white to tan aerial mycelium (Color Plate 74).

On brain heart infusion agar with blood at 37°C, colonies are waxy, wrinkled, and cream to tan colored (Color Plate 75). Conversion to the yeast phase requires 3 to 7 days.

Microscopic: Tease mounts of the room temperature mold colony show mostly hyphae with intercalary and terminal chlamydoconidia. Occasionally conidia resembling *Blastomyces dermatitidis* and *Chrysosporium* sp. are observed. Arthroconidia may form.

The 37°C YEAST phase microscopically appears as large, THICK-WALLED, MULTIPLE BUDDING yeast cells with narrow necks where the daughter cells attach. This form has the likeness of a SHIP'S WHEEL.

Pathogenicity: *Paracoccidioides brasiliensis* causes paracoccidioidomycosis.

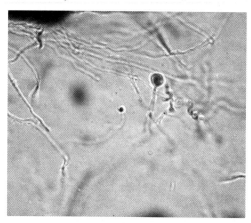

FIGURE 7-6. Conidium, mold phase, *Paracoccidioides brasiliensis*, LPCB stain, ×450.

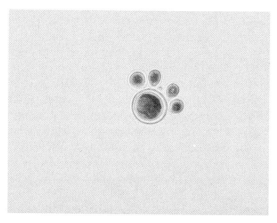

FIGURE 7-7. Yeast phase, *Paracoccidioides brasiliensis*, LPCB stain, ×450.

FINAL EXAM

Matching: Place the letter of the fungus in *Column B* in front of the corresponding description in *Column A.*

Column A	Column B
1. ____ Multiple budding yeasts	A. *Blastomyces dermatitidis* mold phase
2. ____ Spherules	B. *Paracoccidioides brasiliensis* tissue phase
3. ____ Alternating arthroconidia	C. *Histoplasma capsulatum* mold phase
4. ____ Tuberculate macroconidia	D. *Coccidioides immitis* tissue phase
5. ____ Pseudo-encapsulated yeasts inside monocytes	E. *Blastomyces dermatitidis* tissue phase
6. ____ Broad-based, thick-walled, single-budding yeasts	

F. *Histoplasma capsulatum* tissue phase

G. *Coccidioides immitis* mold phase

7. **Discuss four safety precautions that should be met when working with the mold forms of systemic pathogens.**

8. When changing a dimorphic mold to the yeast phase, what are three conditions necessary for complete conversion?

    B. *Coccidioides immitis* and *Geotrichum candidum*

9. Compare and contrast:

    A. *Blastomyces dermatitidis*, *Chrysosporium* sp., and *Scedosporium apiospermum*

STOP HERE UNTIL YOU HAVE COMPLETED THE ANSWERS.

Look up the answers in the back of the book. If you missed more than two, go back and repeat this module. Correctly complete any missed questions.

SUPPLEMENTAL RATIONALE

Blastomycosis (North American Blastomycosis, Gilchrist's Disease; Fig. 7-8)

Blastomycosis, caused by *Blastomyces dermatitidis*, is classically observed south of the Ohio River and east of the Mississippi River. There are, however, cases reported from Canada, Latin America, Africa, and elsewhere. *Blastomyces* are thought to be breathed in, and they produce a mild chronic respiratory infection which gradually worsens over weeks or months. Sputum becomes purulent and blood streaked. The respiratory disease is similar to tuberculosis, coccidioidomycosis, paracoccidioidomycosis, and histoplasmosis; it must be carefully differentiated by cultural and histologic methods. Without treatment the infection usually disseminates to the rest of the body, starting in adjacent subcutaneous tissues. Skin and bone lesions are particularly associated with systemic spread. Skin lesions are ulcerated and crusted or weepy, with small abscesses in the center. The oral and nasal mucosa may be involved. Bone lesions produce pain and loss of function, with the vertebrae and ribs most often affected. In contrast to histoplasmosis and paracoccidioidomycosis, the gastrointestinal tract is rarely infected in blastomycosis. Without therapy the prognosis is poor. See the Introduction to this module for laboratory processing and direct mount results.

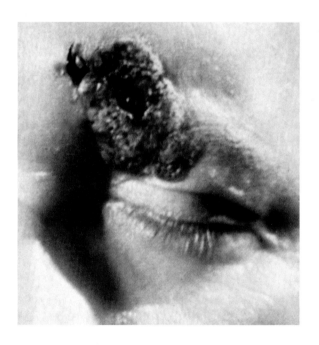

FIGURE 7-8. Blastomycosis of eyebrow. (From Beneke and Rogers: Medical Mycology Manual. Burgess, Minneapolis, 1980, with permission.)

Coccidioidomycosis (San Joaquin Fever; Fig. 7-9)

Coccidioidomycosis, caused by *Coccidioides immitis*, is endemic in the desert areas of the southwestern United States, with some cases reported from Central and

South America. The arthroconidia are very resistant to heat, dryness, and salinity. They reside in the soil; 10 to 14 days after contaminated dust is breathed in, 60 percent of patients with coccidioidomycosis exhibit an asymptomatic respiratory infection. The remaining 40 percent present symptoms of mild or, rarely, severe flu-like respiratory illness (primary pulmonary coccidioidomycosis). The patients recover or, if their immune response is compromised, may succumb to gradual or rapid disseminated disease, with hematogenous spread from the lungs to the bones, joints, skin, subcutaneous tissues, internal organs, and the brain and meninges. The prognosis is good for primary pulmonary disease, but the disseminated mycosis can be fatal. See the Introduction to this module for laboratory procedures.

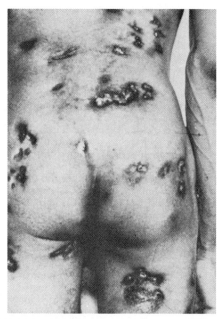

FIGURE 7-9. Disseminated coccidioidomycosis. (From Rippon: Medical Mycology. WB Saunders, Philadelphia, 1982, with permission.)

Histoplasmosis (Darling's Disease; Fig. 7-10)

Histoplasmosis, caused by *Histoplasma capsulatum*, is endemic in the Mississippi river area, Ohio River valley, and along the Appalachian Mountains, although it has been reported in other areas. The organisms multiply in droppings, including chicken and bat guano. Fungi are inhaled, usually producing a subclinical, self-limiting respiratory infection from which the patient quickly recovers. This common type of histoplasmosis has provided a positive skin test to most of the people in endemic areas. In a few instances, a chronic cavitary pulmonary disease occurs, with productive cough and x-ray signs resembling tuberculosis. Also, in a few pa-

tients, the pulmonary illness becomes severe and disseminates via the blood to the spleen, liver, adrenals, kidneys, skin, central nervous system, and other body organs, with a rapidly fatal outcome if not treated. See the Introduction to this module for laboratory procedures.

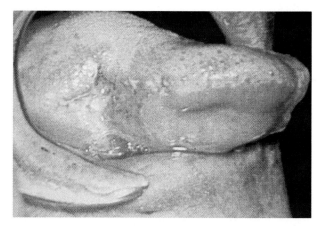

FIGURE 7-10. Histoplasmosis of tongue. (From Beneke: Human Mycoses. Upjohn, Kalamazoo, 1979, with permission.)

Paracoccidioidomycosis (South American Blastomycosis; Fig. 7-11)

Paracoccidioidomycosis, caused by *Paracoccidioides brasiliensis,* is primarily seen in South America, especially Brazil. The most notable clinical sign observed in

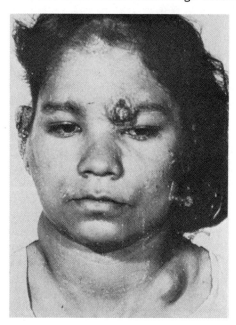

FIGURE 7-11. Cutaneous paracoccidioidomycosis with enlarged lymph nodes. (From Rippon: Medical Mycology. WB Saunders, Philadelphia, 1982, with permission.)

each disease manifestation is lymphatic enlargement. The oral mucosa and gums become infected from trauma caused by chewing contaminated vegetable matter or using fungus-infected vegetation as a tooth-pick. Crusted ulcers develop, which may spread to the tonsils, nasal mucosa, and face (mucocutaneous paracoccidioidomycosis). Organisms from the oral infection or from air are inhaled, producing pulmonary lesions similar to those of tuberculosis and other mycoses (pulmonary paracoccidioidomycosis). Fungi from the oral ulcers or contaminated food are swallowed and cause intestinal manifestations which may spread to the liver and spleen (visceral paracoccidioidomycosis). The patient expires in two or three years from disseminated disease or inability to eat. See the Introduction to this module for laboratory procedures.

Study Questions—Supplemental Rationale

Matching. Place the letter of the answer in Column B in front of the disease in Column A. An answer may be used more than once, as may the disease.

Column A

____ 1. Coccidioidomycosis

____ 2. Histoplasmosis

____ 3. Paracoccidioidomycosis

____ 4. Blastomycosis

Column B
A. Mainly in S. America
B. Conidia in desert soil
C. Assoc. with San Joaquin Valley, Calif.
D. Fungi found in bird droppings
E. Mainly in Mississippi and Ohio River valleys

For the next three questions, refer to this case study.

A 40-year-old woman from Washington, D.C., was admitted to the hospital for investigation of a mass in her right lung. She was on chemotherapy and the cancer seemed to be going into remission. There were no complaints outside those associated with anti-cancer medication, except that she possessed a slight chronic cough. Past history revealed a flulike illness six weeks prior to admission, while she was visiting her sister in California. X-rays showed a well-delineated round density in the right lower lobe. A skin test for tuberculosis was negative. The nodule was surgically removed, and some of the specimen was sent for mycology culture. Within four days, a white fluffy mold grew well on both plain Sabouraud dextrose agar and media with cycloheximide and chloramphenicol.

5. What disease do you suspect? Circle the correct letter.

A. Fungus ball with *Pseudallescheria boydii*

B. Abscess with *Candida albicans*

C. Pulmonary coccidioidomycosis

D. *Trichophyton mentagrophytes* infection

E. Geotrichosis

6. What criteria in the patient's clinical picture and past history would support this diagnosis? List two.

7. Which two procedures must you perform to confirm the diagnosis, and what would be the results?

10. What was the probable mode of exposure to the etiologic agent?

For the next four questions, refer to this case study.

A five-year-old girl from a farm town in Ohio was admitted to the regional hospital for suspected tuberculosis. She possessed a chronic cough with productive sputum, and she complained of breathlessness, tiredness, and weight loss over the last several months. Multiple sputum specimens showed no acid-fast bacilli; her tuberculin skin test was negative. Abnormal hematologic findings were anemia, a low white blood cell count, and some monocytes containing intracellular yeasts with a narrow isthmus between mother and daughter cells. Blood specimens were processed through a membrane filter and placed on brain heart infusion agar with blood at room temperature. After three weeks, tan, fluffy colonies formed. Microscopically, the fungus only produced microconidia along the sides of the hyphae.

11. A contaminant fungus is morphologically similar to the characteristic structures of the causative organism. Name it and provide two ways it may be differentiated from the disease agent in this case study.

8. What disease do you suspect and why? Give two reasons.

9. How would you confirm the identity of this isolate? Present two ways.

STOP HERE UNTIL YOU HAVE COMPLETED THE QUESTIONS.

Look up the answers in the back of the book. If you missed more than three, go back and review this module.

CHART 7-1. Microscopic Morphology of Systemic Pathogens

BLASTOMYCES DERMATITIDIS	PARACOCCIDIOIDES BRASILIENSIS	HISTOPLASMA CAPSULATUM	COCCIDIOIDES IMMITIS

MOLD PHASE

TISSUE PHASE

ORGANISMS CAUSING SYSTEMIC MYCOSES

APPENDIX A
ANSWERS FOR STUDY QUESTIONS AND FINAL EXAMS

Module 1

II.A.4.   Study questions, page 8.

1. F   Plants contain chlorophyll; fungi do not.

2. Yeasts. The sputum came from body temperature (37°C). At 37°C, a dimorphic organism is in a yeast phase.

3. Nodular organs

4. D

II.B.1.c.   Study questions, pages 12-13.

1. A

2. T

3. F   *Candida albicans* forms chlamydospores, which are nongerminating vesicles.

4. D

5. E

6. A. Sporangiospore
   B. Columella
   C. Sporangiophore

IV.   Final exam, pages 16-17.

1. A. Zygosporangium or zygospore (inside zygosporangium)
   B. Blastoconidia
   C. Racquet hyphae
   D. Macroconidium
   E. Verrucose topography
   F. Ascospore
   G. Vegetative hyphae
   H. Sessile chlamydoconidia
   I. Granular or powdery texture
   J. Dimorphism
   K. Basidiospore
   L. Arthroconidia

2. Velvety to woolly texture; umbonate and rugose topography; front color white with a white peripheral ring; reverse colors (starting from the periphery and moving inward) white, orange, yellow-orange, orange-tan, yellow-orange, center orange-tan OR white peripheral rings, with inner rings of varying shades of orange (yellow-orange, orange, and orange-tan). A reasonable facsimile of the above will suffice for an answer.

V.D.   Study questions—Supplemental Rationale, page 18.

1. Subcutaneous

2. *Paecilomyces* sp.

3. D
   G
   C

Module 2

II.C.   Study questions, pages 48-49.

1. Any three of these answers are acceptable:
   —Make sure the specimen is collected from the area most likely to be affected.
   —Use sterile technique in collecting the specimen.
   —The specimen must be adequate.
   —The specimen must be delivered promptly to the laboratory.
   —The laboratory must process the specimen quickly.
   —The specimen must be adequately labelled.

2. T

3. Overnight incubation and multiplication of fungi in the bladder will increase the chance

of isolating them on culture.
4. D
5. F   Alcohol removes surface contaminants; it does not affect fungal pathogens.
6. Organisms are concentrated on a filter rather than diluted in broth.
7. T
8. F   Granules are composed of organisms (bacteria, funguslike bacteria, or fungi) with or without a cementlike matrix or a center of necrotic material. They are the most likely source for isolating the etiologic agent of the infection.

III.H.   Study questions, page 54.
1. Any two of the following answers are adequate:
—A direct exam allows you to send out an immediate preliminary report to the physician, so he or she may initiate treatment or look for other diagnoses.
—With the direct exam results, you will know whether to inoculate any special media.
—The direct exam allows you to observe the yeast phase of dimorphic organisms.
—The direct exam may provide a clue as to the identity of the causative agent, without having to wait for the fungus to incubate.
2. D
3. A
4. F
5. B
6. G
7. E
8. F   All bacteria and fungi will stand out against the black background. Look only for encapsulated organisms.
9. B
10. F   The phenol in LPCB kills any fungus that may be present; thus, it cannot be cultured.

IV.D.   Study questions, page 58.
1. C, D   D is the best answer for specimens contaminated with other fungi. C is all right for pure cultures.
2. A and D   Sabouraud dextrose agar is used so that almost every fungus will grow. Brain heart infusion agar with blood-C&C is used for the fastidious fungi that will not flourish on Sabouraud, while the antibiotics keep down contaminants.
3. B   Dermatophytes grow well on Sabouraud dextrose agar, and the antibiotics hold down contaminants. Dermatophytes are not inhibited by C&C.

4. C   An anaerobic atmosphere is required. *Actinomyces* is inhibited by antibiotics, so do not use D.
5. C   Some strains of *N. asteroides* will not proliferate on Sabouraud dextrose agar. *Nocardia* is inhibited by antibiotics, so do not use D.
6. An intermediate grower is an organism that forms a mature colony in 6 to 10 days.

VII.   Final exam, page 64.
1. A 24-hour collection becomes easily overgrown with bacterial and fungal contaminants.
2. Any two of the following:
Coccidioides immitis
Histoplasma capsulatum
Actinomyces
Nocardia
Candida
Cryptococcus neoformans
Contaminants repeatedly isolated
3. F   Unlike bacteria, fungi do not make the broth cloudy. This necessitates frequent Gram staining.
4. Chitin
5. There are three possible answers for this question, depending on the individual's philosophy and the laboratory's economic situation.

Some laboratories incubate all their cultures at room temperature, so a costly incubator is not required. Fungi will grow at this temperature, but it takes longer for them to mature and thus identify.

If all cultures are put at 30°C, they will grow faster, thus aiding quick results, but an incubator is necessary. A 30°C temperature is recommended in this module.

Some laboratories incubate one set of cultures at 37°C to isolate the yeast phase of dimorphic fungi, and a second set of cultures at room temperature or 30°C for other organisms. This is probably not cost effective, since so few dimorphic fungi are isolated. Also the yeast phase could be immediately observed in specimen direct mounts.

6.   *Advantages*
Tease mount—Quick to make; no incubation period
Slide culture—Beautiful conidial juxtaposition; 2 mounts from one slide culture
Coverslip sandwich—Beautiful conidial juxtaposition; several mounts from one plate

Disadvantages
Tease mount—May destroy conidial juxtaposition
Slide culture—Takes time to set up; incubation period required
Coverslip sandwich—Incubation period required

7. **Specimen site**—Since you know that only certain organisms can be isolated from a particular specimen (Chart 2-1), many fungi are ruled out.
Colonial morphology—Sometimes a colony has such a characteristic morphology, for example, *Penicillium*, that you suspect its identity even before observing the microscopic characteristics.
General microscopic morphology—Since you know that only certain organisms possess hyphae, yeast forms, filamentous bacterial characteristics, or dimorphic attributes (Chart 2-3), many fungi are ruled out.

VIII.C. Study questions—Supplemental Rationale, page 67.
1. T
2. B
3. Negative
4. D
   G
   F
   B
   C

Module 3
III.D. Study questions, pages 90-91.
1. Any five of these answers will suffice:
   —Most fungal contaminants form mature colonies in four to five days.
   —They live in the soil.
   —They become airborne occasionally.
   —They are normally inhaled.
   —Respiratory specimens may normally yield a few colonies of fungal contaminants.
   —Fungal contaminants may be normal skin flora.
   —They may contaminate laboratory cultures.
   —Contaminants are usually nonpathogenic.
   —They are opportunistic pathogens in debilitated patients.
   —Antibiotics in fungal media inhibit fungal contaminants.
   —Fungal contaminants must be repeatedly isolated in large numbers from cultured specimens of the patient to be considered the causative agent of a disease.

2. A. Sporangium
   B. Rhizoids
   C. Stolon
IV.A.8. Study questions, page 95.
1. *Stemphylium* sp.
2. B,D,F,G
3. C
   E
   F
   C
   A
IV.B.10. Study questions, page 101.
1. Any three of the following will suffice:
   —*Gliocladium* forms balls of phialoconidia; the rest produce chains.
   —*Paecilomyces* exhibits tapering conidiophores; the rest do not.
   —*Scopulariopsis* phialoconidia are lemon shaped; the rest are round.
   —*Scopulariopsis* colonies are tan; the rest are usually shades of green.
   —All except *Gliocladium* have been numerously reported as human pathogens.
2. *B* Aseptate
   A,B Vesicles
   C Blastoconidia
   B Merosporangia
   A Foot cells
   A Phialides
3. F   *Acremonium* exhibits unbranching, gradually tapering conidiophores with balls of conidia.
4. B *Chrysosporium*
   B,C, *Sepedonium*
   D,E *Scedosporium apiospermum*
   D *Blastomyces dermatitidis*
   A,C *Histoplasma capsulatum*
V. Final exam, pages 101-102.
1. D
2. F   Dematiaceous organisms exhibit dark-colored hyphae and/or conidia.
3. *A,C* 1.
   A,B 2.
   A 3.
4. Any two of the following:
   —*Epicoccum* has sporodchia, while *Ulocladium* possesses a bent-knee conidiophore, and *Stemphylium* has a straight conidiophore.
   —*Epicoccum* produces orange colonies; the others produce black ones.
   —*Stemphylium* conidial cross septa are constricted; those in the other two fungi are not.
5. F   *Drechslera* possesses the bent-knee conidiophore, while that of

Helminthosporium is straight. Since the poroconidia are so similar, *Dreschslera* was often misidentified as *Helminthosporium* in the past.

    6. T

    7. A. *Curvularia* sp.
       B. *Syncephalastrum* sp.
       C. *Penicillium* sp.
       D. *Mucor* sp.
       E. *Scopulariopsis* sp.
       F. *Acremonium* sp.
       G. *Aspergillus* sp.
       H. *Cladosporium* sp.
       I. *Alternaria* sp.
       J. *Paecilomyces* sp.
       K. *Rhizopus* sp.
       L. *Aureobasidium* sp.

VI.F. Study questions—Supplemental Rationale, pages 105-106.

    1. T
    2. A
    3. F   The cornea is usually resistant to infection; mycotic keratitis primarily begins with trauma to the eye.
    4. Zygomycosis. Uncontrolled diabetes is the typical predisposing factor. Infection characteristically begins in the nasal passages or eye, and aseptate hyphae indicate the fungus must be of the subdivision Zygomycotina.
    5. C
    6. *Rhizopus* sp.
    7. Absolutely not. This disease rapidly erodes into surrounding blood vessels, with systemic spread and death within ten days after the initial sinus/eye symptoms. Treatment should begin as soon as the disease is suspected.

Module 4
II.E. Study questions, page 116.
    1. E
    2. A,D
    3. B,F
    4. C
III.A.6. Study questions, pages 118-119.
    1. D   endothrix invasion
    2. Athlete's foot
    3. *Microsporum*
    4. F   Dermatophytes are intermediate to slow growers.
    5. T
    6. B,C,E
III.B.3.b. Study questions, page 124.
    1. A,C,E
    2. B

    3. C
    4. F   *E. floccosum* macroconidia are club shaped; *T. verrucosum* are rat-tail.
IV. Final exam, pages 125-126.
    1. Superficial mycoses elicit little pathology, while cutaneous mycoses involve more tissue destruction.
    2. T
    3. B
    4. E
    5. Any two of the following will suffice:
    —*T. verrucosum* grows poorly at 25°C; *T. violaceum* grows well.
    —*T. verrucosum* colonies are white to bright yellow; *T. violaceum* colonies are violet.
    —On thiamine enriched media, *T. verrucosum* forms rare rat-tailed macroconidia, while *T. violaceum* does not form macroconidia.
    —Many strains of *T. verrucosum* require inositol as well as thiamine; *T. violaceum* requires only thiamine.
    —*T. verrucosum* produces an ectothrix hair invasion, while *T. violaceum* produces an endothrix invasion.
    6. B
    7. E
    8. C
    9. D
    10. B
    11. B
    12. D
    13. E

Module 5
II.B.2. Study questions, pages 141-142.
    1. C
    2. D
    3. C
    4. F
    5. B
    6. A
    7. *Candida albicans*
III. Final exam, page 149.
    1. F   Most, but not all, isolates of *C. albicans* form germ tubes and chlamydospores.
    2. F   A pseudohypha is constricted; a germ tube is not.
    3. T
    4. F   Zinc artifically reduced the nitrate; the fungus did not produce nitrate reductase.
    5. F   A positive reaction is indicated by gas formation only.
    6. A,D,E,H,I
    7. A,C,D,E

8. A,G
9. A,B,D,F
10. TOC medium is useful for observing germ tubes, chlamydospores, and darkly pigmented colonies. The first two are for identifying *Candida albicans* and *Candida stellatoidea,* and the last is for identifying *Cryptococcus neoformans.* The limitation of this medium is that it cannot be used for microscopic morphology of other filamentous yeasts. Advantages of the medium are that it is a good screening system for the most important yeasts; there is a quick turn around time between inoculation and reading the results; and *Candida tropicalis* does not produce germ tubes or chlamydospores on this medium, thus eliminating confusion in differentiating *C. tropicalis* from *C. albicans.*
11. *Rhodotorula*
12. *Geotrichum candidum*

IV.E. Study questions—Supplemental Rationale, pages 152-153.
1. D
2. Any three of the answers below:
   —Pigeon breeder. *Cryptococcus* is frequently found in pigeon droppings.
   —Patient was immunosuppressed, so his host defenses were lower than normal.
   —Central nervous system symptoms. *Cryptococcus* has a predilection for the brain and meninges.
   —Mucoid yeast. Mucoid colonies are composed of encapsulated organisms.
   —Inhibited by cycloheximide and chloramphenicol.
   How are the other answers ruled out?
   —*Candida.* Organisms would be seen on Gram stain.
   —No disease. *Anything* from CSF should be investigated, whether you think it is a laboratory contaminant or not. In this case, once the yeast is identified, there would be no question as to its significance.
   —*Histoplasma.* Possibly, since it is associated with bird droppings and is endemic in the midwest. However, in CSF, you would see small pseudoencapsulated yeasts *inside* phagocytic cells. Also, at 30°C, *Histoplasma* is a slow-growing mold.
   —*Coccidioides.* This has a predilection for the brain, but in CSF you would observe spherules, and at 30°C a white mold rapidly grows.
3. The capsule around *Cryptococcus* inhibits stain uptake of the yeast itself (Gram stain,

Module 2), thus making it barely visible. When seen, it also resembles debris.
4. Any three of the following: caffeic acid agar, assimilations, urease, India ink prep, mucicarmine stain.
5. B
6. D

Module 6
II.C. Study questions, pages 171-172.
1. B   *C. carrionii* produces black dots or sclerotic bodies; *C. trichoides* causes phaeohyphomycosis, in which no black dots are observed.
2. Similarities. Any three of the following:
   —Black yeasts at first
   —Annellides, although they are not uniformly accepted for *Wangiella*
   —Terminal balls of conidia, which tend to fall down the sides of the conidiophore
   —Clusters of conidia may form on short denticles off the sides of the hyphae.
   —Both decompose (hydrolyze) casein and tyrosine.
   —Both may cause phaeohyphomycosis.
   Differences. Any three of the following:
   —*E. jeanselmei* uses nitrate, while *Wangiella* is negative.
   —*Wangiella* grows at 42°C; *E. jeanselmei* can not.
   —*E. jeanselmei* may cause mycetoma and mycotic keratitis, while *Wangiella* has not been a reported agent of these infections.
   —*Wangiella* does not exhibit annellides as the most distinct, stable, and unique form. (generally accepted opinion).
3. B,D,F
4. A
5. C
6. Cleistothecia with asci and ascospores
IV. Final exam, pages 178-179.
1. C,D (also conidia of B)
2. A
3. B,C
4. B,C
5. A
6. F   Bacteria also may form them.
7. C   The answer cannot be D, because in actinomycosis, granules are yellow.
8. Two of the following:
   —*Sporothrix* colonies turn black with age, especially on potato dextrose agar; *Acremonium* colonies do not.
   —*Sporothrix* possesses a yeast phase; *Acremonium* does not.
   —The mold phase of *Sporothrix* is not as

tightly packed in the flowerette as
Acremonium.

9. E

10. Anaerobic actinomycetes → Casein, tyrosine, xanthine
Aerobic actinomycetes → Gelatin liquefaction
KOH-DMSO prep for sclerotic bodies
Catalase, fermentations

V.G. Study questions—Supplemental Rationale,
pages 182-183.

1. T
2. T
3. T
4. Any two of the following:
—Mycetoma invades bone;
chromoblastomycosis does not.
—Chromoblastomycosis exhibits dry lesions;
mycetoma demonstrates draining sinuses.
—Black sclerotic bodies are seen in
chromoblastomycosis, while in mycetoma,
there are variously colored granules. Black
granules of mycetoma differ from black
sclerotic bodies in that the granules are
composed of chlamydoconidia with
occasional hyphae.
—Different etiologic agents, plus mycetoma,
may be eumycotic or actinomycotic.
5. B   *Actinomyces* is normal flora of the
oral cavity, while the other diseases are
produced by exogenous organisms
introduced by skin puncture with
contaminated thorns and so forth.
6. Sporotrichosis. Any two of these reasons:
—Lesions following the lymphatics
—Cigar bodies in stained sections
—Cream-colored colony at room
temperature, which turned black with age
—Black necrotic lesions
7. C   E is *Acremonium*, which appears
similar but does not possess a yeast phase.
A is wrong because this would be observed
only at 37°C.
8. Since he is a rose gardener, the patient
probably was pricked with a contaminated
thorn.
9. Chromoblastomycosis. Any two of the
following:
—Sclerotic bodies
—Cauliflower lesions
—A slow-growing organism with only this
conidial arrangement is seen exclusively in
chromoblastomycosis.
10. E   It cannot be A because *C. trichoides*
causes phaeohyphomycosis, in which there
are no sclerotic bodies or cauliflower lesions.

Module 7

III. Final exam, pages 194-195.

1. B
2. D
3. G
4. C
5. F
6. E
7. Any four of the following is acceptable:
—Use slanted media in capped tubes rather
than plated media. This minimizes the risk
of conidia becoming airborne.
—Wear mask and gloves.
—Always work under a microbiologic hood.
—Formalinize or wet down mold cultures
before preparing tease mounts.
—Never make slide cultures with the mold
forms of systemic fungi; the conidia are too
easily distributed into the air.
8. Any three of the following will suffice:
—The medium must be enriched.
—The medium must be kept moist.
—The temperature should be 37°C.
—The organism must be subcultured onto
fresh media several times for complete
conversion.
9. A   All three fungi possess conidia on the
sides or tips of the hyphae, resembling
lollipops, and they all have white colonies.
Here are some differences:
—*Blastomyces* is a slow grower, while the
others are rapid and intermediate growers,
respectively.
—*Blastomyces* has a yeast phase, while the
others do not.
—*Chrysosporium* is a nonpathogenic
contaminant, while *Blastomyces* may cause
systemic disease, and *Scedosporium* may
produce subcutaneous problems.
—*Scedosporium* has a rather commonly
observed sexual stage. *Blastomyces*
possesses a sexual stage, but it is not as
routinely observed. *Chrysosporium* does not
exhibit one.
—*Scedosporium* and *Chrysosporium* are

inhibited by cycloheximide and chloramphenicol (C&C); *Blastomyces* mold forms are not.

B   Both organisms produce arthroconidia, are rapid growers, form white colonies, and may produce systemic disease. However, *Coccidioides* forms alternating arthroconidia, is not inhibited by C&C, and has a tissue phase, while *Geotrichum* forms adjacent arthroconidia, is inhibited by C&C, and possesses no tissue phase.

IV.E.   Study questions—Supplemental Rationale, pages 197–198.

1. B,C
2. D,E
3. A
4. E
5. C   All five organisms grow relatively rapidly and are white; however, *Pseudallescheria* and *Geotrichum* are inhibited by cycloheximide, *Candida* is a yeast, and *Trichophyton* would cause dermatomycosis rather than a respiratory infection.
6. Any two of the following:
   —Patient on chemotherapy and therefore immunosuppressed
   —Flu was probably a mild case of coccidioidomycosis
   —California: *Coccidioides* loves the desert soil there.
7. Any two of the following:
   —Perform LPCB tease mounts of the mold, under a microbiologic hood, and search for barrel-shaped arthroconidia with empty cells interspersed.
   —Demonstrate spherules with endospores in histologic sections from the surgical specimen.
   —Serologic studies with known antibodies, to identify the mold
   —Acute and convalescent sera to test for a fourfold rise in antibody titer to *Coccidioides*
8. *Histoplasma capsulatum.* Any two of the following:
   —Ohio, endemic for histoplasmosis
   —Symptoms
   —Typical yeasts on blood differential; they should rule out yeasts of *Blastomyces*
   —Slow grower on nutritious medium
9. Any two of the following:
   —Subculture the isolate to less nutritious medium like Sabouraud dextrose agar to see if the mold produces characteristic macroconidia.
   —Convert the fungus from the mold to yeast phase.
   —Serologic studies with known antibodies, to identify the mold
   —Acute and convalescent sera to test for a fourfold rise in antibody titer to *Histoplasma*
10. Farm town—probably a lot of chickens. *Histoplasma* resides in bird droppings.
11. *Histoplasma* and *Sepedonium* both possess microconidia and macroconidia (some people argue that the microconidia of *Sepedonium* are just immature macroconidia). However, *Histoplasma* is a slow grower and produces a yeast phase, mold forms are not inhibited by cycloheximide and chloramphenicol, and the fungus may elicit systemic disease; but *Sepedonium* is a rapid grower, has no yeast phase, is inhibited by cycloheximide and chloramphenicol, and is a nonpathogenic contaminant.

COMMON SYNONYMS

Synonym	Currently Accepted Name
Acrotheca sporulation	*Rhinocladiella*like conidial formation
Actinomadura	*Nocardia*
Allescheria boydii	*Pseudallescheria boydii*
Bifidobacterium eriksonii	*Bifidobacterium adolescentis*
Blastomyces brasiliensis	*Paracoccidioides brasiliensis*
Candidiasis	Candidosis
Cephalosporium	*Acremonium*
Cerebral chromomycosis	Phaeohyphomycosis
Chromomycosis	Chromoblastomycosis
Cladosporiosis	Phaeohyphomycosis
Cladosporium bantianum	*Cladosporium trichoides*
Cladosporium werneckii	*Exophiala werneckii*
Helminthosporium	misidentified isolates of *Drechslera*
Hormodendrum	*Cladosporium*
Madura foot	Mycetoma
Maduromycosis	Mycetoma
Monilia	*Candida*
Moniliasis	Candidosis
Monosporium apiospermum	*Scedosporium apiospermum*
Mucormycosis	Zygomycosis
North American blastomycosis	Blastomycosis
Petriellidium boydii	*Pseudallescheria boydii*
Phaeomycotic cyst	Phaeohyphomycosis
Phialophora dermatitidis	*Wangiella dermatitidis*
Phialophora gougerotii	*Exophiala jeanselmei*
Phialophora jeanselmei	*Exophiala jeanselmei*
Phycomycosis	Zygomycosis
Pityrosporum orbiculare	*Malassezia furfur*

Pityrosporum ovale	*Malassezia furfur*
San Joaquin Valley fever	Coccidioidomycosis
South American blastomycosis	Paracoccidioidomycosis
Sterigmata (on *Aspergillus, Penicillium*)	Phialides
Streptomyces madurae	*Nocardia madurae*
Streptomyces pelletierii	*Nocardia pelletierii*
Tinea versicolor	Pityriasis versicolor
Torulopsis candida	*Candida famata*
Torulopsis glabrata	*Candida glabrata*
Trichosporon capitatum	*Geotrichum capitatum*
Trichosporon cutaneum	*Trichosporon beigelii*
Trichosporon penicillatum	*Geotrichum penicillatum*

APPENDIX C
GLOSSARY

TERM	DEFINITION	
ACERVULUS (pl. acervuli)	Thick hyphal mat supporting bunches of conidiophores	

ACTINOMYCETE — All genera of the Actinomycetales except the family Myco-bacteriaceae. Representative actinomycetes are *Norcardia, Streptomyces,* and *Actinomyces.*

ACTINOMYCOSIS — Disease caused by the anaerobic funguslike bacteria *Actinomyces, Bifidobacterium,* and *Arachnia.* The most common manifestations are facial (lumpy jaw), pulmonary, and abdominal. Draining sinus tracts contain characteristic sulfur-colored granules.

ACTINOMYCOTIC MYCETOMA — Mycetoma caused by a funguslike bacterium. Granules of various colors may be observed, depending on the etiologic agent.

AERIAL — Above the surface. Aerial hyphae usually support reproductive structures.

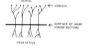

AMPULLA (pl. ampullae) — Swollen conidiogenous cell with conidia developing from a number of different foci on the parent.

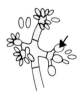

ANAMORPH — Asexual name

ANNELLIDE	Tube- or vase-shaped conidiogenous cell. The first annelloconidium arises holoblastically, while the rest develop enteroblastically, from a tip which exhibits a new ring of material as each annelloconidium passes through. The outer rings provide a saw-toothed appearance at the annellide tip.

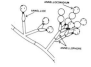

ANNELLOCONIDIUM	Conidium arising from an annellide. The first is holoblastic, but the rest develop enteroblastically. See drawing at ANNELLIDE.
ANNELLOPHORE	Conidiophore, or stalk, which supports annellides
ANNULAR FRILL	Skirtlike remnant of parent material at the base of a conidium

ANTHERIDIUM	Male sexual cell produced by the Ascomycotina
ANTIBODY	Protein synthesized by lymphocytes to help eliminate a foreign material (antigen) from the body
ANTIGEN	Foreign material, including an organism or its extract, which will produce an immunologic response when inoculated into a suitable host.
ARTHRIC CONIDIOGENESIS	Thallic development whereby the daughter cells fragment within the hyphal strand before dispersing. They may be holoarthric or enteroarthric. See thallic conidiogenesis.
ARTHROCONIDIUM (pl. arthroconidia)	Arthric conidium produced by fragmentation of the hyphal strand through the septation points. Arthroconidia may form adjacent to each other or may be separated by disjunctor cells.

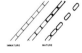

ARTHROSPORE	See arthroconidium.
ASCOCARP	Protective sac which houses asci and ascospores of molds in the Ascomycotina. Asci are extruded from the ascocarp walls into the center of the sac. When the sac is ruptured, asci are released. If the intact sac is completely enclosed, it is called a cleistothecium.

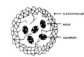

ASCOGONIUM	Female sexual cell produced by members of the subdivision Ascomycotina
ASCOMYCOTINA	Fungal taxonomic subdivision in which asci and ascospores are the sexual method of reproduction
ASCOSPORE	Sexual spore formed by transfer of a male nucleus into a female cell and fusion of the nuclei into a zygote. The mother cell, or ascus, divides by meiosis so that 2, 4, or 8 ascospores develop inside. The asci may be surrounded by a protective outer ascocarp. See drawing at ASCOCARP.
ASCUS (pl. asci)	Sexual mother cell which forms ascospores inside and may be protected on the outside by an ascocarp. Asci are demonstrated in the subdivision Ascomycotina. See drawing at ASCOCARP.

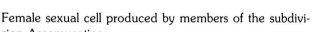

211

ASEPTATE HYPHAE	Hyphae without cross-walls, so that nuclei and cytoplasm move freely between cells. Aseptate hyphae are found in the subdivision Zygomycotina.
ASEXUAL REPRODUCTION	Nuclear and cytoplasmic division, or mitosis, to produce two or more identical cells.
ASPERGILLOMA	Fungus ball caused by *Aspergillus*, especially *A. fumigatus* and *A. niger*
ASPERGILLOSIS	A collection of opportunistic infections caused by various species of *Aspergillus*. The most important disease is invasive pulmonary aspergillosis, which initially demonstrates a lung focus, but later erodes into surrounding blood vessels and disseminates to the rest of the body.
ASSIMILATION	Ability of a fungus to utilize a nutrient in the presence of oxygen
AUXANOGRAPHY	A compound is placed on top of a nutritionally poor agar medium that is seeded with a test organism. If there is growth around the compound after incubation, the organism is using it for growth. In mycology, auxanography is performed for carbohydrate and nitrate assimilation testing for yeasts.
BALLISTOCONIDIUM	Forcibly ejected conidium, usually triggered by a water droplet mechanism. Ballistoconidia, seen in the yeast *Sporobolomyces* sp., develop into individual colonies which satellite around the parent. To test for these projectiles, invert the plate of yeast colonies over a plate of fresh medium. Ballistoconidia will be discharged onto the new medium and form colonies after incubation. 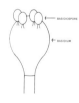
BASIDIOCARP	Protective structure which houses basidia and basidiospores. The mushroom cap is a basidiocarp.
BASIDIOMYCOTINA	Taxonomic subdivision of fungi which produce basidiospores sexually
BASIDIOSPORE	Sexual spore formed by fusion of two compatible nuclei and cells into a zygote. Inside the mother cell, or basidium, the fused nuclei divide by meiosis to form four haploid nuclei, which later travel into four protrusions at the basidium tip to produce basidiospores. The basidium and basidiospores may be protected by an outer basidiocarp. These structures are observed in the subdivision Basidiomycotina.
BASIDIUM (pl. basidia)	Club-shaped mother cell from which basidiospores arise. Both structures are seen only in the subdivision Basidiomycotina. *See* drawing at BASIDIOSPORE.
BLACK DOT	Black sclerotic body found in chromoblastomycosis. This is to be differentiated from the black dot type of tinea capitis, produced by broken off infected hair shafts at the scalp surface.

BLACK PIEDRA	Stony black nodules around scalp hairs. The nodules are caused by *Piedraia hortai*.
BLASTIC CONIDIOGENESIS	Conidium formation whereby the parent cell enlarges, then a septum divides the enlarged portion into a duaghter cell. The daughter begins to develop *before* it is separated from the parent. Blastic conidiogenesis may be holoblastic or enteroblastic.
BLASTOCONIDIUM (pl. blastoconidia)	Holoblastic conidium produced by budding. Yeasts are typical examples of blastoconidia, although some molds (for example, *Cladosporium, Aureobasidium,* and *Nigrospora*) also demonstrate them. 
BLASTOMYCOSIS	Infection with *Blastomyces dermatitidis.* It initially manifests itself as a pulmonary disease, but if the patient is debilitated, infection may disseminate throughout the body, particularly bone and skin.
BLASTOSPORE	See blastoconidium.
CANDIDIASIS	See candidosis.
CANDIDOSIS	Spectrum of diseases produced by the genus *Candida.* Usually infection is opportunistic; an upset in the balance of normal flora by antibiotics, anticancer drugs, debilitating illness, and so forth, enables *Candida* to proliferate where it once was held in check.
CHLAMYDOCONIDIUM (pl. chlamydoconidia)	Thick-walled hyphal survival conidium formed during poor environmental conditions, which will germinate and produce conidia when a better climate occurs. In the past, chlamydospore was the general term; however, a chlamydospore neither germinates nor develops conidia when mature. Chlamydospores are observed in yeasts, while chlamydoconidia are seen in molds.
CHLAMYDOSPORE	Thick-walled vesicle of *Candida albicans* and some other yeasts, which neither germinates nor produces conidia when mature. See chlamydoconidium.
CHROMOBLASTOMYCOSIS	Slow progressing fungal infection of subcutaneous tissues, usually the extremities, with development of dark sclerotic bodies (black dots) on the tissue surfaces
CIGAR BODY	Yeast form of *Sporothrix schenckii,* so called because it resembles the shape of a cigar.
CLAMP CONNECTION	Bridge between two adjacent hyphal cells whereby duplication of compatible nuclei takes place. Clamp connections are seen in the Basidiomycotina as a part of the reproductive process.
CLEISOTHECIUM (pl. cleistothecia)	Completely enclosed ascocarp, containing asci and ascospores 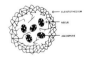

COCCIDIOIDOMYCOSIS	Infection with *Coccidioides immitis*. Initially, the disease presents a flulike respiratory illness, but if the patient is debilitated, it may spread to the rest of the body, particularly the brain.
COLLARETTE	Small ring of remnant material, either at the tip of a phialide or base of a columella.
COLUMELLA (pl. collumellae)	Supporting structure at the tip of a sporangiophore and base of a sporangium. Most, but not all, zygomycetous fungi produce columellae. 
CONDIDIOGENESIS	Conidium formation.
CONIDIOGENOUS CELL	Parent cell from which conidia directly arise. Annellides and phialides are examples of conidiogenous cells.
CONIDIOPHORE	Stalk on which conidia develop. A conidiophore may be a conidiogenous cell or may support conidiogenous cells.
CONIDIUM (pl. conidia)	Nonmotile, asexual reproductive structure which usually separates from the parent. It is not produced by cleavage, conjugation, or free-cell formation. See drawing at CONIDIOPHORE.
COTTONY TEXTURE	Colony with hyphae rising way up in the air, often an inch, before conidia develop. Contaminant fungi may elicit cottony colonies; pathogens usually do not.
CRYPTOCOCCOSIS	Disease elicited by *Cryptococcus neoformans*. The primary illness results from inhalation of the fungus in bird droppings. If the patient is debilitated, infection spreads from the lungs to the brain and rest of the body.
CUTANEOUS MYCOSIS	Fungal disease of the skin, hair, and nail. There is more tissue destruction than with a superficial mycosis.
DEMATIACEOUS	Hyphae and/or conidia in varieties of black, when observed under the microscope. In this text, drawings of dematiaceous organisms are shaded gray.
DENTICLE	Very small, hairlike stalk
DERMATOMYCOSIS	Fungal disease affecting hair, skin, or nail
DERMATOPHYTE	Fungus infecting the dermis (hair, skin, or nail), and belonging to the genus *Epidermophyton*, *Microsporum* or *Trichophyton*

DEUTEROMYCOTINA	Fungal subdivision in which the sexual stage does not exist or is unknown; also called Fungi Imperfecti.
DIMORPHISM	Possessing two different appearances, or phases. In this text, the term will be limited to a mold phase at room temperature and a yeast (tissue) phase at 37°C.

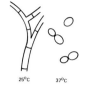

25°C   37°C

DISJUNCTOR CELL	Empty cell between conidia that breaks or dissolves to release the conidia

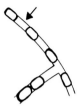

ECHINULATE	Having rough edges; spiny

ECTOTHRIX	Infection around the outside of a hair shaft. Note that fungal invasion initially begins inside the shaft at the root, but arthroconidia develop around the outside further up. The cuticle is destroyed in this type of invasion. Ectothrix properties must be observed in specimen direct mounts, not in hairs that have already been placed on media.

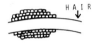

H A I R

ENDOGENOUS	Originating within oneself
ENDOSPORE	Spore produced with a spherule, as in *Coccidioides immitis*

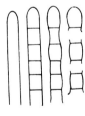

ENDOTHRIX	Infection with arthroconidia inside a hair shaft; the cuticle is not destroyed. Endothrix properties must be observed in specimen direct mounts, not in hairs that have already been placed on media.

H A I R

ENTEROARTHRIC CONIDIOGENESIS	Only inner parent cell wall layers are involved in arthric daughter cell development, for example, in the arthroconidia of *Coccidioides immitis*. See arthric and thallic conidiogenesis.

ENTEROBLASTIC CONIDIOGENESIS	Only inner parent cell wall layers are involved in blastic daughter cell development, for example, in phialoconidia and annelloconidia. See blastic conidiogenesis.

EPIDEMIOLOGY	Geographic location of a disease; also, a study to identify carriers of an infection

ERYTHEMA	Redness
ETIOLOGIC AGENT	Organism causing the disease
EUKARYOTIC	Containing a true nucleus, surrounded by a nuclear membrane
EUMYCOTIC MYCETOMA	Mycetoma caused by a true fungus. Granules of various colors may be observed, depending on the etiologic agent.
FAVIC CHANDELIERS	Blunt, branched hyphae which resemble the antlers of a buck deer. Favic chandeliers may be observed in many old cultures, but *Trichophyton schoenleinii* possesses a predominance of them.
FERMENTATION	Ability of an organism to use a compound in the absence of oxygen
FOOT CELL	In *Aspergillus* sp., a hyphal cell at the conidiophore base; in *Fusarium* sp., the sharply angled end of a macroconidium where it attaches to the conidiophore
FUNGI IMPERFECTI	Those fungi whose sexual stage does not exist or has not yet been discovered. They are classified in the subdivision Deuteromycotina.
FUNGUS (pl. fungi)	Kingdom of organisms that contain true nuclei, are devoid of chlorophyll, and absorb all nutrients from the environment, especially decaying organic matter. Fungi may reproduce asexually and/or sexually.
FUNGUS BALL	Walled-off fungal abscess in the lungs. It may erode into surrounding blood vessels, with subsequent dissemination. Several genera may produce fungus balls, but the most common are *Aspergillus* and *Pseudallescheria*.
FUNGUSLIKE BACTERIUM	A bacterium, 1 μm in diameter, which develops conidia and elicits a funguslike disease
GENICULATE	Bent-knee growth; when one conidium has formed, the growing point of the hyphal strand continues in the opposite direction. The terms sympodial and geniculate usually go hand in hand.
GEOTRICHOSIS	Opportunistic *Geotrichum candidum* infection of various sites, usually caused by imbalance of normal flora so that the etiologic agent proliferates
GLABROUS TEXTURE	Colony containing no aerial hyphae. These are usually yeasts.
GRANULAR TEXTURE	Conidia in a dense profusion on top of the colony, resembling sugar granules

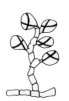

GRANULE | 1–2 mm-wide clump of hyphae and swollen cells in a compact mass, or funguslike bacteria radiating out from a center of necrotic debris. A cementlike matrix may be present. Granules are variously colored, depending on the etiologic agent, and they are observed in tissue from patients with mycetoma.

GRANULOMATOUS | Tumorous

HISTOPLASMOSIS | Infection with *Histoplasma capsulatum.* Initially a subclinical respiratory infection, it becomes systemic and serious if the patient is debilitated.

HOLOARTHRIC CONIDIOGENESIS | All parent cell wall layers are involved in arthric daughter cell development, for example, the arthroconidia of *Geotrichum* sp. See arthric and thallic conidiogenesis.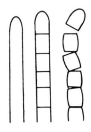

HOLOBLASTIC CONIDIOGENESIS | All parent cell wall layers are involved in blastic daughter cell development, for example, in blastoconidia and poroconidia. See blastic conidiogenesis.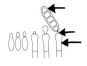

HOLOTHALLIC CONIDIOGENESIS | All parent cell wall layers are involved in thallic daughter cell development, for example, in macroconidia and chlamydoconidia. See thallic conidiogenesis.

HYALINE | Hyphae and conidia lightly pigmented when observed under the microscope. This includes shades of blue and green.

HYPHA (pl. hyphae) | Long strand of cells, with or without crosswalls

IMPERFECT FUNGI | See Fungi Imperfecti

INDURATION | Hardness

INFLAMMATORY | Pus cell response

INTERCALARY | Arising within the hyphal strand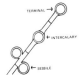

INTERMEDIATE GROWTH RATE | Forming a mature colony in 6–10 days

IN VITRO | Outside the host, as on artificial media

IN VIVO | Inside the host

LUMPY JAW | Hard, swollen area of the jaw caused by infection with *Actinomyces.* It usually occurs after a tooth extraction.

MACROALEURIOSPORE   See macroconidium.

MACROCONIDIUM
(pl. macroconidia)

Holothallic multicelled conidium in which an entire hyphal element converts into a macroconidium. The prefix macro- should be used only when smaller microconidia are also present. Macroconidia may be thick- or thin-walled; smooth or rough; club-shaped, spindle-shaped, or oval; and alone or in clusters.

MEIOSIS

Nuclear and cytoplasmic reduction division in which a diploid zygote produces haploid daughters, each containing genetic information from both parents. This is observed in sexual reproduction.

MEROSPORANGIUM

Tubelike sporangium containing sporangiospores in a row. Merosporangia are observed in *Syncephalastrum* sp.

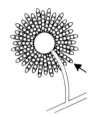

MICROALEURIOSPORE   See microconidium.

MICROCONIDIUM
(pl. microconidia)

Holothallic single-celled (or rarely two-celled) conidium in which an entire hyphal element converts into the microconidium. The prefix micro- should be used only when larger macroconidia are also present. Microconidia are round, oval, or club-shaped, and single or in clusters.

MITOSIS

Nuclear and cytoplasmic division in which the two daughter cells contain the same genetic information as one parent. This occurs with multiplying, nonsexual cells, for example, skin cells in humans. In mycology, besides hyphal proliferation, mitosis is observed in asexual reproduction.

MOLD   Colony growing hyphal (as opposed to yeast) forms

MONILIASIS   See candidosis.

MURIFORM   Divided by horizontal and vertical cross septa

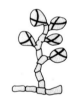

MYCELIA STERILIA

No reproductive structures present, only septate hyphae. These organisms are usually of the subdivision Basidiomycotina; look for clamp connections. With the proper environmental conditions, e.g., different media, temperature, or atmosphere, fruiting structures should develop.

MYCELIUM (pl. mycelia)   Many hyphae intertwined to form a thick mat

MYCETOMA

Slow-growing, subcutaneous lesion, usually on an extremity, characterized by bone deformity and oozing sinus tracts containing granules. Eumycotic mycetoma is caused by true fungi, while actinomycotic mycetoma is elicited by funguslike bacteria.

MYCOLOGY	Study of fungi
MYCOSIS (pl. mycoses)	Disease caused by a fungus
MYCOTIC KERATITIS	Opportunistic fungal infection of the cornea of the eye
NECROSIS	Dead and decaying tissue
NEUROTROPIC	Propensity to invade nervous tissue, particularly the brain
NOCARDIOSIS	Abscess of the lungs with *Nocardia* sp. and subsequent spread to other body sites. Granules are usually not observed.
NODULAR ORGAN	Knot of twisted hyphae seen in older cultures

ONTOGENY	Study of the maturation of an organism
ONYCHOMYCOSIS	Fungal infection of the nail by molds or yeasts. With yeast invasion, the surrounding skin will also be affected. Other names for onychomycosis are tinea unguium and ringworm of the nail.
OPPORTUNISTIC PATHOGEN	Not normally disease producing. When the host is debilitated, as with chronic disease, anticancer therapy, antibiotics, steroids, and so forth, the opportunists proliferate and elicit an infection.
OTOMYCOSIS	Opportunistic fungal infection of the outer ear; the inner ear is not affected.
PARACOCCIDIOIDOMYCOSIS	Infection with *Paracoccidioides brasiliensis.* The most common sites are the oral mucosa, lungs, and intestines. Lymphatic enlargement is characteristic, and with time, the disease becomes systemic.
PATHOGENIC	Producing disease
PENICILLIOSIS	Collection of opportunistic infections caused by the penicillus-containing genera *Penicillium, Paecilomyces,* and *Scopulariopsis.* The most important disease is bronchopulmonary in origin, with later dissemination throughout the body.
PENICILLUS (pl. penicilli)	Conidiophores that branch in multiple layers, providing a brushlike appearance.

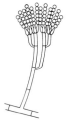

PERFECT FUNGI	Those fungi which reproduce sexually. This includes the subdivisions Zygomycotina, Basidiomycotina, and Ascomycotina.

PHAEOHYPHOMYCOSIS

Formerly called chromoblastomycosis in part, cladosporiosis. Phaeohyphomycosis is a subcutaneous abscess, particularly in the brain, characterized in histologic sections by dark, branched hyphae and occasionally, spherical cells. Sclerotic bodies and granules are absent. The primary etiologic agent is *Cladosporium trichoides*.

PHIALIDE

Tube- or vase-shaped conidiogenous cell. The first phialoconidium is holoblastic and the rest are enteroblastic, arising from a fixed locus in the phialide. The phialide may be ringed at the top by a cup-shaped collarette.

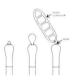

PHIALOCONIDIUM
(pl. phialoconidia)

Conidium arising from a phialide. The first develops holoblastically, but the succeeding conidia are enteroblastically derived. See drawing at PHIALIDE.

PITYRIASIS VERSICOLOR

Formerly tinea versicolor. Pityriasis versicolor is a superficial skin infection characterized by scaly patches of reddish brown, brown, and white, caused by *Malassezia furfur*.

POROCONIDIUM
(pl. poroconidia)

Holoblastic conidium produced through a pore in the parent cell wall

POWDERY TEXTURE

Conidia in profusion on top of a colony, resembling flour

PSEUDOHYPHA

Elongated blastoconidium made by some yeast species. Pseudohyphae are constricted at their point of attachment, while true hyphae are not.

PYCNIDIUM

Asexual sac containing conidia. Pycnidia resemble sexual ascocarps; they must be carefully differentiated by crushing the sacs and examining the contents for conidia rather than asci and ascospores.

RACQUET HYPHAE

Hyphae resembling tennis racquets placed end to end, often seen in older cultures.

RAPID GROWTH RATE

Forming a mature colony within five days

RHIZOID

Rootlike hypha

RINGWORM	Fungus infection caused by *Epidermophyton, Microsporum,* or *Trichophyton*	
RUGOSE TOPOGRAPHY	Furrows radiating out from the colony center	 RUGOSE
SAN JOAQUIN VALLEY FEVER	See coccidioidomycosis.	
SAPROBE	Organism able to live on decaying organic matter in the soil. Most contaminant fungi are saprobes.	
SCLEROTIC BODY	Black, thick-walled cell in tissue which may be divided into horizontal and/or vertical cross septa. Sclerotic bodies are observed in chromoblastomycosis.	
SEPTATE	Containing cross-walls in hyphae, conidia, or spores	
SEPTUM (pl. septa)	Cross-wall in a hypha, spore, or conidium; it usually contains a septal pore, allowing some movement of the cellular contents from one cell to another.	
SEROLOGY	Study of antigen and antibody reactions	
SEROMYCOLOGY	Study of fungal antigens and antibodies	
SESSILE	Arising on the sides of a hypha	
SEXUAL REPRODUCTION	Fusion of two compatible haploid nuclei to form a zygote	
SHIELD CELL	Conidiogenous cell which gives rise to two branches of reproductive structures. Scars at the branch point of attachment give the conidiogenous cell a shield appearance. These cells are observed in *Cladosporium* sp.	
SINUS TRACT	In mycetoma, actinomycosis, and nocardiosis, a tunnel eroded from the infected site to a drainage area, for example, from the lungs to the skin	
SLOW GROWTH RATE	Forming a mature colony in 11–21 days	
SOUTH AMERICAN BLASTOMYCOSIS	See paracoccidioidomycosis.	
SPHERULE	Thick-walled spherical structure produced in tissue or under special in vitro conditions by *Coccidioides immitis.* When young, the spherules are empty; with age, they become filled with endospores.	

SPINDLE-SHAPED	Enlarged in the middle and tapered at the ends, resembling a spindle of yarn on a spinning wheel	
SPIRAL HYPHA	Hypha curved in a spiral, either flat or like a corkscrew	
SPORANGIOLUM (pl. sporangiola)	Small sporangium containing one or a few sporangiospores, as in *Cunninghamella* sp.	
SPORANGIOPHORE	Asexual stalk which supports a sporangium. It may be branched or unbranched.	
SPORANGIOSPORE	Asexual spore formed by cleavage of the sporangium contents. Sporangiospores are produced by the subdivision Zygomycotina. See drawing at SPORANGIOPHORE.	
SPORANGIUM (pl. sporangia)	Asexual saclike structure at the tip of a sporangiophore, and developing sporangiospores inside. See drawing at SPORANGIOPHORE.	
SPORODCHIUM	Hyphal mat densely covered with short conidiophores and conidia	
SPOROTRICHOSIS	Subcutaneous, hard, black, ulcerating lesions, usually on the extremities, caused by *Sporothrix schenckii*. Granules are not observed.	
STERIGMA (pl. sterigmata)	This term is now reserved for the structure which supports a basidiospore on top of a basidium. Regarding *Aspergillus* and *Penicillum*, sterigmata have been replaced by the term phialides.	
STOLON	Hyphal runner connecting groups of sporangiophores, similar to the runner which connects raspberry bushes	
SUBCUTANEOUS MYCOSIS	Fungal disease of the skin, muscle, and connective tissue immediately beneath the skin	
SUPERFICIAL MYCOSIS	Fungal disease of the outermost layers of skin and hair, with little or no pathology evidenced	
SYMPODIAL	First developing a conidium on one side, then further up on the other side, in a repeating fashion	

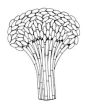

SYNNEMA (pl. synnemata)   Conidiophores bunched together in a parallel fashion as in *Graphium* sp.

SYSTEMIC MYCOSIS   Fungal disease of the deep tissues and organs of the body. In disseminated forms of these infections, subcutaneous and cutaneous areas may also be invaded.

TAXONOMY   Classification of organisms by kingdoms, divisions, subdivisions, classes, orders, families, genera, and species

TELEOMORPH   Sexual name

TERMINAL   At the (hyphal) tip

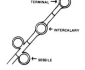

TEXTURE   Term to describe the height of aerial hyphae on a colony

THALLIC CONIDIOGENESIS   A septum forms near the end of a parent, and the growing point ahead of it becomes the daughter conidium. The daughter develops *after* it is separated, though still attached, to the parent. Thallic development may be holothallic or arthric.

THROMBOSIS   Blood clot with subsequent necrosis of surrounding tissue due to lack of oxygen

THRUSH   Candidosis of the oral cavity, usually observed in infants of mothers with vaginal candidosis, and in elderly debilitated patients

TINEA   Ringworm

TINEA BARBAE   Ringworm of the beard; barber's itch

TINEA CAPITIS   Ringworm of the scalp

TINEA CORPORIS   Ringworm of the body

TINEA CRURIS   Ringworm of the groin; jock itch

TINEA NIGRA   Superficial skin infection, usually on the palms of the hands, characterized by nonscaly brown to black patches, and caused by *Exophiala werneckii*

TINEA PEDIS   Ringworm of the foot; athlete's foot

TINEA UNGUIUM   Ringworm of the nail; onychomycosis

TINEA VERSICOLOR   See pityriasis versicolor.

TOPOGRAPHY   Design of hills and valleys observed on fungal colonies

TORULOPSOSIS   Spectrum of opportunistic diseases caused by *Candida (Torulopsis) glabrata*. The lungs and kidney are most often affected, although systemic spread may occur.

UMBONATE TOPOGRAPHY

Buttonlike central elevation on a fungal colony, often accompanied by rugose furrows

VEGETATIVE

Food-absorbing portion of the hyphae, which grow into the agar like roots. Vegetative hyphae may best be seen on the colony's reverse side.

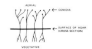

VELVETY TEXTURE

Colonial aerial hyphae arising close and parallel to each other, approximately 1/4 inch high, and resembling the fabric velvet

VERRUCOSE TOPOGRAPHY

Deeply wrinkled, convoluted colony surface

VESICLE

Swollen hypha. It may be the tip of a conidiophore as in *Aspergillus* sp., or the end of a sporangiophore as in *Syncephalastrum* sp.

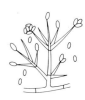

WHITE PIEDRA

Light brown soft nodules around beard and mustache hairs, caused by *Trichosporon beigelii*

WHORL

Several conidia or conidiophores forming around a common axis

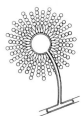

WOOLLY TEXTURE

Colonial aerial hyphae with a slightly matted appearance, approximately 1/2 inch high, resembling wool

YEAST

Single round to oval cell which usually buds to form daughter cells

ZYGOMYCETOUS

Pertaining to the taxonomic subdivision Zygomycotina

ZYGOMYCOSIS

Opportunistic fungal infection caused by genera of the Zygomycotina subdivision. Usually the acute form is elicited in which the initial eye or nasal sinus infection erodes into surrounding tissues, with rapid spread and death.

ZYGOMYCOTINA

Fungal subdivision exhibiting hyphae 6-10 μm wide which are aseptate, except at damaged areas or reproductive structures. Sporangiospores are the typical asexual stage, while zygospores are formed sexually.

ZYGOPHORE

Arm of a hypha which extends toward another compatible arm to produce a zygospore. These are seen in the subdivision Zygomycotina.

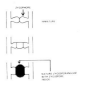

ZYGOSPORANGIUM

Thick outer layer covering a zygospore seen in the Zygomycotina. See drawing at ZYGOPHORE.

ZYGOSPORE

Sexual spore formed by meeting and fusion of two compatible hyphal arms, each containing a nucleus. The resulting zygote becomes a zygospore and is surrounded by a protective zygosporangium. These structures are observed in the subdivision Zygomycotina. See drawing at ZYGOPHORE.

COLOR PLATES

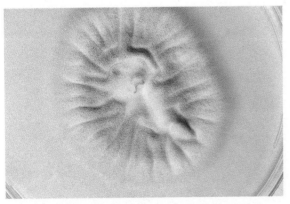

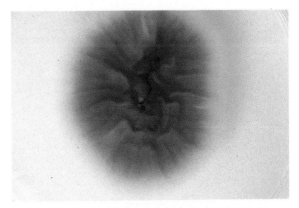

1. Colony front, *Microsporum cookei*, Sabouraud dextrose agar (SDA), 7 days, 25°C.

2. Colony reverse, *Microsporum cookei*, SDA, 7 days, 25°C.

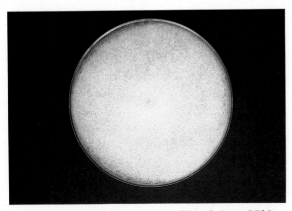

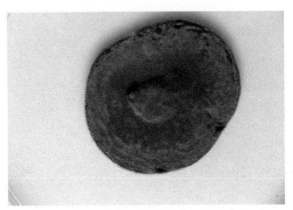

3. Cottony texture, *Rhizopus* sp., SDA, 3 days, 25°C.

4. Velvety texture, *Fonsecaea pedrosoi*, SDA, 16 days, 25°C.

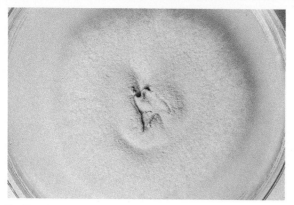

5. Powdery texture, *Microsporum gypseum*, SDA, 7 days, 25°C.

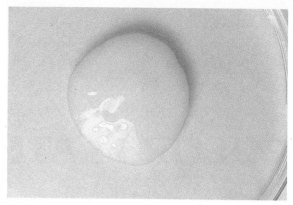

6. Glabrous texture, *Cryptococcus neoformans*, SDA, 17 days, 25°C.

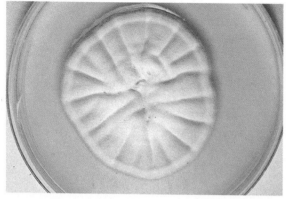

7. Rugose topography, *Epidermophyton floccosum*, SDA, 14 days, 25°C.

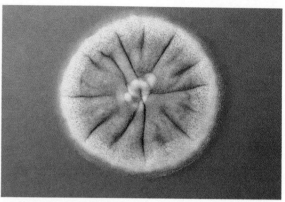

8. Umbonate and rugose topography, *Aspergillus fumigatus*, SDA, 5 days, 25°C.

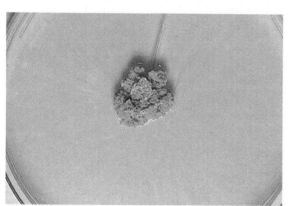

9. Verrucose topography, *Nocardia asteroides*, SDA, 18 days, 25°C.

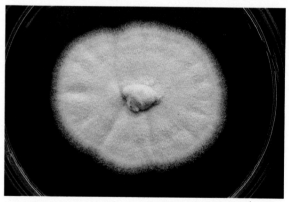

10. Module 1 final exam photograph, colony front.

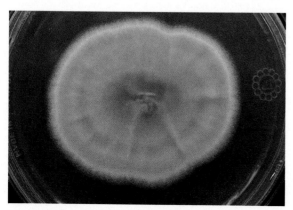

11. Module 1 final exam photograph, colony reverse.

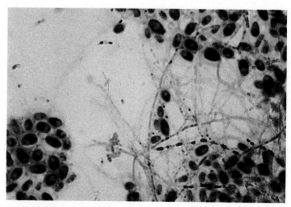

12. Modified Kinyoun carbolfuchsin acid-fast stain, *Nocardia* sp., ×1000.

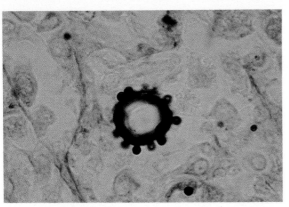

13. Gomori methenamine silver stain, *Paracoccidioides brasiliensis*, ×1000.

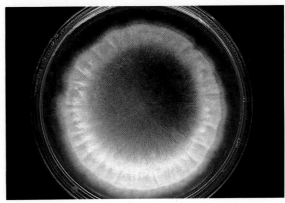

14. *Absidia* sp., SDA, 4 days, 25°C.

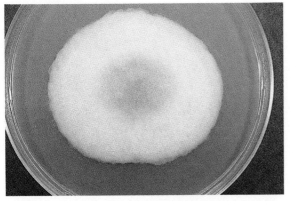

15. *Mucor* sp., SDA, 10 days, 25°C.

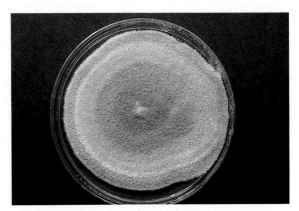

16. *Alternaria* sp., SDA, 9 days, 25°C.

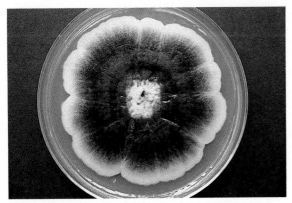

17. *Aureobasidium* sp., SDA, 14 days, 25°C.

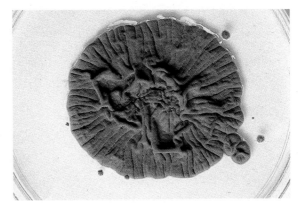

18. *Cladosporium* sp., SDA, 10 days, 25°C.

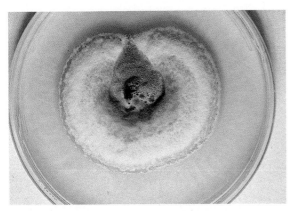

19. *Curvularia* sp., SDA, 6 days, 25°C.

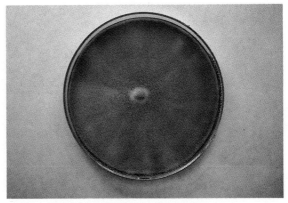

20. *Drechslera* sp., SDA, 14 days, 25°C.

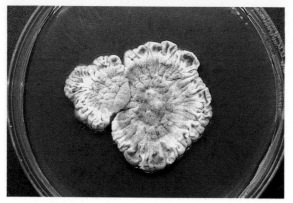

21. *Epicoccum* sp., SDA, 13 days, 25°C.

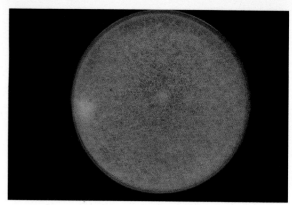

22. *Nigrospora* sp., SDA, 6 days, 25°C.

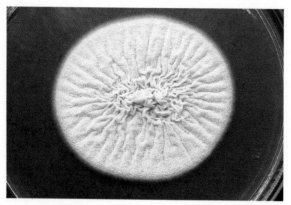

23. *Acremonium* sp., SDA, 13 days, 25°C.

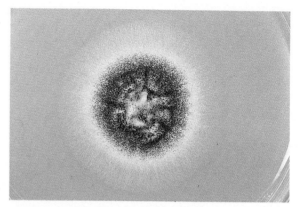

24. *Aspergillus niger*, SDA, 3 days, 25°C.

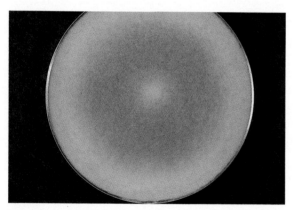

25. *Syncephalastrum* sp., SDA, 5 days, 25°C.

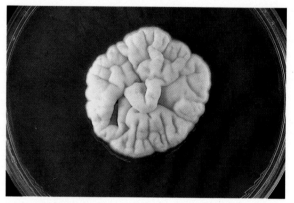

26. *Chrysosporium* sp., SDA, 8 days, 25°C.

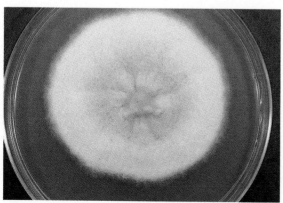

27. *Fusarium* sp., SDA, 9 days, 25°C.

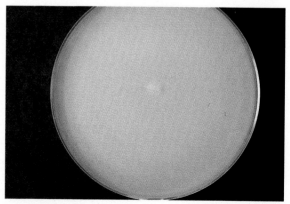

28. *Gliocladium* sp., SDA, 5 days, 25°C.

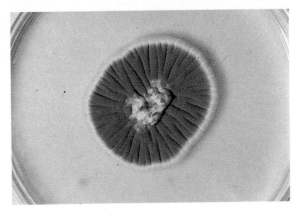

29. *Paecilomyces* sp., SDA, 5 days, 25°C.

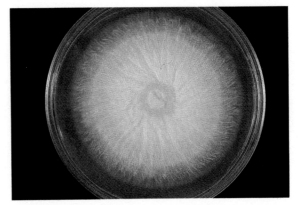

30. *Penicillium* sp., SDA, 6 days, 25°C.

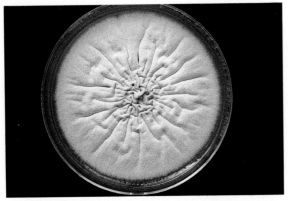

31. *Scopulariopsis*, sp., SDA, 14 days, 25°C.

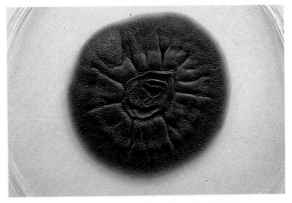

32. *Sepedonium* sp., SDA, 5 days, 25°C.

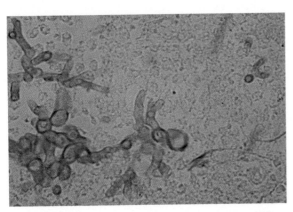

33. Aspergillosis of lung, Gridley fungus stain, ×450.

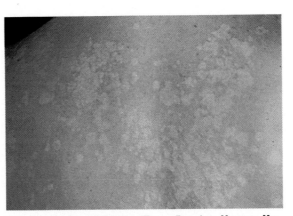

34. *Exophiala werneckii*, SDA, 39 days, 25°C.

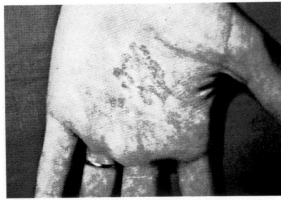

35. Tinea nigra. (From Beneke: Human Mycoses. Upjohn, 1979, with permission.)

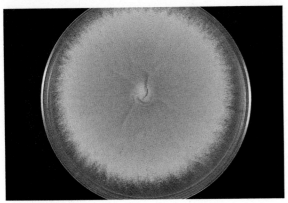

36. Pityriasis versicolor. (From Beneke: Human My-coses. Upjohn, 1979, with permission.)

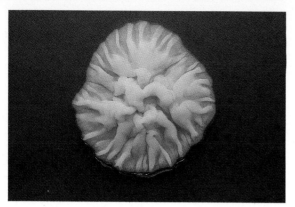

37. *Trichosporon beigelii*, SDA, 10 days, 25°C.

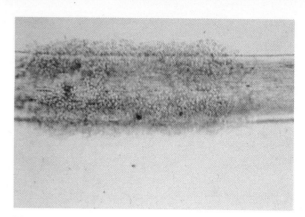

38. White piedra, hair, ×200 (Center for Disease Control).

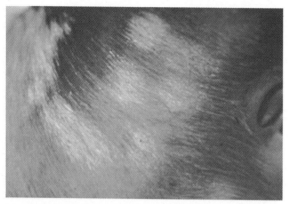

39. Fluorescing hair. (From Dolan et al: Atlas of Clinical Mycology. ASCP, 1976, with permission.)

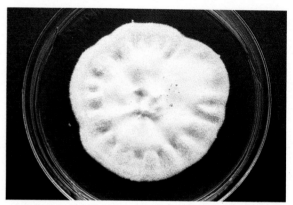

40. *Microsporum audouinii*, SDA, 39 days, 25°C.

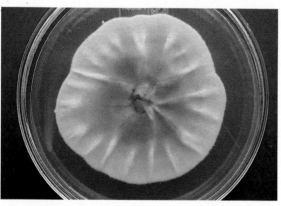

41. Colony reverse, *Microsporum audouinii*, SDA, 39 days, 25°C.

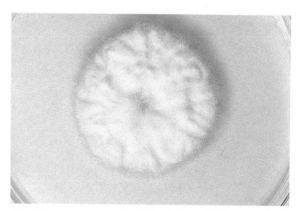

42. *Microsporum canis*, SDA, 7 days, 25°C.

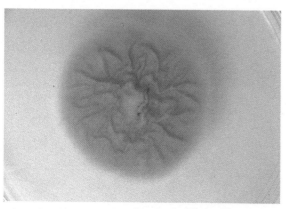

43. Colony reverse, *Microsporum canis*, SDA, 7 days, 25°C.

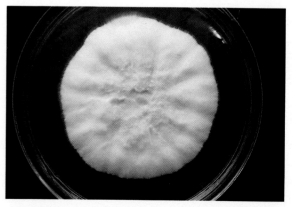

44. Fluffy strain, *Trichophyton mentagrophytes*, SDA, 20 days, 25°C.

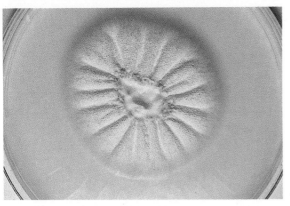

45. Granular strain, *Trichophyton mentagrophytes*, SDA, 10 days, 25°C.

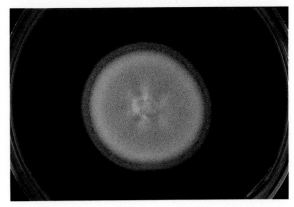

46. *Trichophyton rubrum*, potato dextrose agar, 16 days, 25°C.

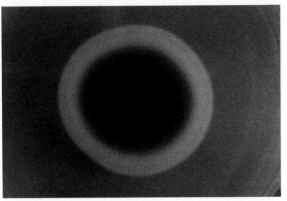

47. Colony reverse, *Trichophyton rubrum*, potato dextrose agar, 16 days, 25°C.

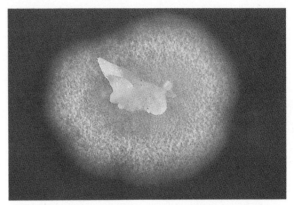

48. *Trichophyton verrucosum*, SDA, 28 days, 37°C.

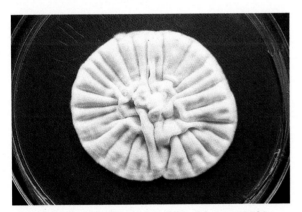

49. *Trichophyton schoenleinii*, SDA, 39 days, 25°C.

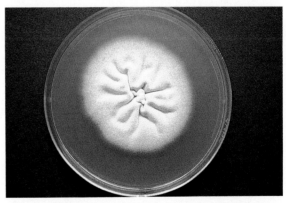

50. *Trichophyton tonsurans*, SDA, 28 days, 25°C.

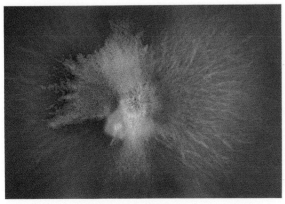

51. *Trichophyton violaceum*, SDA, 28 days, 25°C.

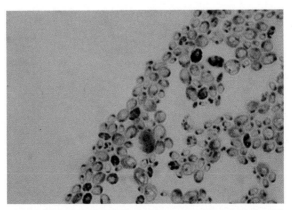

52. Ascus containing two ascospores, *Saccharomyces cerevisiae*, modified Kinyoun acid-fast stain, ×1000.

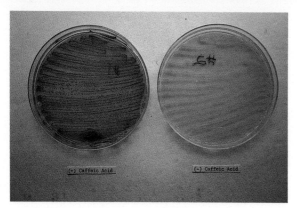

53. Caffeic acid agar: (+) test, *Cryptococcus neoformans;* (−) test, *Candida albicans.*

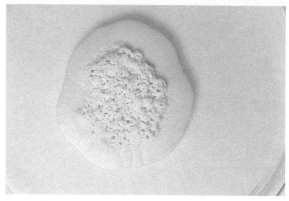

54. *Candida albicans*, SDA, 17 days, 25°C.

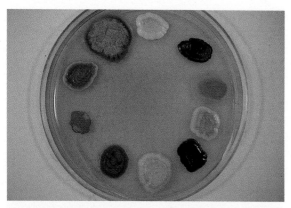

55. Candida BCG agar, 3 days, 25°C (clockwise starting at top): *Candida albicans, Candida (Torulopsis) glabrata, Candida krusei, Candida parapsilosis, Candida pseudotropicalis, Candida tropicalis, Cryptococcus neoformans, Prototheca, Saccharomyces cerevisiae, Trichosporon beigelii.*

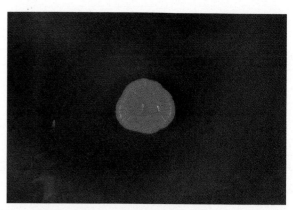

56. Module 5 final exam photograph.

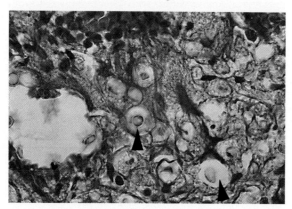

57. Cryptococcosis of lung, hematoxylin and eosin stain, ×450. Arrows indicate the capsule surrounding the organism.

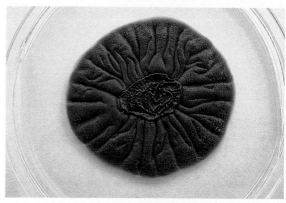

58. *Exophiala jeanselmei*, SDA, 39 days, 25°C.

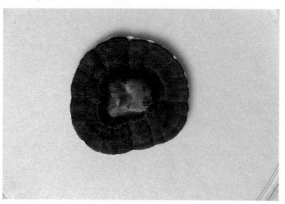

59. *Phialophora verrucosa*, SDA, 20 days, 25°C.

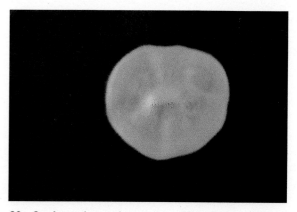

60. *Scedosporium apiospermum*, SDA, 8 days, 25°C.

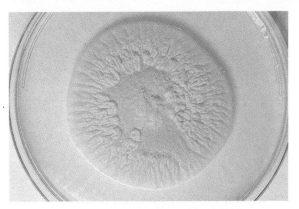

61. *Sporothrix schenckii*, SDA, 23 days, 25°C.

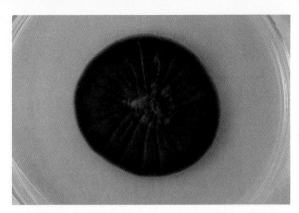

62. *Sporothrix schenckii*, potato dextrose agar, 19 days, 25°C.

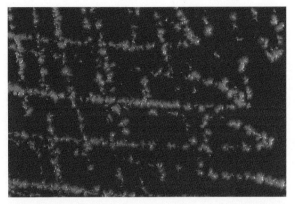

63. *Sporothrix schenckii*, brain heart infusion agar with blood, 14 days, 37°C.

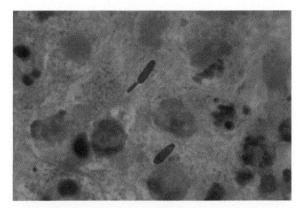

64. *Sporothrix schenckii* yeasts in hand aspirate, periodic acid-Schiff stain, ×1000.

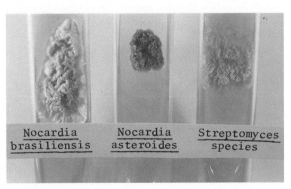

65. *Nocardia brasiliensis, Nocardia asteroides,* and *Streptomyces* sp., SDA, 21 days, 25°C.

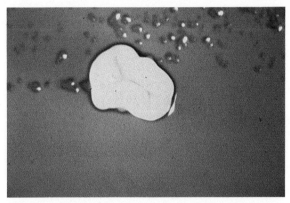

66. Molar tooth colony, *Actinomyces.* (From Dolan et al: Atlas of Clinical Mycology. ASCP, 1976, with permission.)

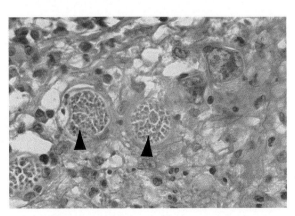

67. *Coccidioides immitis* spherules, hematoxylin and eosin stain, ×450. Arrows indicate spherules.

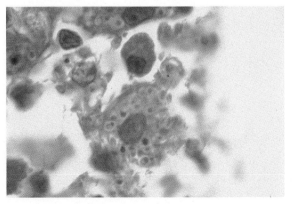

68. Yeasts of *Histoplasma capsulatum* inside spleen macrophage (center of photo), hematoxylin and eosin stain, ×1000.

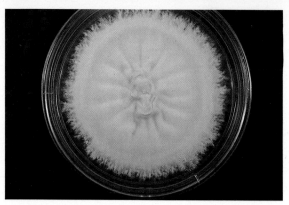

69. *Blastomyces dermatitidis,* SDA, 42 days, 25°C.

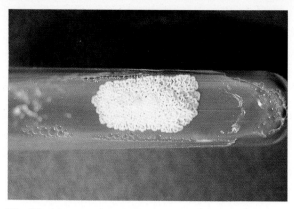

70. *Blastomyces dermatitidis,* brain heart infusion agar with blood, 14 days, 37°C.

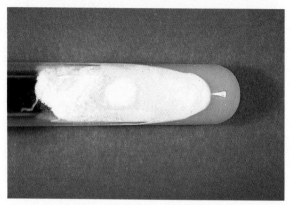

71. *Coccidioides immitis,* SDA, 28 days, 25°C.

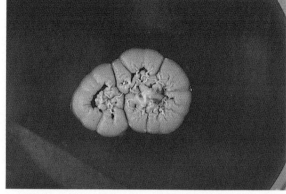

72. *Histoplasma capsulatum,* brain heart infusion agar with blood, 21 days, 25°C.

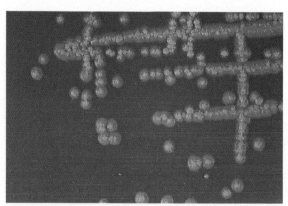

73. *Histoplasma capsulatum,* brain heart infusion agar with blood, 14 days, 37°C.

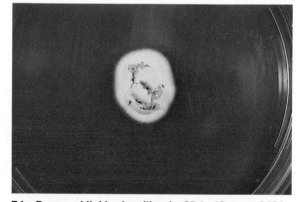

74. *Paracoccidioides brasiliensis,* SDA, 42 days, 25°C.

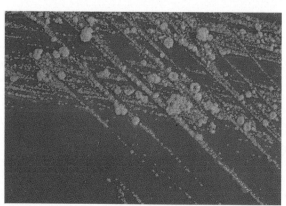

75. *Paracoccidioides brasiliensis,* brain heart infusion agar with blood, 14 days, 37°C.

INDEX

An italic page number indicates an illustration.